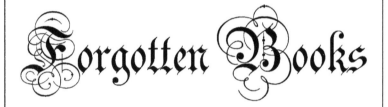

ISBN 978-1-5284-4012-7
PIBN 10916185

1 MONTH OF
FREE
READING

at

www.ForgottenBooks.com

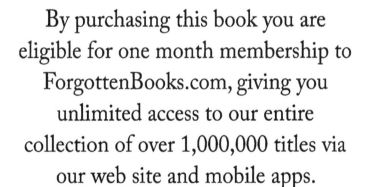

By purchasing this book you are eligible for one month membership to ForgottenBooks.com, giving you unlimited access to our entire collection of over 1,000,000 titles via our web site and mobile apps.

To claim your free month visit: www.forgottenbooks.com/free916185

English
Français
Deutsche
Italiano
Español
Português

www.forgottenbooks.com

Mythology Photography **Fiction**
Fishing Christianity **Art** Cooking
Essays Buddhism Freemasonry
Medicine **Biology** Music **Ancient**
Egypt Evolution Carpentry Physics
Dance Geology **Mathematics** Fitness
Shakespeare **Folklore** Yoga Marketing
Confidence Immortality Biographies
Poetry **Psychology** Witchcraft
Electronics Chemistry History **Law**
Accounting **Philosophy** Anthropology
Alchemy Drama Quantum Mechanics
Atheism Sexual Health **Ancient History**
Entrepreneurship Languages Sport
Paleontology Needlework Islam
Metaphysics Investment Archaeology
Parenting Statistics Criminology
Motivational

TRANSACTIONS

OF THE

SOUTHERN SURGICAL AND GYNECOLOGICAL ASSOCIATION

VOLUME XXVIII

TWENTY-EIGHTH SESSION

HELD AT CINCINNATI, OHIO

DECEMBER 13, 14, AND 15, 1915

EDITED BY W. D. HAGGARD, M.D.

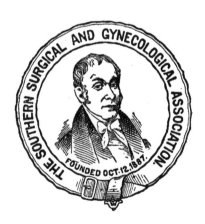

PUBLISHED BY THE ASSOCIATION

1916

The Association does not hold itself responsible for the views enunciated in the papers and discussions published in this volume.

W. D. HAGGARD, M.D., *Secretary,*

NASHVILLE, TENN.

DORNAN, PRINTER
PHILADELPHIA

CONTENTS

CONTENTS

OFFICERS FOR 1915-1916

PRESIDENT

THOMAS S. CULLEN, Baltimore, Md.

VICE-PRESIDENTS

ROBERT S. HILL, Montgomery, Ala.

WILLARD BARTLETT, St. Louis, Mo.

SECRETARY

WILLIAM D. HAGGARD, Nashville, Tenn.

TREASURER

Le GRAND GUERRY, Columbia, S. C.

COUNCIL

J. M. T. FINNEY, Baltimore, Md.

RUDOLPH MATAS, New Orleans, La.

JOHN YOUNG BROWN, St. Louis, Mo.

JOHN WESLEY LONG, Greensboro, N. C.

BACON SAUNDERS, Fort Worth, Texas.

LIST OF OFFICERS

FROM THE ORGANIZATION TO THE PRESENT TIME.

	President	Vice-Presidents	Secretary	Treasurer
1888.	*W. D. Haggard	R. D. Webb J. W. Sears	*W. E. B. Davis	Hardin P. Cochr
1889.	*Hunter M. McGuire	W. O. Roberts *Bedford Brown	*W. E. B. Davis	Hardin P. Cochr
1890.	*George J. Engelmann	*Berthold E. Hadra Duncan Eve	*W. E. B. Davis	Hardin P. Cochr
1891.	Lewis S. McMurtry	*J. McFadden Gaston J. T. Wilson	*W. E. B. Davis	Hardin P. Cochr
1892.	*J. McFadden Gaston	*Cornelius Kollock George Ben Johnston	*W. E. B. Davis	Hardin P. Cochr
1893.	*Bedford Brown	*Joseph Price George A. Baxter	*W. E. B. Davis	Hardin P. Cochr
1894.	*Cornelius Kollock	A. B. Miles J. B. S. Holmes	*W. E. B. Davis	Hardin P. Cochr
1895.	Lewis McLane Tiffany	Ernest S. Lewis Manning Simons	*W. E. B. Davis	*Richard Douglas
1896.	Ernest S. Lewis	Joseph Tabor Johnson *Richard Douglas	*W. E. B. Davis	*A. M. Cartledge
1897.	George Ben Johnston	W. E. Parker Floyd W. McRae	*W. E. B. Davis	*A. M. Cartledge
1898.	*Richard Douglas	*H. H. Mudd James A. Goggans	*W. E. B. Davis	*A. M. Cartledge
1899.	Joseph Tabor Johnson	F. W. Parham W. L. Robinson	*W. E. B. Davis	*A. M. Cartledge
1900.	*A. M. Cartledge	*Manning Simons W. P. Nicolson	*W. E. B. Davis	W. D. Haggard
1901.	*Manning Simons	George H. Noble L. C. Bosher	W. D. Haggard	Floyd W. McRa
1902.	*W. E. B. Davis	J. Wesley Bovée J. W. Long	W. D. Haggard	Floyd W. McRa
1903.	J. Wesley Bovée	Christopher Tompkins Bacon Saunders	W. D. Haggard	Floyd W. McRa
1904.	Floyd W. McRae	George S. Brown J. Shelton Horsley	W. D. Haggard	Charles M. Ross
1905.	Lewis C. Bosher	J. D. S. Davis I. S. Stone	W. D. Haggard	Charles M. Ross
1906.	George H. Noble	Stuart McGuire E. Denegre Martin	W. D. Haggard	Charles M. Ross
1907.	Howard A. Kelly	Rufus E. Fort Hubert A. Royster	W. D. Haggard	Charles M. Ross
1908.	F. W. Parham	Henry D. Fry W. F. Westmoreland	W. D. Haggard	Stuart McGuire
1909.	Stuart McGuire	John Young Brown R. S. Cathcart	W. D. Haggard	Wm. S. Goldsmi
1910.	W. O. Roberts	Joseph C. Bloodgood Lewis C. Morris	W. D. Haggard	Wm. S. Goldsmi
1911.	Rudolph Matas	Guy L. Hunner J. Garland Sherrill	W. D. Haggard	Wm. S. Goldsmi
1912.	J. M. T. Finney	J. E. Thompson W. P. Carr	W. D. Haggard	Wm. S. Goldsmi
1913.	John Young Brown	*Ap Morgan Vance Lomax Gwathmey	W. D. Haggard	Le Grand Guerr
1914.	John W. Long	A. C. Scott James F. Mitchell	W. D. Haggard	Le Grand Guerr
1915.	Bacon Saunders	Thomas S. Cullen S. M. D. Clark	W. D. Haggard	Le Grand Guerr
1916.	Thomas S. Cullen	Robert S. Hill Willard Bartlett	W. D. Haggard	Le Grand Guerr

* Deceased.

HONORARY MEMBERS

1894.—FOY, GEORGE   DUBLIN.

FOUNDER.—HERFF, FERDINAND   SAN ANTONIO, TEXAS.

1894.—JACOBS, CHARLES   BRUSSELS.

1889.—JOHNSON, JOSEPH TABER   WASHINGTON, D. C.

1910.—JONES, ROBERT   LIVERPOOL.

1910.—LANE, ARBUTHNOT   LONDON.

1894.—MARTIN, A.   BERLIN.

1902.—MAURY, RICHARD B.   MEMPHIS, TENN.

1894.—MORISANI, O.   NAPLES.

1910.—MORISON, RUTHERFORD   NEW-CASTLE-ON-TYNE.

1910.—MOYNIHAN, B. G. A.   LEEDS.

1910.—MYLES, THOMAS, SIR   DUBLIN.

1894.—POZZI, S.   PARIS.

1910.—ROBSON, MAYO   LONDON.

FOUNDER.—SCHILLING, NICHOLAS   CEDAR BAYOU, TEXAS.

1910.—STILES, H. J.   EDINBURGH.

1907.—TIFFANY, L. M.   BALTIMORE, MD.

MEMBERS

1908.—ABELL, IRVIN, M.D. Professor of Principles and Practice of Surgery and Clinical Surgery, Medical Department, University of Louisville; Visiting Surgeon, University Hospital, Louisville City Hospital, and St. Mary and Elizabeth Hospital. 1228 Second St., Louisville, Ky.

1911.—ALLEN, CARROLL W., M.D. 1312 Louisiana Ave., New Orleans, La.

1915.—BAER, WILLIAM STEVENSON, F.A.C.S., A.B. Associate Professor Orthopedic Surgery, Johns Hopkins University; Associate in Orthopedic Surgery in charge of Orthopedic Department, Johns Hopkins Hospital; Consulting Orthopedic Surgeon, Home for Incurables; Surgeon-in-chief, Children's Hospital; Visiting Orthopedic Surgeon, Union Protestant Infirmary, Hospital for Women of Maryland, and Robert Garrett Hospital for Children; Consulting Orthopedic Surgeon, Cambridge Hospital, Cambridge, Md. 4 West Madison Street, Baltimore, Md.

1914.—BAILEY, FRED. WARREN, B.Sc., M.D. Assistant Professor of Surgery, St. Louis University School of Medicine; Associate Chief Surgeon, St. John's Hospital; Visiting Gynecologist, St. Louis City Sanitarium. 633 Metropolitan Building, St. Louis, Mo.

1905.—BAKER, JAMES NORMENT, M.D. Visiting Surgeon, St. Margaret's Hospital; Secretary of the Medical Association of the State of Alabama. 719 Madison Avenue, Montgomery, Ala.

1894.—BALBRIDGE, FELIX E., M.D. Huntsville, Ala.

1903.—BALLOCH, EDWARD A., M.D. Professor of Surgery, Medical Department of Howard University; Surgeon to Freedmen's Hospital; Member American Academy of Medicine. 1511 Rhode Island Avenue, N. W., Washington, D. C.

1908.—BARR, RICHARD ALEXANDER, M.D. Professor of Surgery and Clinical Surgery, Medical Department of Vanderbilt University; late Major of First Tennessee Infantry, U. S. A. First National Bank Building, Nashville, Tenn.

1905.—BARROW, DAVID, M.D. Ex-President Kentucky State Medical Society. 148 Market Street, Lexington, Ky.

1905.—BARTLETT, WILLARD, M.D. Surgeon to St. Anthony's Hospital. 4257 Washington Boulevard, St. Louis, Mo.

1901.—BAUGHMAN, GREER D., M.D. Professor of Obstetrics, Medical College of Virginia; Visiting Obstetrician to the Virginia Hospital, Memorial Hospital, and Stuart Circle Hospital, Richmond, Virginia. 26 North Laurel Street.

1907.—BEVAN, ARTHUR DEAN, M.D. Professor of Surgery, Rush Medical College, University of Chicago. 100 State Street, Chicago, Ill.

1908.—BLAIR, VILRAY PAPIN, A.M., M.D. Metropolitan Building, St. Louis, Mo.

1906.—BLOODGOOD, JOSEPH COLT, M.D. Associate Professor of Surgery, Johns Hopkins University; Associate Surgeon, John Hopkins Hospital; Surgeon to the Union Protestant Infirmary; Chief Surgeon to St. Agnes' Hospital. *Vice-President*, 1910. 904 North Charles Street, Baltimore, Md.

1893.—BLOOM, J. D., M.D. Consulting Surgeon, Touro Infirmary; Lecturer on Diseases of Children, Tulane University. New Orleans, La.

1901.—BOLDT, HERMANN J., M.D. Gynecologist to Post-Graduate Hospital, St. Mark's Hospital, German Polyclinic; Consulting Gynecologist to the Beth Israel Hospital and to St. Vincent's Hospital; Professor of Gynecology, Post-Graduate Medical School; Member of the Gynecological Society of Germany; Fellow of the American Gynecological Society; Fellow of the Royal Society of Medicine (London); ex-President of the New York Obstetrical Society; of the German Medical Society of New York; of the Section of Obstetrics of the New York Academy of Medicine. 39 East Sixty-first Street, New York, N. Y.

1902.—BONIFIELD, CHARLES LYBRAND, M.D. Professor of Clinical Gynecology, Medical College of Ohio (Medical Department University of Cincinnati); Member American Association of Obstetricians and Gynecologists; ex-President Cincinnati Academy of Medicine; ex-President Cincinnati Obstetrical Society. 409 Broadway, Cincinnati, Ohio.

1911.—BORDEN, W. C., M.D. Professor of Surgery and Dean, George Washington University; Surgeon-in-Chief to the George Washington University Hospital. 1801 California St., Washington, D. C.

1890.—BOSHER, LEWIS CRENSHAW, M.D. Professor of Practice of Surgery and Clinical Surgery in the Medical College of Virginia; Visiting Surgeon to the Memorial Hospital; Member of American Surgical Association; Member of the American Association of Obstetricians and Gynecologists; Member of Association of American Anatomists; Member of American Urological Association; ex-President of Richmond Academy of Medicine and Surgery. *Vice-President*, 1901; *President*, 1905. 422 East Franklin Street, Richmond, Va.

1895.—BOVÉE, J. WESLEY, M.D. Fellow of American Gynecological Society; President of Washington Obstetrical and Gynecological Society; ex-President Medical and Surgical Society of the District of Columbia; Honorary Fellow Medical Society of Virginia; Professor of Gynecology of George Washington University, Washington, D. C.; Gynecologist to Providence, Columbia, and George Washington University Hospitals; Consulting Physician to St. Ann's Infant Asylum, and Attending Gynecologist to St. Elizabeth's Hospital for the Insane, Washington, D. C. *Vice-President*, 1902, *President*, 1903; Member of *Council*, 1903–1906. The Rochambeau, Washington, D. C.

1905.—BROWN, JOHN YOUNG, M.D. Formerly Surgeon-in-Charge, St. Louis City Hospital; President of the American Association of Obstetricians and Gynecologists, 1906. *Vice-President*, 1909; *President*, 1913. Metropolitan Building, St. Louis, Mo.

1908.—BRYAN, ROBERT C., M.D. Professor of Descriptive Anatomy, University of Medicine, Visiting Surgeon to the Virginia Hospital. First and Main Streets, Richmond, Va.

1910.—BRYAN, W. A., M.D. Professor of Surgery and Clinical Surgery, Vanderbilt University; Professor of Oral Surgery, Dental Department, Vanderbilt University. 146 Eighth Avenue, N., Nashville, Tenn.

1913.—BUIST, A. JOHNSTON, M.D. Professor of Gynecology, Medical College of the State of South Carolina; Visiting Gynecologist, Roper Hospital. 279 Meeting Street, Charleston, S. C.

1907.—BURCH, LUCIUS E., M.D. Professor of Gynecology, Vanderbilt University, Medical Department; Gynecologist, Nashville City Hospital; Captain and Surgeon, N. G. S. T. 706 Church Street, Nashville, Tenn.

1899.—BURTHE, L., M.D. 124 Baronne Street, New Orleans, La.

1900.—BYFORD, HENRY T., M.D. Professor of Gynecology and Clinical Gynecology, College of Physicians and Surgeons (University of Illinois); Professor of Gynecology, Post-Graduate Medical School of Chicago; Surgeon to Woman's Hospital, etc. 122 South Michigan Ave., Peoples Gas Bldg., Chicago, Ill.

1902.—CALDWELL, C. E., A.M., M.D. Clinical Professor of Surgery and Associate Professor of Surgical Anatomy in Medical Department, University of Cincinnati; Surgeon to Cincinnati General Hospital. 1110 Cross Lane, Cincinnati, Ohio.

1910.—CALDWELL, ROBERT, M.D. Professor of Surgical Anatomy, Vanderbilt University; ex-President Nashville Academy of Medicine. 315 Jackson Building, Nashville, Tenn.

1906.—CANNADY, JOHN EGERTON, M.D. Former Surgeon-in-Charge to Sheltering Arms Hospital, Hansford, W. Va.; Fellow of the American Association of Obstetricians and Gynecologists; Non-resident Honorary Fellow of the Kentucky State Medical Society; Fellow of the West Virginia Medical Association, Virginia Medical Society, Tri-State Society of Virginia and the Carolinas, American Association of Railway Surgeons. Coyle and Richardson Building, Charleston, W. Va.

1904.—CAROTHERS, ROBERT, M.D. Professor of Clinical Surgery, Medical College of Ohio, Medical Department Cincinnati University; Surgeon to the Good Samaritan Hospital; 413 Broadway, Cincinnati, Ohio.

1903.—CARR, WILLIAM P., M.D. Professor of Physiology and Professor of Clinical Surgery, Columbian University; Surgeon to the Emergency Hospital and University Hospital; Consulting Surgeon to the Washington Asylum Hospital and the Goverment Hospital for the Insane, Washington, D. C. _Vice-President_, 1912. 1418 L Street, N. W., Washington, D. C.

1899.—CATHCART, R. S., M.D. Professor of Abdominal Surgery, Medical College of the State of South Carolina; Surgeon-in-chief, Roper Hospital, Charleston, S. C.; Surgeon, Atlantic Coast Line Railway, Charleston Consolidated Railway and Lighting Co., The Citadel—the Military College of South

Carolina, and the Confederate Home College, Charleston, S. C. *Vice-President*, 1909. 66 Hasell Street, Charleston, South Carolina.

1904.—CHAMBERS, P. F., M.D. Attending Surgeon, Woman's Hospital; Consulting Surgeon, French Hospital. 49 West Fifty-seventh Street, New York, N. Y.

1907.—CLARK, JOHN G., M.D. Professor of Gynecology, University of Pennsylvania; Gynecologist-in-Chief, University Hospital. 2017 Walnut Street, Philadelphia, Penna.

1907.—CLARK, S. M. D., M.D. Associate Professor Gynecology, Tulane Medical Department; Visiting Surgeon, Charity Hospital. 1435 Harmony Street, New Orleans, La.

1893.—COCRAM, HENRY S., M.D. 108 Baronne Street, New Orleans, La.

1908.—COFFEY, ROBERT C., M.D. Secretary Oregon State Board of Medical Examiners; Councellor Oregon State Medical Association. Stevens Building, Portland, Oregon.

1909.—COLE, HERBERT PHALON, M.D. Instructor in Gynecology and Clinical Diagnosis, Medical Department of the University of Alabama; Gynecologist to City Hospital of Mobile. 202 Conti Street, Mobile, Ala.

1902.—COLEY, WILLIAM B., M.D. Clinical Lecturer on Surgery, College of Physicians and Surgeons; Assistant Surgeon in Hospital for Ruptured and Crippled; Attending Surgeon to General Memorial Hospital; Fellow of the American Surgical Association, New York Surgical Society, and New York Academy of Medicine. 40 East Forty-first Street, New York, N. Y.

1914.—COUSINS, WILLIAM LEWIS, M.D. Surgeon-in-Chief, St. Barnabas' Hospital; Consulting Surgeon, Maine General Hospital. 231 Woodford Street, Portland, Maine.

1907.—CRAWFORD, WALTER W., M.D. Ex-President Southern Medical Association; ex-President Perry County Medical Society; ex-President Mississippi State Medical Association; Surgeon to South Mississippi Infirmary. Hattiesburg, Miss.

1902.—CRILE, GEORGE W., M.D. Professor of Clinical Surgery, Medical College of Western Reserve University; Surgeon to St. Alexis' Hospital; Surgeon to Lakeside Hospital. 1021 Prospect Street, Cleveland, Ohio.

1908.—CRISLER, JOSEPH AUGUSTUS, M.D. Professor of Anatomy and Operative Surgery, College of Physcians and Surgeons, Memphis, Tennessee; Lecturer on Minor Surgery,

S Surg   B

Medical Department, University of Mississippi; ex-Member Mississippi State Board of Health and Medical Examiners; ex-Vice-President Mississippi State Medical Association and Tri-State Medical Association. Memphis Trust Building, Memphis, Tenn.

1906.—CULLEN, THOMAS STEPHEN, M.D. Associate Professor of Gynecology, Johns Hopkins University; Associate in Gynecology, Johns Hopkins Hospital; Consultant in Abdominal Surgery, Church Home and Infirmary. Fellow of the American Gynecological Society; Honorary Member to La Societa Italiana Ostettricia Ginecologia, Rome; Corresponding Member of the Gesellschaft f. Geburtshülfe, Leipzig. 3 West Preston Street, Baltimore, Md.

Founder.—CUNNINGHAM, RUSSELL M., M.D. Professor of Practice of Medicine and Clinical Medicine, Birmingham Medical College; Surgeon to the Pratt Mines Hospital. Ensley, Ala.

1906.—CUSHING, HARVEY, M.D. Professor of Surgery in the Harvard University. 305 Walnut Street, Brookline, Mass.

1907.—DANNA, JAMES A., M.D. Chief Visiting Surgeon, Charity Hospital. Charity Hospital, New Orleans, Louisiana.

Founder.—DAVIS, JOHN D. S., M.D., LL.D. Professor in the Post-graduate School of Medicine of the University of Alabama; Surgeon to Hillman Hospital; ex-President of the Jefferson County Medical Society; Vice-President of the American Obstetricians and Gynecologists, 1909. *Vice-President*, 1905. Avenue G and Twenty-first St., Birmingham, Ala.

1910.—DAVIS, JOHN STAIGE, M.D. Instructor in Surgery, Johns Hopkins University; Assistant Surgeon to the Out-Patient Department of Johns Hopkins Hospital; Visiting Surgeon to the Union Protestant Infirmary, Visiting Surgeon to the Church Home and infirmary. 1200 Cathedral Street, Baltimore, Md.

1900.—DEAVER, JOHN B., M.D. Surgeon-in-Chief to the German Hospital. 1634 Walnut Street, Philadelphia.

1897.—*DORSETT, WALTER B., M.D. Professor of Obstetrics and Clinical Gynecology, St. Louis University; Gynecologist to the Missouri Baptist Sanitarium and to Evangelical Deaconess' Hospital. 5070 Washington Boulevard, St. Louis, Mo.

1896.—DOUGHTY, W. H., M.D. Professor of Special Surgery and Surgical Pathology, Medical Department, University of Georgia; Chief Surgeon to Charleston and Western Carolina Railroad. 822 Greene Street, Augusta, Ga.

1914.—DOWNES, WILLIAM AUGUSTUS, M.D. Assistant Professor of Clinical Surgery, Columbia University, College of Physicians and Surgeons; Attending Surgeon General Memorial and Babies' Hospitals; Associate Attending Surgeon, St. Luke's Hospital and Hospital for Ruptured and Crippled. 37 West Seventy-first Street, New York, N. Y.

1890.—EARNEST, JOHN G., M.D. Professor of Clinical Gynecology, College of Physicians and Surgeons; formerly Professor of Gynecology, Southern Medical College; Visiting Gynecologist to the Grady Hospital. 828 Candler Building, Atlanta, Ga.

1907.—ELBRECHT, OSCAR HERMAN, M.D. Visiting Surgeon, St. Louis City Hospital; Consulting Surgeon to St. Louis Maternity, Bethesda and Missouri-Pacific Railroad Hospitals. 423 Metropolitan Building, St. Louis, Mo.

1891.—ELKIN, WILLIAM SIMPSON, M.D. Professor of Operative and Clinical Surgery, Atlanta College of Physicians and Surgeons; ex-President of the Atlanta Society of Medicine; Surgeon to Grady Hospital. 27 Luckie St., Atlanta, Ga.

1904.—FINNEY, J. M. T., M.D. Associate Professor of Surgery, Johns Hopkins University; Surgeon to Out-patients, Johns Hopkins Hospital. *President*, 1912. 1300 Eutaw Place, Baltimore, Md.

1901.—FORT, RUFUS E., M.D. Chief Surgeon, Nashville Terminal Company; Surgeon to Tennessee Central Railroad; Surgeon to Nashville Hospital; *Vice-President*, 1907. 209 Seventh Avenue, N., Nashville, Tenn.

1905.—FRANK, LOUIS, M.D. Professor of Surgery and Clinical Surgery, University of Louisville; Visiting Surgeon to the Louisville City Hospital. 400 Atherton Building, Louisville, Ky.

1902.—FREIBERG, ALBERT H., M.D. Professor of Orthopedic Surgery in the Medical College of Ohio, Medical Department of the University of Cincinnati; Orthopedic Surgeon to the Cincinnati Hospital and to the Jewish Hospital of Cincinnati. 19 West Seventh Street, Cincinnati, Ohio.

1895.—FRY, HENRY D., M.D. Professor of Obstetrics, Georgetown University; *Vice-President*, 1908. 1929 Nineteenth Street, N. W., Washington, D. C.

1903.—GALE, JOSEPH A., M.D. Surgeon-General Norfolk and Western R. R.; ex-President of Medical Society of Virginia. Roanoke, Va.

1913.—GIBBON, R. L., M.D. Charlotte, N. C.

1897.—GLASGOW, FRANK A., M.D. Professor of Clinical Gynecology of St. Louis Medical College; Gynecologist to St. Louis Mullanphy Hospital; on staff of Martha Parsons Free Hospital; Consulting Surgeon to St. Louis Female Hospital. 3894 Washington Boulevard, St. Louis, Mo.

Founder.—GOGGANS, JAMES A., M.D. Ex-President of the Tri-State Medical Society of Alabama, Georgia, and Tennessee; Senior Councillor of the Medical Association of the State of Alabama; Fellow of the British Gynecological Society. *Vice-President*, 1898. Alexander City, Ala.

1900.—GOLDSMITH, W. S., M.D. *Treasurer*, 1909–1912. 262 Jackson Street, Atlanta, Ga.

1892.—GRANT, HORACE H., M.D. Professor of Surgery in the Hospital College of Medicine; Surgeon to the Louisville City Hospital. 321 Equitable Building, Louisville, Ky.

1905.—GUERRY, LE GRAND, M.D. Surgeon, Columbia Hospital. *Treasurer*. Columbia, S. C.

1896.—GWATHMEY, LOMAX, M.D. Attending Gynecologist to St. Vincent's Hospital and Dispensary, *Vice-President*, 1913. Norfolk, Va.

1896.—HAGGARD, WILLIAM DAVID, M.D. Professor of Surgery and Clinical Surgery, Vanderbilt University. Surgeon to St. Thomas' Hospital, Vanderbilt and City Hospitals. *Treasurer*, 1900; *Secretary*. 184 Eighth Avenue, N., Nashville, Tenn.

1910.—HAGNER, FRANCIS RANDALL, M.D. Professor of Genito-urinary Surgery, George Washington University; Attending Genito-urinary Surgeon, George Washington Univeristy Hospital; Attending Surgeon, Garfield Memorial Hospital. The Farragut, Washington, D. C.

1892.—HALL, RUFUS BARTLETT, A.M., M.D. Professor of clinical Gynecology in the Miami Medical College; Gynecologist to the Presbyterian Hospital; ex-President of the Cincinnati Obstetrical Society; ex-President of the American Association of Obstetricians and Gynecologists; Fellow of British Gynecological Society. 628 Elm Street, Cincinnati, O.

1910.—HANES, GRANVILLE S., M.D. Professor of Surgery of the Rectum and Intestinal Diseases, Medical Department of the University of Louisville; Surgeon to the Louisville City Hospital. The Atherton Building, Louisville, Ky.

1901.—HAZEN, CHARLES M., M.D. Professor of Physiology, Medical College of Virginia. Bon Air (Richmond), Va.

1896.—HEFLIN, WYATT, M.D. Ex-President of the Jefferson County Medical Society. Birmingham, Ala.

1905.—HENDON, GEORGE A., M.D. Professor of Surgery and Clinical Surgery, University of Louisville. 968 Baxter Avenue, Louisville, Ky.

1889.—HILL, ROBERT SOMERVILLE, M.D. Gynecologist to the Laurel Hill Hospital; Senior Councillor of the Medical Association of the State of Alabama; ex-President of the Montgomery County Medical and Surgical Association; former Surgeon of the Second Regiment, Alabama State Militia. Montgomery, Ala.

1902.—HIRST, BARTON COOKE, M.D. Professor of Obstetrics, University of Pennsylvania; Fellow of College of Physicians, Philadelphia; Gynecologist to the Howard, Orthopedic, and Philadelphia Hospitals; Fellow of American Gynecological Society. 1821 Spruce Street, Philadelphia, Pa.

1913.—HODGSON, FRED G., M.D. Assistant in Orthopedics, Atlanta Medical College; Orthopedic Surgeon, Wesley Memorial Hospital and MacVicar Hospital of Spelman Seminary; Junior Orthopedic Surgeon, Grady Memorial Hospital. 72 West Peachtree Street, Atlanta, Ga.

1911.—HOGAN, EDGAR P., M.D. Associate Professor of Gynecology and Abdominal Surgery, Graduate School of Medicine of the University of Alabama; Resident Surgeon and Gynecologist to the Hillman Hospital. 412–14 Empire Building, Birmingham, Ala.

1906.—HOLDEN, GERRY R., M.D. Formerly House Surgeon, Roosevelt Hospital, New York City; formerly Resident Gynecologist, Johns Hopkins Hospital, and Assistant in Gynecology, Johns Hopkins Medical School. 223 West Forsyth Street, Jacksonville, Fla.

1891.—HOLMES, J. B. S., M.D. Ex-President of the Tri-State Medical Society of Alabama, Georgia, and Tennessee; ex-President of the Georgia Medical Association; Fellow of the American Association of Obstetricians and Gynecologists. *Vice-President*, 1894. Tampa Bay Hotel Park, Tampa, Florida.

1900.—HORSLEY, JOHN SHELTON, M.D. Surgeon-in-Charge of St. Elizabeth's Hospital. *Vice-President*, 1904. 617 West Grace Street, Richmond, Va.

1896.—HUNDLEY, J. MASON, M.D. Associate Professor of Diseases of Women and Children, University of Maryland; President Clinical Society of Baltimore. 1009 Cathedral Street, Baltimore, Md.

1903.—HUNNER, GUY LE ROY, M.D. Associate in Gynecology, Johns Hopkins University; Professor of Genito-urinary Surgery, Woman's Medical College of Baltimore; Gynecologist-in-Chief, St. Agnes' Hospital; Visiting Gynecologist, Church Home and Hebrew Hospital, Baltimore, Frederick City Hospital, Frederick, Md., and Hagerstown Hospital, Hagerstown, Md.; Consulting Gynecologist, Brattleboro Memorial Hospital, Brattleboro, Vt. *Vice-President*, 1911. 2305 St. Paul Street Baltimore, Md.

1900.—ILL, EDWARD JOSEPH, M.D. Surgeon to the Woman's Hospital; Medical Director, St. Michael's Hospital; Gynecologist and Supervising Obstetrician, St. Barnabas' Hospital; Consulting Gynecologist to German Hospital and Beth Israel Hospital of Newark, N. J., to All Souls' Hospital, Morristown, N. J., and to Mountain Side Hospital, Montclair, N. J.; Vice-President from New Jersey to Pan-American Congress of 1893. 1002 Broad Street, Newark, N. J.

1908.—*IRWIN, JAMES S., M.D. Danville, Va.

1912.—JACKSON, WILLIAM R., M.D. Professor of Surgery to the Medical Department of the University of Alabama; Consulting Surgeon to the City Hospital and Southern Infirmary, Mobile, Ala. 164 St. Michael Street, Mobile, Ala.

Founder.—JOHNSTON, GEORGE BEN, M.D. Formerly Consulting Surgeon to the Richmond Eye, Ear, and Throat Infirmary; ex-President of the Richmond Academy of Medicine and surgery; ex-President of the Medical Society of Virginia; Member of the American Association of Obstetricians and Gynecologists, and First Vice-President, 1896; Member of the Ninth International Medical Congress; Member of the American Surgical Association; Professor of the Practice of Surgery and Clinical Surgery in the Medical College of Virginia and formerly Professor of Anatomy; Surgeon to Old Dominion Hospital; Consulting Surgeon to the City Free Dispensary. *Vice-President*, 1892; *President*, 1897. 407 East Grace Street, Richmond, Va.

1908.—JONAS, ERNST, M.D. Clinical Professor of Surgery, Medical Department, Washington University; Chief of Surgical Clinic, Washington University Hospital; Gynecologist to the Jewish Hospital; Surgeon to the Martha Parsons Hospital for Children; Fellow of the American Association of Obstetricians and Gynecologists. 4495 Westminster Place, St. Louis, Mo.

1910.—JONES, EDWARD GROVES, A.B., M.D. Professor of Surgery, Medical Department, Emory University (Atlanta Medical College); Surgeon to Grady Memorial Hospital, Georgia Baptist Hospital and Wesley Memorial Hospital. 714 Hurt Building, Atlanta, Ga.

1902.—JORDAN, WILLIAM MUDD, M.D. Surgeon to St. Vincent's Hospital; Gynecologist to Hillman Hospital; formerly Assistant Surgeon, U. S. Marine Hospital Service. Birmingham, Ala.

1912.—JUDD, EDWARD STARR, M.D. Surgeon to St. Mary's Hospital, Rochester, Minn.

1890.—KELLY, HOWARD ATWOOD, M.D. Founder of Kensington Hospital, Philadelphia; Associate Professor of Obstetrics, University of Pennsylvania, 1888–89; Professor of Gynecology and Obstetrics, Johns Hopkins University, 1888–99; Professor of Gynecology, Johns Hopkins University; Gynecologist-in-Chief to Johns Hopkins Hospital; Member Associé Etranger de la Société Obstétricale et Gynécologique de Paris; Correspondirendes Mitglied der Gesellschaft f. Geburtshülfe zu Leipzig; Honorary Fellow, Edinburgh Obstetrical Society, Royal Academy of Medicine (Ireland), and British Gynecological Society; Member Washington Academy of Sciences; Fellow of the American Gynecological Society. *President,* 1907. 1418 Eutaw Place, Baltimore, Maryland.

1907.—KIRCHNER, WALTER C. G., M.D. Formerly Surgeon-in-Charge, St. Louis City Hospital. 508 Metropolitan Building, St. Louis, Mo.

1899.—KOHLMAN, WILLIAM, M.D. 3500 Prytania Street, New Orleans, La.

1913.—LAROQUE, G. PAUL, M.D. Associate Professor of Surgery, Medical College of Virginia; Surgeon, Memorial Hospital. 501 East Grace Street, Richmond, Va.

1914.—LANDRY, LUCIAN, M.D. Assistant Demonstrator in Operative Surgery and Instructor in Clinical Surgery, Tulane University of Louisiana, School of Medicine; Junior Surgeon, Touro Infirmary; Visiting Surgeon, Charity Hospital. 2255 St. Charles Avenue, New Orleans, La.

1894.—LEIGH, SOUTHGATE, M.D. Visiting Surgeon to St. Vincent's and Norfolk Protestant Hospitals; First Vice-President Medical Society of Virginia, 1899–1900. 147 Granby Street, Norfolk.

1912.—LEWIS, BRANSFORD, M.D. Century Building, St. Louis, Mo.

1914.—LEWIS, DEAN, A.B., M.D. Associate Professor of Surgery, Rush Medical College; Attending Surgeon, Presbyterian Hospital; Consulting Surgeon, Anne W. Durand Hospital of the Memorial Institute for Infectious Diseases. 122 South Michigan Avenue, Chicago, Ill.

1893.—LEWIS, ERNEST S., M.D. Professor of Gynecology, Medical Department of Tulane University. *Vice-President,* 1895; *President,* 1896; *Member of Council,* 1896–1903. 124 Baronne Street, New Orleans, La.

1900.—LLOYD, SAMUEL, M.D. Professor of Surgery, New York Post-Graduate Medical School; Attending Surgeon to the Post-Graduate Hospital and St. Francis' Hospital, and Consulting Surgeon to the Benedictine Sanitarium at Kingston, N. Y. 12 West Fiftieth Street, New York, N. Y.

Founder.—LONG, JOHN WESLEY, M.D., F.A.C.S. Emeritus Professor of Gynecology and Pediatrics in the Medical College of Virginia; formerly Gynecologist to the Old Dominion Hospital and the Richmond City Dispensary; Member, ex-Orator, and ex-Vice-President of the North Carolina Medical Society. President of the North Carolina Surgical Club; First Lieutenant, Medical Reserve Corps, U. S. A. *Vice-President,* 1902. *President,* 1914. Greensboro, N. C.

1904.—LUPTON, FRANK A., M.D. 716 North Eighteenth Street, Birmingham, Ala.

1902.—MCADORY, WELLINGTON P., M.D. Surgeon to Hillman Hospital. Birmingham, Ala.

1895.—MCGANNON, M. C., M.D. Professor of Surgery and Clinical Surgery, Medical Department, Vanderbilt University; Chief Surgeon, Woman's Hospital. 118 Eighth Avenue, N., Nashville, Tenn.

1911.—MCGLANNAN, ALEXIUS, M.D. Associate Professor of Surgery, College of Physicians and Surgeons, Baltimore. 114 West Franklin St., Baltimore, Md.

1893.—MCGUIRE, STUART, M.D. Professor of the Principles of Surgery and Clinical Surgery, University College of Medicine; Surgeon-in-Charge, St. Luke's Hospital; Visiting Surgeon, Virginia Hospital; Consulting Surgeon, Virginia Home for Incurables. *Vice-President,* 1906; *Treasurer,* 1908; *President,* 1909. 518 East Grace Street, Richmond, Va.

1891.—McGuire, W. Edward, M.D. Professor of Gynecology, University College of Medicine; Gynecologist to the Virginia Hospital. 411 East Grace Street, Richmond, Va.

1888.—McMurtry, Lewis S., M.D. Ex-President of the American Medical Association; Professor of Abdominal Surgery and Gynecology in the Medical Department of the University of Louisville; Surgeon to the Louisville City Hospital; Gynecologist to St. Mary and St. Elizabeth Hospital; Gynecologist to Gray Street Infirmary; ex-President of the American Association of Obstetricians and Gynecologists; ex-President of the Kentucky State Medical Society; Corresponding Member of the Gynecological Society of Boston; Fellow of the British Gynecological Society; Ordinary Fellow of the Edinburgh Obstetrical Society; Fellow of the American Surgical Society. *President,* 1891. Atherton Building, Fourth and Chestnut Streets, Louisville, Ky.

1888.—McRae, Floyd Wilcox, M.D. Professor of Gastrointestinal, Rectal, and Clinical Surgery, Atlanta College of Physicians and Surgeons; Surgeon to Grady Hospital; ex-President Medical Association of Georgia; ex-Secretary of Section on Surgery and Anatomy, American Medical Association. *Vice-President,* 1897; *Treasurer,* 1901–1903; *President,* 1904. Peters Building, Atlanta, Ga.

1905.—MacLean, Henry Stuart, M.D. Professor of Pathology, University College of Medicine. 406 West Grace Street, Richmond, Va.

1915.—Maes, Urban, M.D. Assistant Professor of Clinical and Operative Surgery, Tulane University of Louisiana School of Medicine; Junior Surgeon, Charity Hospital and Touro Infirmary; Senior Surgeon, New Orleans Dispensary for Women and Children. 1671 Octavia Street, New Orleans, La.

1912.—Malone, Battle, M.D. 1701 Exchange Building Memphis, Tenn.

1891.—Marcy, Henry Orlando, M.D., LL.D. Ex-President of the American Medical Association; President of the Section of Gynecology, Ninth International Medical Congress; late President of the American Academy of Medicine; Corresponding Member of the Medico-Chirurgical Society of Bologna, Italy; Fellow of the American Association of Obstetricians and Gynecologists. 180 Commonwealth Avenue, Boston, Mass.

1899.—Martin, E. Denegre, M.D. Professor of Surgery, Post-Graduate Department, Tulane Medical College; Visiting

Surgeon to Charity Hospital. *Vice-President*, 1906. 741 Carondelet St., New Orleans, La.

1909.—MARTIN, FRANK, M.D. Clinical Professor of Surgery at the University of Maryland. 1000 Cathedral Street, Baltimore, Md.

1913.—MARTIN, FRANKLIN H., M.D. Professor of Gynecology, Post-Graduate School; Consulting Staff, St. Luke's Hospital. Editor, Surgery, Gynecology, and Obstetrics.. 30 North Michigan Avenue, Chicago, Ill.

1904.—MASON, J. M., M.D. Gynecologist to St. Vincent's Hospital. 1915 Sixteenth Avenue, S., Birmingham, Ala.

1899.—MASTIN, WILLIAM M., M.D. Fellow of the American Surgical Association; Member of the American Association of Genito-urinary Surgeons; Surgeon to the Mobile City Hospital. Joachim and Conti Streets, Mobile, Ala.

1893.—MATAS, R., M.D. Professor of Surgery, Medical Department of Tulane University; Fellow of the American Surgical Association. *President*, 1911. 3523 Prytania St., New Orleans, La.

1896.—MATTHEWS, WILLIAM P., M.D. Professor of Anatomy Medical College of Virginia; Orthopedic Surgeon to the Old Dominion Hospital. Richmond, Va.

1902.—MAYO, CHARLES H., M.D. Attending Surgeon, St. Mary's Hospital; Fellow of American Surgical Society; ex-President, Western Surgical and Gynecological Association and of Minnesota State Medical Society. Rochester, Minn.

1899.—MICHINARD, P. E., M.D. 624 Gravier Street, New Orleans, La.

1888.—MILLER, C. JEFF., M.D. Visiting Surgeon to Charity Hospital of Louisiana; Professor of Clinical Obstetrics and Clinical Gynecology in the Tulane University of Louisiana; Chief of the Division of Obstetrics, Gynecology and Abdominal Surgery of the Presbyterian Hospital. 1638 Joseph Street, New Orleans, La.

1907.—MITCHELL, JAMES F., M.D. Surgeon to Providence Hospital. *Vice-President*. 1344 Nineteenth Street, Washington, D. C.

1901.—MIXTER, SAMUEL JASON, M.D. Surgeon, Massachusetts General Hospital; Consulting Surgeon, Massachusetts Charity Eye and Ear Infirmary; Instructor of Surgery, Harvard Medical School. 180 Marlborough St., Boston, Mass.

1910.—MOORE, JAMES E., M.D. Professor, and Chief of the Department of Surgery in the College of Medicine and Surgery of the University of Minnesota; Fellow and ex-Vice-President of the American Surgical Association; Member and ex-President of the Western Surgical Association; Member and ex-Chairman of the Surgical Section of the American Medical Association; Honorary Member of the American Orthopedic Association. 212 Millard Hall, University of Minneapolis, Minneapolis, Minn.

1911.—MOORE, JOHN THOMAS, M.D. Kress Medical Bldg., Houston, Texas.

1904.—MORAN, JOHN F., M.D. Professor of Obstetrics, Georgetown University; Obstetrician to Georgetown University Hospital and Columbia Hospital for Women. 2426 Pennsylvania Avenue, Washington, D. C.

1902.—MORRIS, LEWIS C., M.D. Professor of Anatomy and Associate Professor of Gynecology, Birmingham Medical College; Councillor of Medical Association, State of Alabama; Vice-President of Tri-State Medical Society of Alabama, Georgia, and Tennessee. *Vice-President*, 1910. 716 North Eighteenth Street, Birmingham, Ala.

1900.—MORRIS, ROBERT TUTTLE, M.D. Professor of Surgery, New York Post-Graduate Medical School and Hospital. 616 Madison Avenue, New York, N. Y.

1901.—MULLALLY, LANE, M.D. Professor of Obstetrics and Diseases of Children, Medical College, State of South Carolina; Visiting Physician in Obstetrics and Pediatrics, Roper Hospital. Charleston, S. C.

1894.—MURPHY, J. B., M.D. Ex-President American Medical Association; Professor of Surgery, Northwestern University, Professor of Surgery, Post-Graduate School and Hospital; Attending Surgeon, Cook County and Mercy Hospitals. 2526 Calumet Avenue, Chicago, Ill.

1889.—NICOLSON, WILLIAM PERRIN, M.D. Professor of Anatomy and Clinical Surgery, Atlanta College of Physicians and Surgeons; Visiting Surgeon to Grady Hospital; Senior Surgeon to Wesley Memorial Hospital; Senior Surgeon, St. Joseph's Hospital. *Vice-President*, 1900. Healey Building, Atlanta, Ga.

1890.—NOBLE, GEORGE H., M.D. Dean and Professor of Abdominal Surgery and Clinical Gynecology, Atlanta School of Medicine; Gynecologist of Grady Hospital; Senior

Gynecologist, Wesleyan Memorial Hospital, Atlanta; Fellow of the American Gynecological Association and the American Association of Obstetricians and Gynecologists; ex-President of the Medical Association of Georgia; ex-Secretary of the Section of Obstetrics, American Medical Association. *Vice-President*, 1901; *President*, 1906. 131 South Pryor Street, Atlanta, Ga.

1911.—NORRIS, HENRY, M.D. Rutherfordton, North Carolina.

1901.—OCHSNER, A. J., M.D. Adjunct Professor of Clinical Surgery, College of Physicians and Surgeons; Surgeon-in-Chief, Augustana and St. Mary's Hospital. 2106 Sedgwick Street, Chicago, Ill.

1903.—OCHSNER, EDWARD H., M.D. Surgeon to Augustana and St. Mary's Hospital. 2106 Sedgwick Street, Chicago, Illinois.

1904.—OECHSNER, JOHN F., M.D. Professor of Orthopedic Surgery and the Surgery of Children, Post-Graduate Medical Department, Tulane University of Louisiana; Visiting Surgeon, Charity Hospital. Macheca Building, New Orleans, Louisiana.

1902.—OLIVER, JOHN CHADWICK, M.D. Dean and Professor of Operative Surgery, Miami Medical College; Surgeon to the Cincinnati, Christ, and Presbyterian Hospitals. 628 Elm Street, Cincinnati, Ohio.

1888.—PARHAM, F. W., M.D. Professor of Surgery in the New Orleans Polyclinic. *Vice-President*, 1899; *President*, 1908. 1429 Seventh Street, New Orleans, La.

1910.—PAYNE, ROBERT LEE, JR., M.D. Assistant Gynecologist to St. Vincent's Hospital; Surgeon to the Southern Railway; Consulting Surgeon to the Seaboard Air Line Railway. 300 Freemason St., Norfolk, Va.

1899.—PERKINS, W. M., M.D. Chief of the Clinic Chair of General Clinical and Operative Surgery, New Orleans Polyclinic; Assistant Demonstrator of Operative Surgery, Medical Department, Tulane University of Louisiana; Visiting Surgeon to the Charity Hospital. 830 Canal Street, New Orleans, La.

1908.—PETERSON, REUBEN, A.M., M.D. Professor of Obstetrics and Gynecology, University of Michigan; Obstetrician and Gynecologist-in-Chief to the University of Michigan Hospital. Ann Arbor, Mich.

1899.—PLATT, WALTER BREWSTER, M.D. Surgeon to the Robert Garrett Hospital for Children. 802 Cathedral Street, Baltimore, Md.

1889.—POLK, WILLIAM M., M.D. Dean and Professor of Obstetrics and Gynecology, Cornell University Medical College; Gynecologist to Bellevue Hospital; Consulting Surgeon to St. Luke's, St. Vincent's, New York Lying-in, and Trinity Hospitals; ex-President of American Gynecological Society, and New York Obstetrical Society. 310 Fifth Ave., New York.

1900.—PORTER, MILES F., M.A., M.D. Surgeon to Hope Hospital; Professor of Surgery, Indiana University School of Medicine. 47 West Wayne Street, Fort Wayne, Ind.

1900.—RANSOHOFF, JOSEPH, M.D., F.R.C.S. Professor of Anatomy and Clinical Surgery, University of Cincinnati; Surgeon to Cincinnati, Good Samaritan, and Jewish Hospitals; Member American Surgical Association. 19 West Seventh Street, Cincinnati, Ohio.

1911.—REDER, FRANCIS, M.D. Surgeon, St. Louis City and St. John's Hospitals and Missouri Sanatorium. Delmar Building, St. Louis, Mo.

1890.—REED, CHARLES ALFRED LEE, M.D. Ex-President of the American Medical Association; Professor of Gynecology and Abdominal Surgery in the Cincinnati College of Medicine and Surgery; Surgeon to the Cincinnati Free Hospital for Women; Fellow of the American Association of Obstetricians and Gynecologists; Fellow of the British Gynecological Society; ex-Chairman of the Section on Obstetrics and Diseases of Women of the American Medical Association; Secretary-General of the Pan-American Medical Congress, 1893; Honorary Member of the Medical Society of the State of New York. 19 W. Seventh Street, Cincinnati, Ohio.

1914.—RHODES, GOODRICH BARBOUR, A.B., M.D. Assistant Clinical Professor of Surgery, Ohio-Miami Medical College of the University of Cincinnati; Junior Attending Surgeon, Cincinnati and Good Samaritan Hospitals and Episcopal Hospital for Children. 4 West Seventh Street, Cincinnati, Ohio.

1912.—RICHARDSON, EDWARD P., M.D. Surgeon to Out-patients, Massachusetts General Hospital, and Surgeon to the Robert B. Brigham Hospital for Chronic Diseases. 224 Beacon Street, Boston, Mass.

1888.—ROBERTS, WILLIAM O., M.D. Professor of Principles of Surgery and Clinical Surgery, Medical Department of the

University of Louisville; formerly Secretary of the Surgical Section of the American Medical Association. *President*, 1910; *Vice-President*, 1889. Atherton Building, Louisville, Ky.

1901.—ROBINS, CHARLES RUSSELL, M.D. Professor of Gynecology, Medical College of Virginia; Gynecologist to the Memorial Hospital; Surgeon to the Atlantic Coast Railroad. 8 West Grace Street, Richmond, Va.

1906.—ROGERS, CAREY PEGRAM, M.D. Chief of Surgical Staff, St. Luke's Hospital; Consulting Surgeon, Seaboard Air Line Railway. 221 Laura Street, Jacksonville, Fla.

1901.—ROGERS, MACK, M.D. Professor of Anatomy, Birmingham Medical College. 212 Twentieth Street, Birmingham, Ala.

1901.—ROSSER, CHARLES M., M.D. Professor of Surgery, Baylor University, College of Medicine; Consulting Surgeon, Parland Hospital; Attending Surgeon, Texas Baptist Memorial Sanitarium; ex-Vice-President Texas State Medical Association; Vice-President, Tri-State Society of Texas, Louisiana and Arkansas. *Treasurer*, 1904–07. 432 Gaston Avenue, Dallas, Texas.

1899.—ROYSTER, HUBERT ASHLEY, A.B., M.D. Surgeon to Rex Hospital; Surgeon-in-Chief, St. Agnes' Hospital; Surgeon to Southern Railway. *Vice-President*, 1907. 423 Fayetteville Street, Raleigh, N. C.

1909.—RUFFIN, KIRKLAND, M.D. Surgeon-in-Charge of St. Christopher's Hospital. 218 York Street, Norfolk, Va.

1901.—RUNYAN, JOSEPH P., M.D. 302 West Second Street, Little Rock, Ark.

1908.—RUSSELL, WM. WOOD, M.D. Associate Professor of Gynecology, Johns Hopkins University; Associate in Gynecology, Johns Hopkins Hospital; Gynecologist to Union Protestant Infirmary, Baltimore. 1208 Eutaw Place, Baltimore, Md.

1893.—SAUNDERS, BACON, M.D. Professor of Surgery and Clinical Surgery and Dean of Faculty of Medical Department, Fort Worth University; ex-President, Texas State Medical Association. *Vice-President*, 1903; *Member of Council*, 1908. Ninth and Houston Streets, Fort Worth, Texas.

1910.—SCHACHNER, AUGUST, M.D. 844 Fourth Avenue, Louisville, Ky.

1907.—SCOTT, ARTHUR CARROLL, M.D. Senior Surgeon, Temple Sanatorium. *Vice-President*, 1914. Temple, Texas.

1915.—SEELIG, MAJOR G., A.B., M.D. Professor of Surgery, St. Louis University School of Medicine; Attending Surgeon, Jewish and St. Louis City Hospitals; Chief of Surgical Out-Patient Department, Jewish Hospital. Wall Building, St. Louis, Mo.

1899.—SHANDS, A. R., M.D. Professor of Orthopedic Surgery in the Medical Department of the George Washington University and in the University of Vermont; Orthopedic Surgeon to the George Washington University Hospital, the Emergency Hospital, and Central Dispensary; Charter Member Washington Academy of Sciences; Member American Ortho-pedic Association; and Honorary Member of Medical Society of Virginia. 901 Sixteenth Street, N. W., Washington, D. C.

1914.—SHANDS, HARLEY R., A.A., M.D. Visiting Sur-geon, Mississippi State Charity and Baptist Hospitals. Cen-tury Building, Jackson, Miss.

1902.—SHERRILL, J. GARLAND, M.D. Professor of Surgery and Clinical Surgery, University of Louisville; Consulting Surgeon to Louisville Hospital. *Vice-President*, 1911. Ather-ton Building, Louisville, Ky.

1900.—SIMPSON, FRANK FARROW, M.D. Assistant Gyne-cologist, Mercy Hospital; Gynecologist to Out-patient Depart-ment, Mercy Hospital. Jenkins Arcade Bldg., Pittsburgh, Pa.

1913.—SIMPSON, JAMES KNOX, M.D. Attending Gyne-cologist St. Luke's Hospital; Associate Gynecologist Duval County Hospital, Jacksonville, Fla.

1899.—SMYTHE, FRANK DAVID, M.D. Gynecologist to St. Joseph's and City Hospitals; Professor of Gynecology, Didactic and Clinical, in the Memphis Hospital Medical College; ex-President West Tennessee Medical and Surgical Association; formerly Member of the Mississippi State Board of Health and State Board of Medical Examiners of Missis-sippi. Porter Building, Memphis, Tenn.

1904.—STOKES, JAMES ERNEST, M.D. Salisbury, N. C.

Founder.—STONE, ISAAC SCOTT, M.D., Sc.D. Professor of Gynecology, Georgetown University; Gynecologist to Columbia and Georgetown University Hospitals; Fellow of the American Gynecological Society; Fellow of the Royal Society of Medicine, London, England. *Vice-President*, 1905. 1618 Rhode Island Avenue, N. W., Washington, D. C.

1894.—TALLEY, DYER F., M.D. Associate Professor of Surgery, Birmingham Medical College; Attending Surgeon to Hillman Hospital; Surgeon to the Talley and McAdory Infirmary; ex-President of the Jefferson County Medical Society; Member of the Southern Medical Association; Member of the Pan-American Medical Association; Member of the Alumni Association of the Charity Hospital of Louisiana; Member of the Board of Censors of the Jefferson County Medical Society; Member of the Alabama State Board of Censors, Committee of Public Health and Examiners; Fellow of the American Association of Obstetricians and Gynecologists. 1801 Seventh Avenue, Birmingham, Ala.

Founder.—TAYLOR, HUGH M., M.D. Professor of Practice of Surgery and Clinical Surgery, University College of Medicine; Surgeon to the Virginia Hospital; ex-President of the Virginia Board of Medical Examiners. 6 North Fifth Street, Richmond, Va.

1898.—TAYLOR, WILLIAM WOOD, A.B., M.D. Gynecologist to the Lucy Brinkley and the Memphis City Hospitals. 206 Randolph Building, Memphis, Tenn.

1892. THOMPSON, J. E., M.D. Professor of Surgery in the University of Texas. *Vice-President*, 1912. Galveston, Tex.

1908.—TORRANCE, GASTON, M.D. Member Surgical Staff Hillman's Hospital; also the Sister's Hospital and St. Vincent's; Fellow of the American Association of Obstetricians and Gynecologists. 328 Woodward Building, Birmingham, Ala.

1909.—TROUT, HUGH HENRY, M.D. Surgeon-in-Chief of Jefferson Surgical Hospital, Roanoke, Va. 1303 Franklin Road, Roanoke, Va.

1888.—TUHOLSKE, HERMAN, M.D. Professor of Surgery, Medical Department, Washington University; Consulting Surgeon, St. Louis City Hospital; Surgeon to St. Louis Polyclinic Hospital. 465 North Taylor Street, St. Louis, Missouri.

1912.—TURCK, RAYMOND C., M.D. Consolidated Building, Jacksonville, Fla.

1905.—*VANCE, AP MORGAN, M.D. Surgeon to St. Mary and Elizabeth Hospital; Consulting Surgeon, Louisville City Hospital. *Vice-President*, 1913. 921 Fourth Street, Louisville, Ky.

1893.—VANDER VEER, ALBERT, M.D. Professor of Clinical, Didactic, and Abdominal Surgery, Albany Medical College; ex-President of the American Surgical Association; ex-President of the American Association of Obstetricians and Gynecologists; ex-President of the Medical Society of the State of New York. 28 Eagle Street, Albany, New York.

1909.—VAUGHAN, GEORGE TULLY, M.D. Professor of Surgery and Head of Department of Surgery in Georgetown University; Chief Surgeon in Georgetown University Hospital; Visiting Surgeon, Tuberculosis Hospital; Consulting Surgeon, St. Elizabeth's Hospital; Consulting Surgeon, Washington Asylum Hospital. 1718 I Street, Washington, D. C.

1891.—WALKER, EDWIN, M.D., PH.D. Gynecologist to the Evansville City Hospital; ex-President Mississippi Valley Medical Association; President of the Indiana State Medical Society; Fellow of the American Association of Obstetricians and Gynecologists. 712 Upper Fourth Street, Evansville, Indiana.

1912.—WALKER, GEORGE, M.D. Associate in Surgery, Johns Hopkins University. 1 E. Centre St., Baltimore, Maryland.

1911.—WARING, T. P., M.D. Savannah, Ga.

1905.—WATHEN, JOHN R., A.B., M.D. Professor of Principles and Practice of Surgery and Clinical Surgery, University of Louisville; Surgeon to St. Anthony's, Louisville City, and University of Louisville Hospitals. 628 Fourth Avenue, Louisville, Ky.

1898.—WATKINS, ISAAC LAFAYETTE, M.D. Ex-President of the Montgomery County Medical and Surgical Society. Montgomery, Ala.

1907.—WATTS, STEPHEN H., M.D. Professor of Surgery University of Virginia; Surgeon-in-Chief and Director of the University of Virginia Hospital. University of Virginia, Charlottesville, Va.

1901.—WERDER, X. O., M.D. Gynecologist, Mercy Hospital, Pittsburgh: Professor of Gynecology, West Pennsylvania Medical College; Consulting Surgeon to the South Side Hospital, Allegheny General Hospital, St. Francis Hospital, etc. 524 Pennsylvania Avenue, Pittsburgh, Pa.

1888.—WESTMORELAND, WILLIS F., M.D. Professor of Surgery, Atlanta College of Physicians and Surgeons. *Vice-President*, 1908. 241 Equitable Building, Atlanta, Ga.

1904.—WHALEY, T. P., M.D. Lecturer on Genito-urinary and Renal Surgery, Charleston Medical School; Lecturer on Diseases of Skin, Medical College of State of South Carolina; Surgeon to Sherra's Dispensary; Visiting Surgeon, Charleston City Hospital. 13 Wentworth Street, Charleston, South Carolina.

1913.—WILLIAMS, ESPY MILO, M.D. Surgeon, St. Mary's Hospital. Main Street, Patterson, La.

1900.—WILLIAMS, J. WHITRIDGE, A.B., M.D. Professor of Obstetrics, Johns Hopkins University; Obstetrician-in-Chief, Johns Hopkins Hospital; Gynecologist to the Union Protestant Infirmary. 1128 Cathedral Street, Baltimore, Md.

1907.—WILLIS, A. MURAT, M.D. Instructor in Abdominal Surgery, Medical College of Virginia; Junior Surgeon to Memorial Hospital, Richmond, Va. 405 East Grace Street, Richmond, Va.

1913.—WINDELL, JAMES TOLBERT, M.D. 715 West Jefferson Street, Louisville, Ky.

1905.—WINSLOW, RANDOLPH, M.D., LL.D. Professor of Surgery, University of Maryland; Chief Surgeon, University Hospital; Consulting Surgeon, Hebrew Hospital, and to Hospital for Crippled Children. 1900 Mt. Royal Terrace, Baltimore, Md.

1905.—WITHERSPOON, T. CASEY, M.D. Formerly Professor of Operative and Clinical Surgery, Medical Department, St. Louis University; Member of American Association of Anatomists. 307 West Granite Street, Butte, Mont.

1900.—WYSOR, JOHN C., M.D. Surgeon-in-Charge, Chesapeake and Ohio Hospital. Clifton Forge, Va.

1900.—YOUNG, HUGH H., M.D. Chief of Clinic, Genitourinary Surgery, Johns Hopkins Hospital. 330 North Charles Street, Baltimore, Md.

1802.—ZINKE, GUSTAV E., M.D., F.A.C.S. Professor of Obstetrics and Clinical Midwifery in the Ohio-Miami Medical College, University of Cincinnati, 1896–1916; Emeritus Professor of Obstetrics, 1916; Honorary Chief of Staff and Obstetrician and Gynecologist to the German Hospital; President of the Cincinnati Obstetric Society, 1887; President, Academy of Medicine of Cincinnati, 1894; Member and Chairman of Section on Obstetics, Gynecology and Abdominal Surgery, American Medical Association, 1914; Fellow (and Secretary) of American Association of Obstetricians and Gynecologists; Honorary Member, Jackson County Medical Society, Kansas City, Mo.; Honorary Member, Cincinnati Obstetricians and Gynecologists, 1908. 4 West Seventh Street, Cincinnati, Ohio.

CONSTITUTION

ARTICLE I

The name of this Association shall be THE SOUTHERN SURGICAL AND GYNECOLOGICAL ASSOCIATION.

ARTICLE II

The object of this Association is to further the study and practice of surgery and gynecology among the profession of the Southern States.

ARTICLE III

This Association shall adopt and conform to the Code of Ethics of the American Medical Association.

ARTICLE IV

SECTION 1. Any reputable physician who practises surgery or gynecology, and who is vouched for by two members of the Association and recommended by the Council, shall be eligible to membership in this body.

SEC. 2. The honorary members shall not exceed twenty-five in number, and shall enjoy all the privileges of other members, excepting to vote or hold office, but shall not be required to pay any fee.

ARTICLE V

SECTION 1. The officers of this Association shall be a President, two Vice-Presidents, a Secretary, a Treasurer, and a Council, elected by ballot.

SEC. 2. The President and Vice-Presidents shall be elected for one year, and the President shall not be eligible for reëlection at any time; the Secretary and Treasurer, each, for five years; and the Council as provided for in the By-laws.

ARTICLE VI

SECTION 1. It shall be the duty of the President to preside at all meetings of the Association; to give the casting vote; to see that the rules of order and decorum be properly enforced in all deliberations of the Association; to sign the approved proceedings of each meeting, and to approve such orders as may be drawn upon the Treasurer for expenditures ordered by the Association.

SEC. 2. In the absence of the President the first Vice-President shall preside, and in his absence the second Vice-President shall preside.

SEC. 3. In the absence of all three, the Association shall elect one of its members to preside *pro tem*.

SEC. 4. It shall be the duty of the Secretary to keep a true and correct record of the proceedings of the meetings; to preserve all books, papers, and articles belonging to the archives of the Association; to attest all orders drawn on the Treasurer for moneys appropriated by the Association; to keep the account of the Association with its members; to keep a register of the members, with the dates of their admission and places of residence. He shall collect all moneys due from the members and pay to the Treasurer, taking his receipt for the same. He shall report such unfinished business of previous meetings as may appear on his books requiring action, and attend to such other business as the Association may direct. He shall also supervise and conduct all the correspondence of the Association, and edit the TRANSACTIONS under the direction of the Council.

SEC. 5. It shall be the duty of the Treasurer to keep a correct record of all moneys received from the hands of the Secretary, giving his receipt for the same; pay them out by order of the Association as indorsed by the President and attested by the seal in the hands of the Secretary.

SEC. 6. It shall be the duty of the President of the Association to appoint an Auditing Committee, consisting of three members of the Association, whose duty it shall be to examine the books of the Secretary and Treasurer, and report on the same on the last day of the session.

ARTICLE VII

Vacancies occurring in the offices of the Association shall be filled by appointment of the President until the next meeting. He shall also have the appointment of all committees not otherwise provided for.

ARTICLE VIII

This Constitution shall take effect immediately from the time of its adoption, and shall not be amended except by a written resolution, which shall lie over one year, and receive a vote of two-thirds of the members present.

ARTICLE IX

The membership of the Association shall be limited to two hundred.

BY-LAWS

ARTICLE I

The Southern Surgical and Gynecological Association shall meet annually on the Tuesday of the week preceding the week in which Christmas occurs, at 10 A.M., at such place as may be designated at the preceding meeting.

ARTICLE II

The members present shall constitute a quorum for business.

ARTICLE III

The annual dues of each member shall be $10, paid in advance.

ARTICLE IV

The usual parliamentary rules governing deliberative bodies shall govern the business workings of this Association.

ARTICLE V

All questions before the Association shall be determined by a majority of the votes present.

ARTICLE VI

The President shall deliver an annual address at each meeting of the Association.

ARTICLE VII

The Secretary of the Association shall receive at each annual Session a draft from the President, drawn on the Treasurer, for the sum of $500, for services rendered the Association, and to this shall be added the necessary expense incurred in the discharge of his official duties.

ARTICLE VIII

It shall be the duty of the Secretary, one month prior to the annual meeting, to notify the members of the Association and urge their attendance.

ARTICLE IX

The authors of papers shall notify the Secretary, six weeks prior to the meeting, of the titles of their essays, so that they may be incorporated in the preliminary programme.

ARTICLE X

COUNCIL

The Council shall consist of five members; and of those elected at the primary meeting, the first shall serve five years, the second four, and the third three, the fourth two, and the fifth one year; so that subsequently one member of the Council shall be elected annually to serve five years. No member of the Council shall be eligible for reëlection. The President and Secretary shall be *ex-officio* members of the Council.

This Council shall organize by electing a Chairman and Secretary, and shall keep a record of its proceedings.

The duties of this Council shall be—

1. To investigate applications for membership and report to the Association the names of such persons as are deemed worthy.

2. To take cognizance of all questions of an ethical, judicial, or personal nature, and upon these the decision of the Council shall be final; *provided*, that appeal may be taken from such decision of the Council to the Association, under a written protest, which protest shall be sustained by the Association, and the matter shall then be referred to a special committee, with power to take final action.

3. All motions and resolutions before the Association shall be referred to the Council without debate, and it shall report by recommendation at as early an hour as possible.

ARTICLE XI

The President shall appoint at each annual meeting a Committee of Arrangements.

ARTICLE XII

The Council shall have full power to omit from the published TRANSACTIONS, in part or in whole, any paper that may be referred to it by the Association, unless specially instructed to the contrary by the Association, which will be determined by vote.

ARTICLE XIII

Any member failing to pay his dues for more than one year shall be dropped.

ARTICLE XIV

No paper shall be read before this Association which does not deal strictly with a subject of surgical or gynecological importance.

ARTICLE XV

No paper read before this Association shall be published in any medical journal or pamphlet for circulation, as having been read before the Association, without having received the endorsement of the Council.

ARTICLE XVI

The readings of papers shall be limited to twenty minutes each, except by permission of the Association.

MINUTES OF THE PROCEEDINGS

AT THE

TWENTY-EIGHTH ANNUAL MEETING

OF THE

SOUTHERN

SURGICAL AND GYNECOLOGICAL

ASSOCIATION

HELD AT THE

GIBSON HOTEL

Cincinnati, Ohio

DECEMBER 13, 14 AND 15, 1915

TWENTY–EIGHTH ANNUAL MEETING

FIRST DAY.—*Monday, December* 13, 1915.

The following named members were present:

ABELL, IRVIN
BAILEY, FRED WARREN
BALLOCH, EDWARD A.
BARR, RICHARD ALEXANDER
BARROW, DAVID
BARTLETT, WILLARD
BLAIR, VILRAY P.
BLOODGOOD, JOSEPH C.
BOLDT, HERMAN J.
BONIFIELD, CHARLES L.
BOVEE, J. WESLEY
BROWN, JOHN YOUNG
BRYAN, ROBERT C.
BUIST, A. JOHNSON
BYFORD, HENRY T.
CALDWELL, C. E.
CALDWELL, ROBERT
CANNADAY, JOHN EGERTON
CAROTHERS, ROBERT
CARR, WILLIAM P.
COLE, HERBERT PHALON
COUSINS, WILLIAM LEWIS
CRISLER, JOSEPH AUGUSTUS
CULLEN, THOMAS S.
DANNA, JAMES A.
DAVIS, JOHN D. S.
DOWNES, WILLIAM A.
ELBRECHT, O. H.
FINNEY, J. M. T.
FORT, RUFUS E.

FRANK, LOUIS
FREIBURG, ALBERT H.
GOLDSMITH, W. S.
GRANT, HORACE H.
GUERRY, LE GRAND
HAGGARD, WILLIAM DAVID
HAGNER, FRANCIS R.
HALL, RUFUS B.
HANES, GRANVILLE S.
HEFLIN, WYATT
HENDON, GEORGE A.
HILL, ROBERT SOMERVILLE
HODGSON, FRED G.
HORSLEY, J. SHELTON
HUNDLEY, J. MASON
ILL, EDWARD JOSEPH
JACKSON, WILLIAM R.
JOHNSTON, GEORGE BEN
JONAS, ERNST
JUDD, EDWARD STARR
KELLY, HOWARD ATWOOD
KIRCHNER, WALTER C. G.
LEWIS, BRANSFORD
LEWIS, DEAN
LONG, JOHN W.
MCGLANNAN, ALEXIUS
MCGUIRE, STUART
MCMURTRY, LEWIS S.
MCRAE, FLOYD WILCOX
MALONE, BATTLE

MARTIN, FRANK

MARTIN, FRANKLIN H.

MAYO, CHARLES H.

MILLER, C. JEFF

MITCHELL, JAMES F.

MOORE, JAMES E.

MOORE, JOHN THOMAS

MORRIS, ROBERT TUTTLE

OCHSNER, A. J.

OLIVER, JOHN C.

PARHAM, F. W.

PAYNE, ROBERT LEE

RANSOHOFF, JOSEPH

REED, CHARLES A. L.

RHODES, GOODRICH B.

RICHARDSON, EDWARD P.

ROBERTS, WILLIAM O.

ROBINS, CHARLES RUSSELL

ROSSER, CHARLES M.

ROYSTER, HUBERT A.

RUSSELL, WM. WOOD

SAUNDERS, BACON

SCHACHNER, AUGUST

SCOTT, ARTHUR CARROLL

SHANDS, HARLEY

SHERRILL, J. GARLAND

SIMPSON, FRANK F.

SMYTHE, FRANK D.

STOKES, JAMES ERNEST

TALLEY, D. F.

TROUT, HUGH H.

WATHEN, JOHN R.

WATTS, STEPHEN H.

WINDELL, J. T.

WINSLOW, RANDOLPH

WYSOR, JOHN C.

ZINKE, E. GUSTAV

Letters and messages of regret were received from a number of Fellows who were unable to attend the meeting.

Morning Session. The Association met in the ball-room of the Gibson Hotel and was called to order by the Chairman of the Committee of Arrangements, Dr. Charles A. L. Reed, Cincinnati, Ohio, who said:

Fellows of the Southern Surgical and Gynecological Association: As Chairman of your Committee of Arrangements, it affords me extreme pleasure and satisfaction not only in behalf of myself, but more especially in the name of my colleagues, the resident Fellows of the Association, and profession of this city, to welcome you to our city and to extend to you its hospitality.

There is but very little to say or to do on this occasion. I might indulge in what is, more or less usual, a recapitulation of the achievements of this Association and of the devotion of the City of Cincinnati to the causes and purposes which you have in view. I feel, however, in doing so I would only be carrying coals to Newcastle. In other words, you are familiar with the master motives and with the consecration of this city to the same scientific and humane objects; therefore, I come to the specific discharge of the duties of my office as Chairman of Committee of Arrangements.

By turning to the official program you will notice that at 12.45 today there is to be a luncheon at the Sinton Hotel. At 2 P.M., following this luncheon, the members of the Association will take the street cars and visit the Cincinnati General Hospital. A theater party has been provided for the ladies this evening, while the Association will have an evening session. With these announcements I feel I have discharged my duties for the time being, except to say that every member of the committee, whose name appears upon the program is at your disposal to do anything that you may wish to have done. If you do not see anything you want, ask for it.

It only remains for me to turn the meeting over to the officers and to present to you your distinguished President, Dr. Bacon Saunders, of Fort Worth.

President Saunders, in calling the twenty-eighth annual meeting together for the transaction of its scientific work, said: It is extremely pleasing to me, as I know it is to the Fellows, to see such a representative attendance at this opening session. I am glad to recall, as I am sure many of the members do, the extremely pleasant and profitable meeting we had here in this city a number of years ago, and I know that the Fellows are all glad to come back. I feel that we all realize that, notwithstanding the inclemency of the weather, this meeting is not only going to be a pleasant, but a profitable one.

With the characteristic energy of this Association, we will now proceed with the regular program. (Applause.)

Papers were read as follows: 1. "An Experimental and Clinical Study on the Transplantation of Fascia in the Treatment of Postoperative Ventral Hernia," by Dr. Willard Bartlett, St. Louis, Missouri.

2. "The Moscowitz Operation—Inguinal Route for Femoral Hernia," by Dr. John D. S. Davis, Birmingham, Alabama.

These two papers were discussed together by Drs. Brown, Cullen, Sherrill, Mayo, Boldt, Blair, and discussion closed by the essayists.

3. "High Degrees of Heat *versus* Low Degrees of Heat as Palliative Treatment for Advanced Cases of Cancer of the Uterus, With an Autopsy Report on a Case Treated by the Long Application of Low Heat as Advocated by Dr. J. F. Percy," by Dr. Herman J. Boldt, New York City.

On motion of Dr. W. D. Haggard, the gentlemen whose

names are herewith given were extended the privileges of the floor: Dr. H. J. Sherk, Pasadena, California; Dr. Edward C. Moore, Los Angeles, California; Dr. A. C. Stokes, Omaha, Nebraska; Dr. E. D. Newell, Chattanooga, Tennessee; Dr. W. M. McCabe, Nashville, Tennessee; Dr. Joseph S. H. Gallagher, Nashville, Tennessee; Dr. Gordon K. Dickinson, Jersey City, New Jersey; Dr. Charles W. Hibbett, Louisville, Kentucky; Dr. E. L. McKenney, Louisville, Kentucky; Dr. C. H. Harris, Birmingham, Alabama; Dr. M. H. Fletcher, Asheville, North Carolina, and Dr. E. A. Ill, Newark, New Jersey.

The paper of Dr. Boldt was discussed by Drs. Cullen, Bovée, Mayo, Horsley, Blair, McGlannan, Byford, Robins, Miller, and Carr, after which the discussion was closed by the essayist.

4. "Adenomyoma of the Round Ligament; Early Tuberculosis of the Cervix," by Dr. Thomas S. Cullen, Baltimore, Maryland; discussed by Dr. Jackson.

5. "Pulsating Exophthalmos; Report of a Case Cured by Ligation of Common Carotid Artery," by Dr. Goodrich B. Rhodes, Cincinnati, Ohio, which was discussed by Drs. Blair, McGlannan, Hendon, Finney, and discussion closed by the essayist.

6. "Thymic Findings in One Hundred Fatal Cases of Goitre; A Clinical and Pathological Analysis" (by invitation), by Dr. J. M. Blackford and Dr. R. S. Freligh, Rochester, Minn.

Dr. Alexius McGlannan moved that the discussion of this paper be postponed until after the reading of the paper of Dr. Judd.

Seconded and carried.

On motion the Association adjourned until 8.00 P.M.

NOTE. No afternoon session was held on account of the visit to and inspection of the Cincinnati General Hospital.

Evening Session. The Association reassembled at 8.00 P.M. and was called to order by the First Vice-President, Dr. Thomas S. Cullen.

7. "Results of Operations for Exophthalmic Goitre," by Dr. E. Starr Judd, Rochester, Minnesota.

There was no discussion of the papers of Drs. Blackford and Judd.

8. President's Address: "The Great Professional Problem of the Present Decade," by Dr. Bacon Saunders, Fort Worth, Texas.

Dr. Charles L. Bonifield, Cincinnati, moved that a rising vote of thanks be extended to President Saunders for his splendid address.

Seconded and carried unanimously.

9. "Unilateral Hematuria Associated with Varicosities and Multiple Microscopic Calculi of the Papilla," by Dr. R. L. Payne, Jr., Norfolk, Virginia.

10. "Pancreatic Cyst As a Cause of Unilateral Hematuria; Report of a Case," by Dr. Joseph Ransohoff, Cincinnati, Ohio.

These two papers were discussed together by Drs. Hagner, Cullen, Bailey, Lewis, Moore, and discussion closed by Dr. Payne.

11. "A case of Exstrophy of the Bladder in Which the Urine was Diverted into the Lower End of the Ileum," by Dr. V. P. Blair, St. Louis, Missouri.

12. "Report of a Case of Exstrophy of the Bladder Operated Nearly Thirty Years Ago, with Subsequent History," by Dr. Randolph Winslow, Baltimore, Maryland.

These two papers were discussed together by Drs. Jonas, Haggard, and discussion closed by Dr. Winslow.

13. "Giant Ureteral Calculus," by Dr. Irvin Abell, Louisville, Kentucky.

Discussed by Drs. Cullen, Smythe and Moore.

On motion, the Association adjourned until 9.00 A.M., Tuesday.

SECOND DAY.—*Tuesday, December* 14, 1915.

Morning Session. The Association met at 9.00 A.M., and was called to order by the President.

14. "The Advantages of Separate Suture of the Mucous Membrane in Gastric Surgery," by Dr. Richard A. Barr, Nashville, Tennessee.

Discussed by Dr. Jackson, and discussion closed by the essayist.

15. "In Cases of Symptoms Without Gall-stones, What Disposition Shall be Made of the Gall-Bladder?" By Dr. Le Grand Guerry, Columbia, South Carolina.

16. "Cholecystostomy *versus* Cholecystectomy," by Dr. Charles H. Mayo, Rochester, Minnesota.

These two papers were discussed together by Drs. Jackson, Carr, Sherrill, Crisler, Cullen, Finney, McGuire, Long, Ochsner, and discussion closed by Drs. Guerry and Mayo.

17. "Report of the Use of Caudal Anesthesia for Urological Work, With Lantern Slides," by Dr. Bransford Lewis, St. Louis, Missouri.

18. "Some Observations on Local Anesthesia," by Dr. H. P. Cole, Mobile, Alabama.

These two papers were discussed by Drs. Crisler, Moore, Caldwell, Jackson, Stokes, and discussion closed by Drs. Lewis and Cole.

The President appointed Dr. C. Jeff. Miller, Dr. John D. S. Davis, and Dr. J. Garland Sherrill, as a Committee to audit the accounts of the Secretary and Treasurer.

19. "Echinococcus Cysts of the Liver," by Dr. George Ben Johnston, Richmond, Virginia (no discussion).

20. "Intussusception in Infants," by Dr. Lewis S. McMurtry, Louisville, Kentucky.

This paper was discussed by Drs. Watts, Royster, Parham, Morris, Sherrill, Abell, and discussion closed by the author of the paper.

On motion of Dr. Brown, the Association adjourned until 2 P.M.

Afternoon Session. The Association reassembled at 2 P.M., and was called to order by Dr. F. W. McRae, who occupied the Chair *pro tem.*

21. "Chronic Obstruction *versus* Intestinal Stasis," Illustrated by a Case, by Dr. F. W. Parham, New Orleans, Louisiana.

22. "Colon Resection and Report of Cases," by Dr. Frank Martin, Baltimore, Maryland.

23. "The Operative Treatment of Pyloric Obstruction in Infants, with a Review of Sixty Personal Cases," by Dr. William A. Downes, New York City.

These three papers were discussed together by Drs. Mitchell, Lewis, Brown, McGlannan, Ochsner, and discussion closed by Drs. Martin and Downes.

24. "Focal Infections," by Dr. Robert T. Morris, New York City.

25. "A Further Study of the Use of Iodin in Combating the Peritonitides," by Dr. J. A. Crisler, Memphis, Tennessee.

Discussed by Drs. Morris, Sherrill, Jackson, Royster, Lewis, Frank, and discussion closed by Dr. Crisler.

26. "Typhoid Perforation Peritonitis; Report of an Unusual Case," by Dr. Frank D. Smythe, Memphis, Tennessee.

Discussed by Dr. Jackson, and in closing by the essayist.

27. "Salpingitis Secondary to Appendicitis," by Dr. James E. Moore, Minneapolis, Minnesota.

Discussed by Drs. Elbrecht, Bovée, Cullen, and Morris.

28. "Rupture of Pseudomucinous Ovarian Cyst and Pseudomyxomatous Appendix," by Dr. Fred. W. Bailey, St. Louis, Missouri.

29. "Plastic Operations for Acquired Deformities of the Face," with lantern slides, by Dr. J. Shelton Horsley, Richmond, Virginia.

30. "Elephantiasis Following Extirpation of the Inguinal Gland," by Dr. J. T. Windell, Louisville, Kentucky.

On motion the Association adjourned until Wednesday, 9 A.M.

THIRD DAY.—*Wednesday, December 15, 1915.*

The Association met at 9 A.M., and was called to order by the President.

31. "Ulcer of the Jejunum, with Report of a Case," by Dr. Robert T. Bryan, Richmond, Virginia.

Discussed by Drs. Ochsner and Jackson.

32. "Estimation of Patient's Resistance Prior to Operation," by Dr. A. C. Scott, Temple, Texas.

Discussed by Drs. Horsley, Morris, Hagner, Rhodes, Carr, Parham, Long, Royster, and discussion closed by Dr. Scott.

33. "Sarcomata in Unusual Situations," with lantern slides, by Dr. Hubert A. Royster, Raleigh, North Carolina.

34. "Radium in the Treatment of Lymphosarcoma." by Dr. Howard A. Kelly, Baltimore, Maryland.

These two papers were discussed by Drs. Moore, Morris, Ransohoff, Jonas, Talley, Oliver, Jackson, Ochsner, McGlannan, and discussion closed by Dr. Kelly.

THE PRESIDENT.—It is now in order to have a report from the Auditing Committee.

Dr. C. Jeff Miller reported that the Auditing Committee had examined the accounts of the Secretary and Treasurer and found them to be correct, and that there is a cash balance in bank of $779.73.

(Signed)   C. JEFF. MILLER,
J. GARLAND SHERRILL,
JOHN D. S. DAVIS.

Dr. Randolph Winslow moved that the report be accepted. Seconded and carried.

The Secretary read the report of the Council as follows:

Report of the Council. Gentlemen of the Southern Surgical and Gynecological Association: The Council recommends:

1. That the Association endorses the organization of National Board of Medical Examiners as outlined by the President of the American Medical Association in his address at the San Francisco meeting; and, furthermore, that the President of this Association appoint a committee of one member from each State represented in this membership, to secure the approval of State boards and to coöperate with any other committee working to a similar purpose.

2. That this Association be represented on the Board of Governors of the American College of Surgeons by Dr. R. E. Fort, Dr. Guy L. Hunner, and Dr. Louis Frank.

3. That a committee of three be appointed by the President to make an independent survey of the problem of first-aid work with the Board of Standardization and its secretary.

4. That the resignation of Harvey Cushing be accepted.

5. That the deaths of our esteemed Fellows, Dr. W. B. Dorsett and Dr. Ap. Morgan Vance, be suitably recorded in the Transactions.

6. That the three vacancies on the membership roster be filled by Dr. M. G. Seelig, of St. Louis; Dr. William S. Baer, of Baltimore, and Dr. Urban Maes, New Orleans.

7. That a committee of three, consisting of Drs. Stuart McGuire, Chairman, J. W. Long, and J. M. T. Finney, be appointed to report on the best method of rendering the list of members more elastic; to recommend any needed changes in the Constitution and By-laws, and to consider the question of dues and suggestions to the committee from the members are respectfully requested by the Council.

8. That the next place of meeting be the Greenbrier Hotel at White Sulphur Springs, West Virginia.

9. That the vacancy on the Council occurring from the expiration of service of Dr. Stuart McGuire be filled by the retiring President, Dr. Bacon Saunders.

10. The following officers are nominated for the ensuing year: President, Dr. Thomas S. Cullen, Baltimore, Maryland;

Vice-Presidents, Drs. Robert S. Hill, Montgomery, Alabama, and Dr. Willard Bartlett, St. Louis, Missouri.

The offices of Secretary and Treasurer hold over.

Respectfully submitted,

(Signed)   STUART McGUIRE,
            JOHN YOUNG BROWN,
            F. W. PARHAM,
            J. M. T. FINNEY,
            JOHN W. LONG,
            BACON SAUNDERS.

Dr. F. W. McRae moved that the report be accepted and adopted.

Seconded and carried.

THE PRESIDENT.—I will appoint Dr. Ochsner and Dr. Winslow to escort the newly elected President to the Chair. (Applause.)

Dr. Cullen, in accepting the Presidency, said: Fellow members: I deeply appreciate the honor you have conferred upon me. Several years ago the Southern Surgical and Gynecological Association met in Baltimore. A few of us were asked to take part in the proceedings, and that afternoon we were surprised to find that we had been elected members of the Association. I personally deeply appreciate the confidence you have reposed in me. I have attended the meetings regularly since that time, and consider it a great advantage to know so many members of the Association. Last year you were good enough to honor me by making me a Vice-President, and I considered that more than sufficient for anything I have ever done; but to be elected President, to be included in a group of men who have been Presidents and Past Presidents, is a signal honor of which any man might be proud.

"I want to express my appreciation personally to Dr. Haggard for all that he has done for this Association and for the splendid program of this year.

"I want to assure the President, Dr. Saunders, that we will with his assistance and the assistance of the various members, try and put ginger into our work next year as he has done this year. Once more, please accept my best thanks for this great honor" (Applause.)

DR. SAUNDERS.—"Fellows of the Association: It will be remembered I said last year—if not publicly—privately, that after being elected to this exceedingly honorable position, I scarcely knew whether to laugh or to cry. It has been the most pleasing episode of my life to have the honor of being officially connected in this way with this very distinguished body. I want to thank every individual Fellow of this Association. I want especially to thank our esteemed Secretary, Dr. Haggard, for his great activity and zeal in making this perhaps a record-breaking meeting. (Applause.)

"In conclusion, let me say, one of the greatest pleasures in retiring from this office is to be aware of the fact that I place into the hands of such a competent man this emblem (referring to gavel) of authority."

35. "Remarks on the Employment of Subcutaneous Dermic Fistula in the Treatment of Ascites," by Dr. Walter C. G. Kirchner, St. Louis, Missouri.

Discussed by Drs. Caldwell, Horsley, Jackson, Watts, and discussion closed by the essayist.

36. "Conservative Pelvic Surgery," by Dr. Floyd W. McRae, Atlanta, Georgia.

Discussed by Drs. Morris, Bovée, Hill, Royster, Robins, Cullen, and discussion closed by the essayist.

On motion the Association adjourned until 2 P.M.

Afternoon Session. The Association reassembled at 2 P.M., and was called to order by Dr. Saunders.

37. "American First-aid Conference," by Dr. Joseph C. Bloodgood, Baltimore, Maryland.

38. "Report of Gangrenous Abscess of the Lung," by Dr. D. F. Talley, Birmingham, Alabama.

Discussed by Drs. Bloodgood, Carr, Winslow, Jackson, and discussion closed by the essayist.

39. "Fracture of the Neck of the Femur," by Dr. Alexius McGlannan, Baltimore, Maryland.

40. "Treatment of Fractures," by Dr. W. P. Carr, Washington, D. C.

41. These two papers were discussed together by Drs. Rosser, Malone, Caldwell, Trout, Freiburg, Robins, Jackson, Moore, Morris, Scott, Carothers, and the discussion closed by Drs. McGlannan and Carr.

42. "Cysts of the Appendix," by Dr. John T. Moore, Houston, Texas.

On motion of Dr. Haggard, which was duly seconded and carried, Dr. John Wesley Long, Greensboro, North Carolina, described "A New Method of Shortening the Round Ligaments."

Dr. Joseph C. Bloodgood, Baltimore, showed some slides of Cancerous Breast Tumors.

Dr. Charles M. Rosser, Dallas, Texas, offered the following resolution, which was unanimously adopted by a rising vote:

Resolved, That an expression of sincere appreciation be tendered the profession and the public of Cincinnati for a repetition of the splendid cordiality with which they received us on the occasion of our former meeting, the pleasure of which has at no time been forgotten. In these expressions we would also include the institutions and newspapers which have placed their facilities at our command, each helpful to our enterprises and our desired usefulness.

To the ladies of this community we would especially make our most profound acknowledgements for the many kindly courtesies they have so generously extended.

On motion, the Association then adjourned to meet at White Sulphur Springs, West Virginia, December 11, 12, and 13, 1916.

WILLIAM D. HAGGARD, M.D.,

Secretary.

THE GREAT PROFESSIONAL PROBLEM OF THE PRESENT DECADE

By Bacon Saunders, M.D.
Fort Worth, Texas

PERMIT me to acknowledge, first, the sincerest and most heartfelt appreciation of the distinguished honor conferred on me a year ago by the Fellows of this Association. Not to do so would be tantamount to conviction by default of a base ingratitude against which every better impulse within me would rise in mutinous revolt. To be counted by the Fellows of this the greatest association of this country, for any reason and even to a limited degree, fit to occupy the position that has been made honorable by the great men who have filled it, and by whose presence among us at our annual assemblies we are still blessed; and which, too, has been made illustrious and hallowed by the memory of those others, the immortals, who occupied it while sojourning in the activities of this life, and by the magnetism of their very presence made the countenance of every Fellow to glow as with the effulgence of the new day, but have crossed over the river and are now resting peacefully "under the shade of the trees" in the elysian fields of the blessed beyond, is indeed a signal and in the present instance, I fear, unmerited honor. Being assured that the regular official scientific program would present its usual unsurpassed variety of subjects together with ample scope for profitable discussion, it has seemed worth while, and possibly wise, to step aside from the course usually pursued by my predecessors and suggest, very briefly, for your consideration, as *apropos* to both the time and the occasion, certain present conditions that are not in any sense technical or scientific in character but which intimately and materially touch the welfare of every member of every branch of the medical profession.

Stupendous and all-important as these interests are if they alone were at stake, it might be possible, without fatal disregard of duty, to overlook them under the plea of sectarian or partisan origin. If, however, the science of medicine is not simply a cult, hoary and bended with the exploded and exploding theories of the ages, but is in demonstrable verity what it claims to be, and what we hope and steadfastly believe it will continue to be, and the arts of medicine and surgery are to attain and maintain the splendid perfection their loyal subjects believe they have already reached, these same devotees, looking the while with expectant eyes toward a future, big with the promise of greater and better service to the human race and reflexly to themselves, there is no person or people living today or that may come tomorrow whose welfare must not be taken into account. If such cursory and of necessity limited discussion of the subject shall, peradventure, cause a perfectly full and frank admission to ourselves and among ourselves that the conditions are real, and not only real but a militant and forceful power for evil, and evil only to the best and dearest interests of life, and have already disseminated the germs of their toxic, miasmatic breath into the nostrils of every profession, calling, and avocation of mankind's activities, from the pulpit to the hewers of wood and drawers of water, and are not the idle fancy of a distempered brain nor the disturbing nightmare, the distress sign of some beleagured stomach, the transcendant importance of giving them careful consideration, will come home, and those heretofore little concerned, both people and profession, may be aroused from lethargic indifference to active, wide-awake realization of the demands of the times.

Every period of history, every phase of human activity has had its own problems peculiar to it and arising out of the circumstances and environments of the social and economic life of the world at that particular time, which had to be met and naturally could only be met by the people directly concerned in those activities. And as with them, so with us, the effective agencies in the solution of the problems of yesterday will perhaps, have entirely lost relation to those of tomorrow. The problems of today are our own, devised to us by the teeming, pushing, often scrambling world we were born into, without our knowledge or consent, and we ourselves must solve them, often in fear and trembling, but always with truth, vigor, valor, and a clear conscience. Otherwise, and if this had not been the fate of the human family throughout all history, the course of life would often have run differently from what it did. The leafy bowers and flower-decked paths of Eden might have shielded father Adam and mother Eve in quite another solution of the simple problem of their lives, and thus have changed the whole sequence of human events.

The application of scientific discoveries and ingenious inventions to all the varied activities of modern life have wrought such wonderful changes in the social and economic conditions and even the avocations of both men and women it is not a matter for surprise that in the whir and whirl of life's panorama a considerable number of people should have become dizzy and mentally hazy and so demoralized and confused in their point of view and their moral vision so blurred, that for the time being they do not see accurately the outlines of the finer and higher ethical standards. They do not fail to see themselves loom big and important in life's mirror, but have lost the power, and possibly even to a

great extent, the inclination or desire and do not feel the
necessity to weigh carefully moral and ethical values. The
atmosphere of the times seems to have dulled the edge of
conscience and stunted the moral perception of the world
as the salt sea corrodes the keenest steel and shrivels vege-
tation beyond the uses of either beauty or utility. To
describe the condition in terms entirely professional, and
with apologies to our oculist friends, not a few of the
people have been for some time affected; some very acutely,
others moderately, with well-marked moral strabismus
and ethical astigmatism. If it were not that they attract
attention by the noise they make and their general misfit
in respectable surroundings they would without doubt
be a much greater menace to public welfare than they are.
It could not be expected that the medical profession would
prove entirely immune to this widespread moral infection.
And more's the pity. Not a few who have sat in the San-
hedrim of the elect are now the victims of this virulent
infection, and have developed signs and symptoms of such
loathsomeness as should make the ghosts of the ancient
worthies of medicine rise from their graves and point the
finger of scorn at them as unfit to sit in the councils of
representative medicine.

While volumes might be written of the dangers and even
tragedies of this tendency in its ultimate results as applied
to the common welfare, the feature of it that first and directly
concerns us now is its damnably debasing conscience-searing
effect on a considerable number of the ancient and world-
acclaimed honorable profession of medicine. It is not
intended to even intimate that the members of the medical
profession are of any poorer moral fiber or any less resistant
than those of any other guild or avocation, but rather that
their position in the social world, by reason of their calling,
brings them into contact with every stratum of life and in the
limelight of this publicity the obliquities they may have
seem all the greater. This responsibility they assume at

the portals of the medical career and is part of the high office they enter. We hear much said politically and sociologically of the white man's burden. This is the medical profession's burden and what we are going to do with it is easily and far away the most important and vital problem of our time.

Nearly a third of a century ago, during the first decade of this Association, the circumstances and the average attainments of medical practitioners throughout the country in general, and particularly in the recently devastated States of the South, were so widely different from those of today that the stupendous obstacles they had to overcome in solving the problem of the time are almost forgotten if indeed some of us have ever known them. Medical organization was in its infancy. The American Medical Association itself then scarcely numbered more hundreds on its membership rolls than it now does thousands. The problem then was to get men of a common vision and purpose together; the slogan of the times was recruits and more recruits to enlist under one flag, a virile, cohesive, enthusiastic force, a solid phalanx, if you please, with which to attack the cohorts of ignorance in both professional and public ranks. There were malingerers, deserters, and camp-followers and even contemptible night-prowling jackals in those days as now. Then, too, there was that other class of God-forsaken human rubbish who stand aloof from every effort for improvement or progress, fold their arms, and with the impotence that is the legitimate child of cowardice, say, "What's the use?" Such minus quantities never helped to work out the problems of any age, any condition, or any people. If we had waited on them there would be no Panama Canal, no electric telegraph or telephone, no yellow-fever ridden Cuba or any other of the epoch-making feats that have made our times and civilization illustrious. They were but the barnacles that cumber and lessen the speed but cannot stop the ship of progress.

No medieval crusade not even that of the Holy Grail manifested greater devotion and more unswerving purpose than did the true evangels of universal progress, professional efficiency, and uplift, the medical profession of those days. The higher standard of education and qualifications of today is the result of the determined, uncompromising singleness of purpose of that and the succeeding decade. And thus was the phenomenal occurrence brought to the attention of the world, of a conscience-striken profession, by sheer force of determined effort, in a righteous cause, compelling its own better equipment for greater efficiency in the work it had set forth to do. But as it was with them so it will be with us. Our conscience-smiting and heart-racking problem is no less persistent and loudly insistent for the right answer. Not to respond to this imperative need of the hour is to acknowledge ourselves what, in truth, we are, moral weaklings who know our duty but are too cowardly to do it. Whatever other misfortune betide us in these times of stress and strain may an evergracious Providence protect us from doctors that are moral cowards and shy even at a thin shadow of responsibility.

Whether inspired wholly by a spirit of genuine altruism or conceived to a degree in the hope of self-conservation, the good already accomplished by the patriots of that campaign affords one of the most beneficent and soul "inspiring" episodes of all history. None can now be found with the temerity to raise a voice to question either the wisdom of the undertaking or the efficiency of the result, though there were not wanting in the beginning, doubting Thomases, shouting with puerile voices, impossible, to meet and vanquish the entrenched minions of ignorance in open conflict. Insistent professional demand reinforced by the active approval of an enlightened public opinion have now so definitely settled that question that nothing short of a cataclysm to modern civilization can change it. It would be a consummation devoutly to be hoped for if all other questions of public weal and professional conscience could be so satisfactorily fixed. Will we, of this decade, be strong enough, brave enough, and true enough to duplicate the wonderful spectacle in the solution of our problem?

Mention has been made of the educational and scientific qualifications required by the present-day standard and the strenuous efforts that have been made and are still being made to bring everything up to the level of these requirements. Is such a thing possible, or mayhap even probable, that in focussing every effort, concentrating the entire thought and energy on the development of the intellectual faculties and the perfection of manual skill in the individual, we are perforce, of the very intensity of such activity leaving the weightier matters of the heart, soul and conscience untutored and undeveloped as little worth, while in our scheme of scientific exaltation and thus while heroically pulling against a sea of ignorance have subconsciously dropped into a whirlpool of ethical and moral deficiency. If such has been or is a factor in the present state of affairs it may be pertinent to inquire what does it profit either the world or the profession to develop a scientific giant that is a pigmy in morality and an ethical derelict? Think about it. It is worth more, too, than just a glimpsing thought.

In view of this, and after all is said and done, then the most important, because the one absolutely essential factor in the solution of our problem is as it always has been and always will be, the personal equation. This Association, and all other associations combined may meet and pass resolutions in "convention assembled," as the formula goes, couched in elegantly worded periods and continue to meet and resolve until the crack of doom for all the good it will do unless exemplified, energized, and electrified by the every-day personal lives of the Fellows. There is no neutral ground on this proposition. Under present conditions the medical man who is not whole-souled, flat-footed, squared-toed for outspoken daily-lived professional honesty, square-dealing and "do unto others as he would be done by" in the broadest, most catholic sense is at heart opposed to them, and to use a common but expressive solecism, "His room is better than his company." Of this we may rest quite sure that on this question "he that is not for us is against us," and should be so "nominated in the bond." We have undeniably reached the time when the continued respectable position of the medical profession in the estimation of right-thinking people and by the same token, the proper safeguarding of the public good, demands that the line must be drawn, and to use a biblical figure, the sheep separated from the goats. There will be some who, for a time, will masquerade in sheep's clothing but in spite of the well-groomed and shining fleece, if they *look* like goats, *act* like goats and *smell* like goats, according to the rules and regulations "in all such cases made and provided," *they are goats*. What a strange characteristic of this form of animal life, too, that it is always the goat that complains at the line before drawn, never the sheep.

While the problem that demands solution at our hands is personal to every one of us it is also nation wide, yes world wide, in potentiality for weal or woe to all human kind. Let us not deceive ourselves. We are in this respect in the largest and very best sense our brother's keeper. We cannot simply lift immaculate skirts and Pharisee-like disdainfully "pass it by on the other side." No pestilence will be overcome by running from it nor a cesspool drained and cleansed with a pitchfork. Unanimity of professional sentiment and personal intercourse of its members, that is like Cæsar would have his wife, "not only virtuous, but above suspicion," will as certainly command the enthusiastic public conviction and endorsement that is necessary to a final perfect and triumphant solution of this vexatious question as the morrow's sun dispels the shadows of night. Public opinion when aroused by its own unrequited welfare will become a mighty irresistable force that brooks no interference with its righteous mandate.

These comments are by no means intended to promulgate the claim to being the prophet of a new vision. Those on the watchtowers looking with zealous eye for whatever might asperse the name and sully the fair reputation of medicine and be inimical to public welfare long since heralded the approach of the pestilential visitation. A large and ever-increasing army of the triple allies of truth, justice, and human beneficience is already in the field and doing yeoman service.

The requisites for fellowship in the great American College of Surgeons has already done a tremendous amount of good in emphasizing the crying need for higher and juster professional ideals, and is destined to wield a still greater influence and power as time goes on. A plank in the platform of principles of the college that has not been given the serious attention it deserves, and which is not second in importance to any of its undertakings, is that referring to the standardization of hospitals. The prodigious and portentous spread of so-called "private sanitariums" that, mushroom-like, spring up by night in every village and almost at every cross-roads is disturbing and most distressing to public welfare and professional righteousness. That this is a delicate and touchy subject because of the multiplicity of interests implicated, I am well aware. But the time has come in the widespread over-growth of this fad that indicates a very serious and harmful pathological condition has developed and makes it necessary to tell the simple unvarnished truth about it though vials of wrath be poured on the devoted head of the relator.

Many, very many private sanitariums are conducted on the highest scientific plane in the most sanitary, efficient, and ethical manner, and are, therefore, beyond the pale of criticism. But unfortunately it is also true, be it said to the everlasting shame of men and women boasting of the insignia and parading in the habiliments of medicine, that probably somewhere from 30 to 50 per cent. of the *privately* owned and *secretly operated pseudo sanitariums* are hot-beds of dishonesty and veritable culture fields of immorality. In short, fit hibernating places for his satanic majesty and all his devilish hosts. I wonder if those in power realize what a travesty on public benefaction it is when in almost every state of this glorious union of ours anybody, no matter who, so he goes by the sobriquet of "doctor," can get a charter under the great seal of the State for anything and no questions asked, provided the bantling is called by the name of "sanitarium." In the fulness of time when the great heart of medical men really and sincerely beats for human welfare and happiness there will come some power whose duty it will be to see that this disgraceful state of affairs is made impossible.

It is utter foolishness and waste of time to hope that the interests that thrive on ignorance, malevolence, and duplicity will cease their devilish practices of their own volition. The devil with his corps of angels has been at work in the world since Eden, and so far as we have any right to believe will remain with us until the millenium. 'Tis said the way to fight his satanic majesty is with fire. There is nothing quite so unbearably and roasting hot to him as knowledge, wisdom, and courageous right living. Did I hear anybody say, "That's all very well, but it sounds a little too much like the meeting-house for me." Nevertheless, the elementary principles of justice, honesty, and right-living do not depend on church relation or religious faith. Murder, theft, and oppression are essentially and morally wrong without reference to religious or political affiliation or social conditions. A very able man of affairs said publicly a few years ago that the best way to get the people in a more favorable attitude to corporations was for the corporations to first *be good themselves.* This is undoubtedly not only the correct but the very wisest philosophy of life. We may advise our neighbors to do right by exhortations, resolutions, and promises, but the thing that will knock the last prop from under them is to do right ourselves. The thing for you and for me as individuals is to work out this problem in the right way—the only way by which it can be effectually done. Some there will be among us who will love rather the onions, the garlic, and the flesh pots of a crooked life than the milk and honey of "good-will to all and offence toward none." As in the ancient time the prophet found seven thousand souls that had not bowed the knee to Baal, so there are in medical Israel a thousand times seven thousand who "have not cringed the knee that thrift may follow fawning," who panoplied with the loftiest altruism, with the sword of scientific truth unsheathed, shielded by the breast plate of a clear conscience, shod with the gospel of more happinesss and longer life to mankind, and inspired by unfaltering faith in justice and humanity, are now going forth from victory to victory, conquering and to conquer.

REPORT OF A CASE OF GANGRENOUS ABSCESS OF LUNG

By D. *F.* Talley, M.D.
Birmingham, Ala.

In many cases it is hard to distinguish between abscess and gangrene of the lung.

An abscess of the lung may become gangrenous, and gangrene of the lung may become localized into an abscess.

It is not my purpose, in this short paper, to discuss the etiology and pathology of this condition, but to mention briefly some of the salient points in the treatment of a disease which under expectant management has been attended by a frightful rate of mortality.

In the past decade wonderful strides have been made in surgery of the chest, but there is much yet to learn. The profession at large should realize that abscess and gangrene of the lung are conditions to be dealt with surgically, and not to be treated expectantly with a death rate running from 75 to 95 per cent.

G. Picot, in his Paris thesis of 1910, reports 133 cases of gangrenous abscess treated expectantly with only 10 recoveries—a mortality of about 93 per cent. He also reports 149 cases treated surgically with 105 recoveries—a mortality of less than 30 per cent. Lenhartz and Körte in a series of 65 operated cases report equally as good results.

Garré reports 400 cases of abscess, gangrene, and bronchiectasis treated surgically with 300 recoveries; where the pus was not fetid a recovery was obtained in 87 per cent. of cases.

The case I am to report occurred in a young married woman after the birth of her first child.

During the course of labor she had several convulsions, after which the attending physician decided to give a general anesthetic and deliver with forceps. Ether was administered and the child delivered with little trouble.

In twenty hours after delivery the patient's rectal temperature registered 103.4° F.

In forty hours after delivery she commenced coughing. Sixty hours after delivery cough aggravated and rust-colored sputum expectorated; the temperature at this time registered 102° F. and pulse 134.

She now complained of lancinating pains in the right side, and there was considerable abdominal distention. In twelve days after delivery she began to expectorate a large quantity of pus which was fetid, and it soon became so decided in its odor that it was very disagreeable to remain in the room while she was coughing. This condition continued with fetid expectoration, high temperature and pulse for six weeks after delivery, when I was consulted with reference to the advisability of an operation.

It was quite evident that an operation offered her the only chance for recovery, and yet she was weak and had gone through such a long siege of sepsis it was probable that an operation attended with any considerable amount of shock might prove fatal. With the aid of a skiagraph and careful physical examination the abscess was fairly well located under the seventh rib posteriorly between the spinal column and the angle of the scapula.

The tissues were infiltrated with a weak solution of novocain and adrenalin, the rib exposed and a section of about two inches removed.

A small round needle was introduced through the layers of the pluræ and no up-and-down movement was imparted, which was fair evidence that the two layers were adherent.

Not being entirely satisfied with this test alone, a careful dissection was made through the layers, which showed positively that dense adhesions were present; this simplified further procedure, a long needle attached to an aspirating bottle was introduced into the lung; the first puncture missed but the second entered the abscess and a small amount of pus showed in the tube; immediately before the operation the patient sat up and leaned forward in which position the abscess best emptied itself.

The needle, which entered the abscess at a depth of about three inches, was left in position and the long point of a Percy electric cautery passed down by its side into the abscess cavity. A split-rubber tube, wrapped with gauze, was introduced and furnished satisfactory drainage.

Patient's temperature dropped to normal in a few hours after operation—the first time she had been found free of fever in more than six weeks. In twenty-four hours her temperature rose again, due to infection of the external wound which was closed with a few sutures of silkworm gut. This infection was rather severe and all the sutures were removed in three days, after this the infection soon subsided and temperature dropped to near normal.

The rubber tube caused some discomfort when the patient lay on her back, so it was removed and gauze introduced which completely plugged the wound and stopped all drainage, causing temperature to rise. The rubber tube was replaced and allowed to remain four weeks, during which time patient rapidly improved. In two weeks after the removal of the drain the wound was healed.

It is now more than ten months since the operation and patient is in perfect health.

By a careful physical examination it cannot be detected that her lung was ever damaged.

All cases of abscess and gangrene of the lung should be opened and drained, unless the abscesses are multiple and inaccessible.

Tuffier cured two cases by lung compression by packing

in fat and omentum extrapleurally over the diseased area, but this method seems inadequate for most cases, as there is need for actual drainage, and there may be a sequestrum of necrotic lung that must come away before the abscess can close.

DISCUSSION

DR. JOSEPH C. BLOODGOOD, Baltimore, Maryland.—Some years ago, after Sauerbruck came out with his publication, I became interested in surgery of the lung, went over autopsies, and found about a thousand or more localized single abscesses in the lung that seemed operable at the time. In discussing the subject with my medical colleagues at the time they agreed with me that abscesses were operable, but how could we diagnose them? Since then the x-ray has come in, and I believe it is going to be helpful to us in the recognition of abscess of the lung in a period when operation promises a cure. I am afraid we are going to be slow in our developing and diagnostic interpretations or interpretation of x-rays of the lung if we wait for the x-rays in the cases we operate on, and as Dr. Hugh is going to take up this branch of surgery at the Hopkins, I made this suggestion to him: In the hospital, in all cases about to die, medical or surgical, that an x-ray be made of the chest. In a conveniently arranged x-ray room, it is not an ordeal for a patient to be taken there on a stretcher, even though she or he is dying, taking a number of pictures of the chest, and if there is an autopsy you remember altogether what you see in the x-ray and what is found at autopsy, otherwise we will be slow in interpreting the x-ray. Up to the present time I have seen a large number of x-rays of the chest, perhaps hundreds, and I do not believe I have seen six röntgenograms of the cases in which I have opened the chest or have seen the autopsy afterward. I know, however, that there is no difference. I have had one case in which the shadow was absolutely dense, and yet it was clear fluid. There is apparently no difference in the shape of the shadow of clear fluid and that of the solid lung. If in the lung area a distinctly recognizable dense shadow comes in you know there is something there, and from the other clinical pictures you may conclude what it is. Before operating on any case there should be two studies made, one by the *x*-ray and the other by the fluoroscope. Not long ago I had an *x*-ray made of the chest of a woman who I thought had metastasis. The *x*-ray showed a distinct area in the upper right mediastinum that all of us took for a solid growth, yet when we looked at it with the fluoroscope it pulsated. The difficulty attending the diagnosis has greatly changed with the advent of the *x*-ray, but unless we autopsy other cases than those we are going to operate upon, our interpretations of *x*-ray of the chest will be a slow process.

DR. W. P. CARR, Washington, D. C.—I want to congratulate Dr. Talley on his good result in this case and his judgment in doing this operation, and I want to say in reference to what Dr. Bloodgood has said regarding *x*-ray pictures, that they ought to be stereopticon pictures. They show so much better than the simple plain picture any condition in the chest or in the skull. After looking at some very beautiful stereopticon *x*-ray pictures lately taken by Dr. Groover, of Washington, I have been able to see things both in the chest and in the skull I never dreamt could have been seen before.

There is just one other point, namely, in all these cases of infection, where we have time, we ought to make a culture of the pus or a culture from the sputum in a case like the one Dr. Talley has reported and see if we can't make a proper vaccine. I have seen many cases of various kinds of infection saved by making a culture, developing a vaccine, and using it. Not long ago one of my colleagues was about to amputate an arm for an infection, and I asked him to wait a few minutes. We found a staphylococcus infection, and knowing how well a vaccine acts in staphylococcus infection, I got him to wait another day. We injected this patient with a stock vaccine, the infection cleared up rapidly and the arm was saved. I have done this repeatedly. I have seen abscess cavities both around the kidneys and in the pleura, and in other places that would drain indefinitely, and seem not to improve at all until a proper vaccine was given.

In staphylococcus infections a vaccine often acts like a charm. It acts almost as well as diphtheria antitoxin does for diphtheria in most cases. In mixed infections it is not so good, but when we have infection with both staphylococcus and streptococcus, if we can get rid of the staphylococcus we do great good. As a rule, in mixed infections the staphylococcus is in greater abundance than the streptococcus, and when we get rid of them, the rest of the infection runs a quick and more favorable course. The stock vaccine for streptococcus has not been of any value in my experience, but when we can get an autogenous vaccine I think it will do much good.

Dr. RANDOLPH WINSLOW, Baltimore, Maryland.—I do not propose to take much of the time of the Association in discussing this paper. I simply wish to say that the most important feature about these conditions of the lung is that of diagnosis.

The x-ray is probably going to be of great benefit in clearing up the diagnosis in these cases. I have gone several times into a lung upon the specific basis that a cavity was present which was accessible to operation. In one case I failed to find the abscess or the cavity, and the man subsequently died, which he probably would have done anyway, on account of tuberculosis. In another case a man had the symptoms of abscess of the lung; he would have cough with the expectoration of pus, but the expectoration would come on at certain times, which seemed to imply that an abscess cavity had filled up, and then he would suddenly regurgitate half a pint to a pint or more of pus at a time. He had other physical signs of trouble in the chest, and I entered his lung also, hoping to find an abscess. He died. We made a postmortem examination on him and did not find any abscess whatever. There was, however, bronchiectasis, and doubtless the bronchial tubes would become distended with pus, and at certain periods, like the geysers, would become ready for eruption and the pus would be expelled. In one case I recall to mind very definitely at present, a man had the symptoms of an abscess; he had dullness upon percussion and other physical signs. I explored his chest, found an abscess cavity, evacuated the material, drained the cavity, and he made a good recovery, so that I think abscesses of the lung, like abscesses of the brain or abscess in the buttocks or anywhere else, should be treated in the same manner. An abscess is an abscess, and pus is pus, and it should be emptied wherever we can get at it.

I have another case in mind also in which I did the same thing and evacuated the abscess with recovery of the patient. I am not absolutely certain that it was an abscess of the lung. It might possibly have been an encapsulated collection of pus in the pleural cavity. However, I am inclined to think that it was in the lung itself. People with abscess of the lung will die, although occasionally they may recover by expectorating the pus, but we should not leave them with that possibility or improbability. They should be operated on the same as for any other condition, and doubtless with a fair probability of a successful issue.

DR. WILLIAM R. JACKSON, Mobile, Alabama.—I wish to thank the doctor for his instructive paper. It is rare that we have the report of a successful case of gangrene of the lung operated upon, and I am glad to have heard this report.

Lung abscess is a frequent condition, and when we have unresolved pneumonia existing for three weeks we should aspirate to see whether or not pus is present. In all probability it is. If, after three weeks of pneumonia, we fail to find by aspiration the presence of pus, we may suspect that there is pneumonia of a tuberculous nature persisting. I understood the doctor to say that he found pus present. But he did not say how much gangrenous lung tissue came through the tube or throat. Sometimes we have empyema from a ruptured abscess of the lung taking place, and *vice versa*, and a bronchial fistula announcing the presence of an abundance of putrid pus, but we do not know whether it came from the lung or pleura. In other words, it may be a pleuritis pulmonalis resulting in a pneumonia abscess, ruptured through a bronchial fistula and followed by pulmonary vomiting of putrescent pus, a sudden emptying, with hyperresonance of the chest. But a case of distinct gangrene of the lung means a serious thing, because with such a condition of the lung the patient has sapremia followed by death, as a rule.

DR. D. F. TALLEY, Birmingham, Alabama (closing).—I realize that one great difficulty in doing this kind of work would not be so much in diagnosing the condition as in locating it. Mistakes are sometimes made between collections of pus in the pleura and in the lung, but this was in the lung. In the first place, I had to go down about three inches before I was able to reach the abscess. In the next place, when the patient coughed, after it was opened up, he whistled through the wound. It involved a good-sized bronchus.

There are a few points I did not bring out in my short paper that I think should be emphasized somewhat, and one of them is we should try to make the diagnosis earlier and try to get in and drain the lung earlier without subjecting the patient to five, six or eight weeks of sepsis.

Another important thing is to do this operation with a local anesthetic. Of course, we are getting to do more and more work in this country with local anesthesia, and it should go on.

Another point is we should be sure that the pleura is not opened so that we will get pleural infection. In a case such as I had pleural infection would have probably proved fatal.

Another point of importance is the use of the cautery in opening through into the lung, for several reasons. In the first place, you have no loss of blood; in the second place, you seal the lung tissue as you go through it and this makes a channel for the pus to go through. The lung tissue is sealed so that you do not get infection into the lung surrounding the drainage tract.

Another thing is the inefficiency of gauze drainage. Where you have gauze in a small sinus it will plug the wound up, it will not drain it, hence the necessity in these cases of instituting drainage by means of a tube.

PULSATING EXOPHTHALMOS, WITH REPORT OF A CASE CURED BY LIGATION OF THE COMMON CAROTID ARTERY

By Goodrich B. Rhodes, M.D.
Cincinnati, Ohio

THE subject of pulsating exophthalmos has been studied by many writers, notably Sattler, Eysen, and de Schweinitz and Holloway, whose monographs cover the reported cases to 1908. Sattler has collected 106 cases, Eysen 167, and de Schweinitz and Holloway 69, a total of 342. A study of these cases, however, reveals the fact that a number of cases are duplicated in Eysen's and de Schweinitz's and Holloway's lists, reducing the actual number to 256. Since de Schweinitz's and Holloway's study there have appeared in the literature 52 cases of pulsating exophthalmos. These I have collected and made, together with my own case, the basis of this study.

The symptom-complex of pulsating exophthalmos has been shown by operation and autopsy to be caused by one or more of the following lesions: aneurysm of the ophthalmic artery inside or outside of the skull, pulsating orbital tumors, aneurysmal dilatation of the internal carotid artery in the cavernous sinus, thrombosis of the cavernous sinus and ophthalmic vein, arteriovenous aneurysm of the orbit, pressure on the sinus by an external growth, and rupture of the internal carotid into the cavernous sinus. This paper will concern itself solely with those cases probably due to rupture of the internal carotid into the cavernous sinus, whether caused by trauma or occurring spontaneously. I say probably, for the diagnosis is not always certain, as Wilder found no lesion of the carotid in six clinically characteristic cases which came to autopsy. There were no postmortems made in my series.

In this series of 53 cases 37 were found to be traumatic in origin, 9 occurred spontaneously, while in 7 the cause was not given.

The average age of the patients was 36. The youngest was 15, and the oldest, a spontaneous case, was 84.

There were 31 males and ten females, the sex not being mentioned in the other 12 cases.

In the traumatic cases the time elapsing from the receipt of injury to the appearance of the first symptom, bruit, clings remarkably closely to an average of twenty-one days. To this fairly constant latent period certain cases present a marked exception, 6 cases occurring immediately upon receipt of the injury, while the cases of Lystad, Orloff, and Hildebrand show intervals of two years, six months and four months respectively.

The left eye was affected in 15 cases and the right in 23. A bilateral involvement occurred in 4 cases, 2 of them being spontaneous in origin, 1 due to trauma and the fourth having no cause mentioned.

Upon the classic tripod of exophthalmos, orbital pulsation and a bruit audible both to patient and examiner is built up a superstructure of phenomena which can be divided into those due to the aneurysm itself, and those caused by nerve lesions either traumatic in origin or resulting from prolonged circulatory disturbances set in motion by the reversal of circulation. The exophthalmos, bruit, and pulsation are obviously due to the aneurysm, and are among the first to appear, and of these the first and most constant in its appearance is the bruit. Exophthalmos occurred at later periods, varying from a few days to a month after the bruit. Pulsation is a still later symptom, appearing within a few days after exophthalmos has been noticed. The subjective character of the bruit is variously described by the patients. We read of noises like escaping steam, rattle of machinery, chirping of birds, and other comparisons expressing sounds entirely unlike. Objectively the bruit is the typical arteriovenous aneurysmal bruit, with systolic accentuation, usually heard with greatest intensity over the orbital cavity or the temporal area, and along the course of the vessels in the neck. In some cases it was of interest to note that the only place where the bruit could be heard was along the lateral sinus.

Certain nerve lesions are commonly noticed which can be explained by a study of the anatomy of the region. The most serious lesion is atrophy of the optic nerve, either due to immediate laceration from basal fracture, pressure, or slow development from continued circulatory disturbance. Paralyses of the motor mechanism of the eyeball is in some cases due to extreme exophthalmos, in which cases the globe is immovable, and in others due to lacerations or pressure upon individual nerves, among which the abducens is most common. This nerve was paralyzed in 9 cases, among which was one spontaneous, namely, that of Hird and Haslam. It has been claimed by some authors that paralysis of the abducens is characteristic of the traumatic variety exclusively and is indicative of basal fracture, but this individual presented a slowly developing external rectus paralysis beginning six days after admission to the hospital with spontaeous pulsating exophthalmos.

Loss of pupillary reflex with persistent dilatation of the pupil occurs in many of the cases, both spontaneous and traumatic, and is due to laceration of the carotid plexus of the sympathetic. Injury to the superior petrosal nerve carrying facial nerve fibers is said by some to be responsible for the absence of tear secretion, but was observed only in the case of Lystad.

Various minor symptoms are encountered with great frequency. Among these are diplopia, hemorrhages, or edema of the retina, tortuosity and dilatation of the retinal veins. Almost all cases show an increase in ocular tension, but only two cases developed an absolute glaucoma.

Facial paralysis is a rare symptom, occurring most often in the traumatic type of the disease, but like abducens paralysis can no longer be said to be confined purely to that variety.

Any study of the forms and effects of treatment must necessarily be complicated by many factors. It is not to be expected that gross nerve injuries occurring primarily will be cured by any method at our command, nor will cases coming late to operation with complete degeneration of the optic nerves be restored to vision by a cure of the aneurysm. By a cure we understand, then, those cases in which the exophthalmos, pulsation, bruit, and chemosis have been permanently stopped. In addition we find that several methods of treatment have been frequently employed in the same case. These have been classified as a failure for the first form of treatment employed, but if a cure resulted after other methods were used in addition it was recorded as a cure of the combined treatment. A carotid ligation in itself may be a failure, but may produce enough change to enable a subsequent ligation of the ophthalmic vein to perfect the cure.

The methods of treatment employed in these 53 cases embrace practically all the known procedures which have been advanced, with the exception of electropuncture.

1. Ligation of the common carotid alone: 15 cures, 3 improved, and 4 failures. One of these failures, reported by Buchtel, resulted in death, from what cause is not mentioned. Another one, that of Barbieri, died from secondary hemorrhage. Thus we have a mortality of 9.1 per cent. for this method. Previous estimates of the mortality are given by Eisen, 6.2 per cent; Orlow, 8.3 per cent.; and de Schweinitz and Holloway, 11.7 per cent. Averaging these percentages we have a general mortality of all reported cases of 7.8 per cent. for carotid ligation. It must be remembered, however,

that a considerable number of these patients died from secondary hemorrhage, as a result of operation in the pre-aseptic period, so we are faced by the fact that our mortality at the present day is greater by far than the mortality from the first 113 cases reported, in which there was only 1.9 per cent. The mortality from carotid ligation should be merely the mortality of the disease for which the ligation is done, therefore a percentage of 7.8 per cent. would seem to be entirely too high. The mortality of carotid ligation for all causes in 172 cases as compiled by Siegrist from 1881 to 1897 is 20.5 per cent.

In a certain number of instances the bruit and pulsation are stopped when the common carotid of the same side is compressed. Others are unaffected by this. Common carotid ligation effected a cure in 10 cases in which digital compression over the carotid absolutely stopped the bruit and pulsation. In one such case carotid ligation failed to cure. On the other hand, in 3 cases in which pressure failed to check pulsation and bruit failure resulted from carotid ligation alone. May it not be possible to derive from this a prognosis of the probable result of operation by ligation of the carotid. To make a more complete study of this point I have reviewed the 106 cases of Sattler, and I find 33 of these in which observation is made. The results are as follows: Cures when digital pressure completely stopped the bruit, 19 cases; failures when digital pressure did not completely stop the bruit, 6 cases; no cure when digital pressure completely stopped bruit, 4 cases; cures when digital pressure failed to completely stop the bruit, 4 cases.

By combining these figures deduced from Sattler's statistics with mine it will be noticed that 38 out of 47 cases, or roughly 80 per cent. will support a prognosis which may be expressed as follows: pulsating exophthalmos in which digital pressure on the common carotid of the same side stops the bruit completely will probably be cured by ligation of that common carotid alone. Or this might better be expressed, that pulsating exophthalmos in which digital pressure on the common carotid fails completely to stop the bruit will probably not be cured by simple ligation of the common carotid. Emphasis is laid on the bruit because it is the most persistent symptom and yet the one which is detected with the greatest delicacy by the patient.

2. In 1897 Schimanowsky first ligated the superior ophthalmic vein, after unsuccessful ligation of the common carotid. This orbital operation, commonly known as Sattler's operation, was performed as a primary procedure in three cases in this series with two successes and one failure. One of the successful cases was operated on by the temporary resection of the outer wall of the orbit.

3. Continuous compression of the common carotid was resorted to in eight cases. Only one of these, that of Claiborne, was cured, after wearing a constant pressure bandage for eighteen months.

4. Injections of gelatinized serum after the method of Lancereaux and Paulesco were carried out in 6 cases. Two were cured, two improved and two received no benefit. The treatment consists in the intramuscular injection of 2 per cent. solution of gelatin in serum. Five per cent. or more is very painful and causes a rise of temperature. Less than 2 per cent. is without effect.

5. In one case Cunningham produced a cure by the use of Neff's gradually contracting clamp (catgut and rubber band) applied to the common carotid.

6. Ligation of internal carotid: This method is the operation most highly recommended by various writers. Of the 4 cases so treated one was cured and three were improved. No failures resulted.

7. Ligation common carotid combined with ligation of superior ophthalmic vein, angular vein, inferior ophthalmic vein or any other orbital vein which is found dilated or pulsating. Three cases were cured and one failed by this method.

8. Weinkauff reports one spontaneous cure in a woman, aged eighty-four years, apparently a case produced spontaneously.

9. Ligation of common carotid and superior thyroid. Two cases were cured. No failures.

10. One ligation of the external carotid was employed with a successful result.

11. Ligation of the common carotid followed by ligation of the internal carotid resulted in improvement in one case.

12. Ligation of both the external and internal carotid together with the internal jugular vein in one case resulted in failure. This same case subsequently treated by the orbital operation was greatly improved.

13. Zeller has proposed the following operation: Ligation of the internal carotid close to the skull in the neck combined with ligation of the artery just proximal to the origin of the ophthalmic artery. Cadaver experiments showed him that it is possible only in exceptional cases to see the origin of the ophthalmic artery and to put a ligature proximal to it around the internal carotid without pulling on the latter vessel. In the single case in which this method was tried the ligature sawed through the artery before it was tied. The patient died of hemorrhages.

14. Enucleation of the orbit was resorted to in two cases in which absolute glaucoma developed.

The total number of cures by all methods is 26; 9 were improved and 10 resulted in complete failure.

It is hard to draw any general conclusions as to the best method of treatment from so small a collection of cases, but the total number of reported cases is so small that we must be guided more by a study of the individual ones than by statistical deductions in arriving at any conclusion. Ligation of the common carotid is undoubtedly the classical operation, first performed by Travers in 1803, and is probably the safest method. But even in this procedure deaths have occurred, and in this series cerebral complications occurred in 2 cases, paralysis of forearm and hand and difficulty of speech in the one instance, and in the other aphasia and facial paralysis occurred one month after ligation, so it is only fair to assume that it was due to extension of the clot into some small branches of the middle cerebral. The orbital operation while yielding good results, exposes the patient to great danger from hemorrhage in some cases. No method has proved free from danger. Even the gelatinized serum injections of Lancereaux-Paulesco have resulted in apoplectic attacks probably due to embolism or thrombosis.

In the case of immediate failure by any one method what shall be done? Cures have resulted from various ligations after long periods, but shall we await that result or shall a second operation be made within a few days or weeks? This would seem to depend entirely upon the condition found by the oculist, who should work in conjunction with the surgeon. If the optic nerve is completely atrophied it might be well to await result of the first ligation, but if the nerve is not entirely gone the case should be kept under constant supervision by an oculist, and a second operation performed when in his opinion permanent damage to the nerve is seen to be threatening. The second operation which gives the best results would appear to be the orbital ligation. Ligation of the other common carotid was only practiced in one case, resulting in failure, and would not seem to possess any more advantages, and to present greater dangers than the orbital operation.

AUTHORS' CASE.—W. W., male, aged twenty-seven years, was struck October 29, 1914, on right side of head by a thug. He was knocked over to the left side and struck the left side of his head against a pile of granite blocks. No visible wound. Unconscious for a short period, but was able to walk to his home, suffering intense pain and vomiting frequently. Within twenty-four hours he noticed a throbbing noise in his head. This, with headache, steadily increased and persisted, followed by prominence of the left eye with intense venous congestion of the conjunctiva of both eyes. Vision of left eye blurred. December applied for treatment to Dr. Robert Sattler, to whom I am indebted for the privilege of operating upon this case. Exophthalmos of fully 2 cm. of left eye. Orbital pulsation. Bruit heard most distinctly over the eye and adjacent temporal region. Patient complains of constant rhythmic loud noise in the head which allows him little sleep. Pronounced chemosis present.

Ophthalmic examination by Dr. Sattler showed marked venous stasis with enormous dilatation and tortuosity of the branches of the central retinal vein and general edema of the retina. Orbital venous stasis of right eye. Compression of the left common carotid silences both the subjective and objective bruit and reduces the orbital tension. Exophthalmos is lessened, but does not entirely disappear. Pulsation ceases immediately.

Operation, January 22, 1915. Ligation of common carotid with two silk ligatures. No symptoms were noticed when ligature was tied. The patient had immediate and permanent relief from the bruit and pulsation while the exophthalmos receded very gradually, being still noticeable four months later. Vision returned to normal and remained so April 10, 1915, three months after operation, he developed an intense chemosis of the lids of the right eye, but no exophthalmos nor pulsation. This subsided after several weeks, aided by a plastic operation performed by Dr. Sattler, and was thought to be due to the extension of the clot into the orbital veins. He is now perfectly cured.

CASES FROM THE LITERATURE

Cunningham.

White man, aged thirty-nine years, no previous disease except dysentery (Philippines). Four years ago in a fight was struck on left cheek. Spat blood and felt sick. Two days later roaring in head began and gradually grew worse. Could not sleep lying down and spent nights in chair. Two months later sudden pain in right temple, and eye protruded to a marked degree. Diplopia and dilatation of superficial veins over eye and temple. While returning from work he became temporarily unconscious. Taken to hospital.

Decided to try Neff's clamp (*Jour. Am. Med. Assn.*, August 26, 1911, p. 700), catgut, and rubber band. Applied so that faint pulsation was noticed distal to clamp. Visible pulsation disappeared in orbit. Bruit lessened. Four days later both had entirely disappeared. Left hospital on tenth day.

September 30. Exophthalmos lessened. No bruit or pulsation, or roaring in head.

October 9. Clamp removed. Found to have cut its way through artery. Dysphagia by pressure on trachea. Improved spring pressure clamp (described) to lie parallel to vessel, and not press on surrounding tissues.

Beauvois, A.

1. Woman, aged forty-one years, fracture of base of skull from falling down stairs. Month later, right exophthalmos, no pain. Systolic murmur. Later, right-sided abducens paralysis, diminished vision. Ocular and carotid compression without result. Common carotid ligated three months after accident. Murmur ceased, slight aphasia and left lid paresis. Exophthalmos persisted, but less. Gradual loss of vision. Ten days later murmur reappeared, but could be stopped by compression of left carotid. Injected 5 c.c. of 1 per cent. gelatinized serum into thigh every other day. After three injections (Lancereaux-Paulesco) injection increased to 20 c.c., then 50 c.c., at last to 100 c.c. Exophthalmos disappeared, but paralysis of both abducens and slight dilatation of pupil persisted. Three months after beginning treatment a local cure.

2. Woman, aged fifty-three years, received severe blow beneath right eye with the handle of a pump, ten years before. First seen December, 1905. August, 1905, intense pain in the right side of head. At end of December, 1905, diplopia, exophthalmos conjunctival reddening, systolic murmur. Fundus slightly congested. Vision: R., 0.4; L., 0.6; paralysis of right abducens. Visual field slightly diminished. Injection in thigh 2½ per cent. gelatin every five days. After twenty-two injections exophthalmos reduced one-half, with normal motion and complete disappearance of diplopia.

Zeller.

Case report of one operation: patient died of hemorrhage caused by ligature sawing through the artery before it was tied. Zeller's procedure—ligation of internal carotid as near as possible to the skull in the neck and also the ligation of the artery just proximal to the origin of the ophthalmic artery. Cadaver experiments showed him that it is possible only in exceptional cases to see the origin of the ophthalmic artery and to put a ligature proximal to it without pulling on the carotid. The possibility of a clot caused by the ligature obliterating the ophthalmic artery must be considered. No danger to the eye is to be expected, collateral circulation is very free. No danger to brain.

Becker.

Soldier, wounded by explosion of his gun. Four wounds on the right side of face, two on nose, one at corner of mouth, and another in right eye. Ten days later, left eye protruded, increasing steadily in next few days. Retina showed hemorrhages and the ocular movements became more and more limited until entirely lost. On eighteenth day pulsation appeared. Compression of carotid caused diminution of pulsation. X-ray showed fragment of bone 2 x 1.5 cm. in the neighborhood of cella turcica and cavernous sinus. Internal carotid ligated one and one-half months after accident. Relief for four weeks, then return of former symptoms, but in eight weeks great improvement. After three months further improvement. Lateral movements of eyeball normal. Vision with a + 4, 5/15.

Jacques.

Man, aged twenty-five years, injured in motor-cycle accident by falling against the wheel, striking on right side of head. Base fracture. Three weeks later pulsating exophthalmos. Intense epistaxis nine times in six weeks from right nostril occurring after any strong effort. Ligature of right common carotid. Three days later improvement, but later return of all symptoms. Still later operative exposure of the inner portion of orbit. A polyp was found in the sphenoidal sinus which communicated with the cavernous sinus. Sphenoidal sinus packed with iodoform gauze which was removed on the sixth day without hemorrhage.

Pooley.

Negro, aged thirty years, was struck on back of head with a blackjack. Three scalp wounds, one on parietal bone near junction with occipital, one farther forward, and another on the temple. Unconscious. Noise in head distressing on recovering consciousness. Two days later all symptoms of arteriovenous aneurysm except pulsation. Exophthalmos, injected conjunctiva, and lids, blowing murmurs heard over eye and a continuous whirring rumbling sound. Eye could be pushed back. Carotid compression diminished but did not stop bruit. No change in fundus and vision is unimpaired. Treated for a few days by pressure bandage and carotid compression. Later, ptosis, exophthalmos, enormous dilatation of conjunctival vessels and lids, pulsation, especially at inner canthus, papillitis with enormous dilatation of retinal vessels. One vein in the lower temporal region seemed to be obstructed above and below the obstructed part was greatly distended. Noises in head had become greatly aggravated. Occasional violent pain in orbit. No impairment of hearing. Patient refused operation.

Knapp (discussion of Pooley's paper).

Three cases in all of which the common carotid was ligated. Bruit, exophthalmos, and chemosis relieved, but the optic nerve went on to atrophy.

Claiborne (discussion of Pooley's paper).

Case like Pooley's. Applied pressure bandage, which was kept up for eighteen months. Mixed treatment internally. Perfect cure.

Barrett and Orr.

Male, aged fifty years, ten weeks before observation fell while intoxicated. Unconscious from twenty-four to thirty-six hours. In hospital three weeks. No evidence of organic lesions. Six weeks after injury complained of buzzing in the ears, and a few days later exophthalmos. V. 6/36. Lower lid everted, marked exophthalmos in middle line, conjunctiva of lower lid engorged and swollen, fundus veins dilated. External canthus divided and orbit explored, finger pushed behind eye where a pulsating mass was felt. Later a marked bruit was heard over temporal bone and the eye synchronous with the pulse. Two days later eye became stationary with many hemorrhages and distended veins in the fundus. Progressed. Ligation of common carotid. Steady improvement, exophthalmos diminished.

Rubel.

Young man. Three and one-half years ago almost lost vision in left eye and the hearing in both ears following a severe blow on the head. Some months later developed the complete picture of pulsating exophthalmos (left).

Ophthalmic findings: Arteries normally full, veins dilated, stasis. Atrophy of pailla. Numerous yellowish flecks on fundus from papilla to periphery. Patient observed for two weeks. Then left common carotid ligation by Kraske. Tension of globe (Schiotz) on both sides before operation 20 mm. Hg. No difference noted on successive days. Immediately after ligation the tension (left) fell to

8 mm. At close of operation 11 mm. Nine days later, left 15 to 17 mm. Hg; seventeen days later, left 15 mm., right 16 mm. Hg. Retinal changes cleared up with disappearance of exophthalmos. Nine and one-half months later all right except for optic atrophy.

E. Eliot, Jr.

Man, aged, fifty-one years, was admitted October 15, 1909. Moderately alcoholic. Ten years ago a piece of steel entered the right cornea, resulting in ulceration and partial loss of sight in that eye. Five weeks before admission he was assaulted, receiving a blow on the left zygoma with some heavy instrument. Was unconscious for a short time, bleeding from mouth and fractured nose. Walked home. Left eye was swollen and nearly shut, got gradually better and seventeen days after injury he had some use of eye. Two weeks ago he noticed protrusion of left eyeball, and during past week eversion of lower lid. Throbbing pain in eye with each heart beat and a murmur or buzzing sound could be heard distinctly in left ear. Severe pains shooting from left to right side of head. Dizzy at times. No vomiting.

Examination: Marked exophthalmos, left eye. Eyelids swollen, between them a ridge of red conjunctiva one inch long and one quarter inch wide. Eye reacted to light and slightly to accommodation. Pulsations could be seen and felt. Continuous blowing murmur could be heard over entire skull and vessels of left side of neck. This sound was exaggerated with every heart beat, and loudest over left eye. Ophthamic examination showed marked swelling of papilla and edema of retina. Veins enlarged and tortuous. Arteries small. Operation: Ligation of common carotid, just above omohyoid. No sign of interference with cerebral circulation. Intracranial murmur ceased and exophthalmos disappeared rapidly, at ten days little remained. Three years later, eyesight has gradually improved. Continued use in reading results in headache. No exophthamos.

Gibson.

Showed photographs of a case where he had ligated carotid in 1904. There had been some intracranial operation, during which some trauma was inflicted, and further operative measures were abandoned on acccount of severe hemorrhage. On admission both eyes were bulging, and the sight of one eye was lost. Common carotid tied and in course of time patient recovered entirely as far as appearance of eyes was concerned.

Flemming and Johnson.

Man, aged, forty-seven years, previously good health. September, 1907, fell on back of head. Unconscious for few moments. No reason for fall. Walked home. Well until November, when he noticed he could not see objects placed on left side. Found to be suffering from hemianopia. No proptosis then, but soon afterward beating noise. April 19, 1908, noticed that left eye was prominent and inflamed. This increased. April 29, left side proptosis, lids swollen and congested. Chemosis, especially lower fornix. Pupils equal and reacted normally to light and accommodation, all movements of left eyeball are limited. Pulsation of eyeball, bruit, etc. Pulsation and bruit arrested by compression of common carotid. No cranial nerve affected, except optic (left hemianopia), and right hypoglossal, the tongue deviating slightly to right. May, 14, left common carotid ligated with silk in continuity, at level of cricoid. Pulsation immediately arrested, and never returned. Proptosis gradually disappeared. June 10 sat in chair and June 11 became aphasic, with right facial paralysis, tongue deviating strongly to right, and weakness in right arm. Better next day and gradually improved. September 29, still slight proptosis. No pulsation detected. Faint systolic murmur heard over eye. Conjunctival vessels injected. Left eye vision, 6/6. Hemianopia unchanged. No facial weakness, but tongue still deviated to right. Weakness of right hand Late onset of cerebral symtoms supposed to be due to extension of clot into some small branches of middle cerebral.

Gwynne Williams.

No operation. Male, aged twenty-nine years, has had dilated veins over left eye ever since he was a baby. Fell on head when nine and had concussion. Left eye "weak," but became prominent only in last eleven months. Has twice had subconjunctival hemorrhages, when eighteen and twenty-five years old. Exophthalmos, chemosis, eye pushed forward and outward, all motions limited. No diplopia. Bruit, systotic. Eyeball pulsates. Pressure on common carotid diminishes swelling and stops pulsation. No pulsation seen in veins of retina.

Lazarew.

Lazarew's case was sixth in Russian literature, among 150 known. Patient seventeen years old. Three years ago noticed that right eye was becoming more prominent, with noticeable swelling at inner angle and pulsation. Came on suddenly on arising in the morning. No trauma. Common carotid ligated. Pulsation stopped immediately, but the exophthalmos persisted. In the evening the patient complained of pain in the teeth of the lower jaw, and a slight pulsation in the eye began again. No improvement after five days so Lazarew ligated the superior ophthalmic vein. Lazarew believes that he is the first to perform this operation. Cerebral disturbances followed, but subsided after 14 days. Cure complete.

Savariaud.

Small girl had head squeezed between a large plank and a boat; had hemorrhage from right ear and nose. Later, paralysis of the abducens on the right side, exophthalmos, and continuous murmur with systolic emphasis. Slight pulsation. Injections of gelatin after Lancereaux's method failed.

Bedell.

Man, aged thirty-nine years, was riding on an open street car, May 31, 1913. Derailed and thrown against a tree, he was thrown to the ground and struck his head. Next day was dazed, with all signs of true fracture of the base of the skull, bleeding from nose, ears, and mouth, and vomiting. No paralysis of face, all reflexes normal. Mind cleared in about four days and memory gradually returned. Hearing on left side lost and slight ptosis of left upper eyelid. Constant dizziness and headache. Five days after accident the patient felt something "like electricity" in the upper angle of the left orbit, which was found to be a definite pulsation and bruit. At that time there was marked diplopia, dilated pupil, and beginning proptosis.

May 7, 1914. Patient complains of constant noise in head and terrible headache. Right eye, V. 20/30. Decidedly proptosed. Outward motion limited. Veins of lids especially at inner corner of upper lid, prominent and tortuous. Pupil active and normal. Retinal vessels overfull, veins especially. Congestion of disk. No pulsation of globe.

Left eye, V. 20/30. Proptosis more marked than right. Extremely large mass of tortuous and dilated veins on the upper lid. In the upper and inner corner of the orbit is a large dilated vessel (2 cm. in diameter), transmitting a distinct bruit. Visible pulsation of globe. Pupil normal. Entire conjunctiva congested. Retinal veins congested and tortuous. No hemorrhages. Field of motion limited. Eyeball turned in 30 degrees; abducens paralysis. Bruit most intense over the supraorbital ridge, although felt over the entire head. Systolic blowing murmur heard over the same area is stopped by carotid pressure. Left ear, thin gray retracted membrane. Hearing greatly reduced. Large perforation of septum of the nose. Wassermann and Noguchi negative.

March 29. Pressure on the left eye partially reduces it, causes strong pulsation, and patient complains of dizziness. Carotid pressure or pressure on the ophthalmic vein deep in left orbit stops pulsation and bruit. Lying down increases headache but does not affect exophthalmos. Diplopia.

October 4. No improvement. Patient refuses operation.

G. J. Palen.

Woman, aged sixty-five years. October 18, 1908, complained of pain in the right eye extending into the head, photophobia, and lacrimation. In forty-eight hours there occurred a vesicular eruption along the course of the supraorbital nerve (right). This eruption disappeared in three or four days.

October 21. Pain, which had recurred at intervals, became more intense, and she was unable to open the right eye. No inflammation of the eye at this time. Had interstitial nephritis, atheroma, and hypertrophy of heart for some time.

November 9. Marked ptosis, proptosis. Pupil dilated and eyeball deviated outward and somewhat downward. Vision below normal; optic disk swollen; veins tortuous and engorged. For sometime prior to her attack she had had a very intense noise in the head which was continuous but seemed increased at every heart beat. "A rushing sound like rushing water." This did not cease until onset of pain October 18. At age of eight she was struck on head by the handle of a pump, but had no trouble from it. Had scarlet fever, whooping cough, varioloid, and grip three times. No acute illness prior to this condition. Condition rapidly became worse. Bruit heard plainest over eyeball and right antrum, less intensely so over the right side of the head, and with diminished intensity downward along the side of the neck. Had sound of tubular breathing with marked systolic accentuation. Pressure on right carotid checked bruit and eye could easily be pushed into the orbit. Pressure on the left carotid gave no result. No pulsation at this time. Refused operation. In bed, recumbent, carotid compression used.

November 13. The eye protruded markedly and was fixed in medium position. Marked chemosis, complete ectropion of lower lids, cornea insensitive and dull, swelling of disk very intense. At the inner upper angle was a soft compressible tumor, and the veins above and to the temporal side were engorged. Distinct pulsation felt over this tumor, and beginning pulsation of eyeball noticed. Condition became much worse. Bruit heard over entire head, loudest over right orbit and right and left mastoid regions, and much louder than before. KI in increasing doses. No result from digital compression   Slight improvement, but vision was gone. Treatment continued at home. Proptosis lessened and pulsation disappeared about latter part of January.

March 1. Had severe hemorrhage from left nostril after which eyeball receded greatly. Bruit still heard over entire head, loudest over lateral sinus.

January 24. Bruit disappeared, still partial ptosis, slight increase in ocular movements. Vision O; optic nerve atrophy. No engorgement of veins about orbit or at inner angle.

The peculiarity of this case was the intensity of the bruit along the course of the lateral sinus. The intensity of the bruit lessened markedly above and below this line.

Matthewson::

Man, aged thirty-two years, thrown from top of car October 8, 1910, fracturing the base of the skull.

November 5. Left eye proptosed with complete ptosis. Considerable swelling of conjunctiva and restricted motion of globe. Fundus negative. Vision fingers eight feet in upper field; lower field lost. No pulsation of globe.

December 20. Veins of upper lid much dilated, ball pulsated, slight pallor of nerve, slight dilatation of retinal veins, no bruit, occasional headache.

March 11. Vision almost gone.

August 1. Condition more marked. Loud blowing murmur heard over greater part of skull.

September 5. Common carotid tied. Month later, little proptosis, no bruit or pulsation.

Barbieri.

Italian man, aged forty-three years. April 24, 1907, had intense pain in the temporal region. Next day exophthalmos, and one month later the right eye pulsated. Injection of 5 per cent. gelatin tried without result.

October 21. Ligature of right common carotid. Exophthalmos and pulsation continued.

January 8, 1908. The left common carotid was tied.

April 4. When last seen exophthalmos present; movements of eyeball moderately free; pupil inactive to light; slight headache; subjective noises continued.

Mayor Spencer.

Gunner, aged twenty-three years, struck by fist in the right eye.

June 12, 1906. Black eye, skin not broken. Three weeks later began to have buzzing noises in head, becoming worse. On examination six weeks after trauma, pulsating swelling, with thrill and murmur, detected in the orbit. Treated by compression of carotid and calcium chloride internally, but swelling increased in size. Marked proptosis, with some swelling of lids and lacrimation Pulsating swelling about size of hazel nut projected under upper eyelid. Expansile pulsation, distinct thrill and loud musical whirring murmur, and it seemed that the main bulk of the tumor was deep in the orbit, while the small swelling was only an offshoot. Vision, 6/6 in each eye; slight diplopia on looking upward and to the right. Fundus and conjunctiva normal.

December 5. Right common carotid ligated. Pulsation entirely diasppeared on tightening the ligature, but a slight thrill could still be felt over the right eyebrow. Pulsation in the small swelling reappeared slightly six days later, nor deep in orbit. Excised, fusiform dilated vessel. All pulsation and thrill at once disappeared. Since well and no recurrence (March 1907). No trace remains except a slight fullness in right orbit.

Orloff.

Pulsating exophthalmos developed six months after a deep wound in the region of the left parietal and temporal bones in a thirty-year-old patient. Successful result obtained after ligating the ophthalmic vein in the depths of the orbit after temporary resection of external wall of orbit.

Buchtel.

Operated August 13, 1912. Male, struck on head with a pitch-fork three months before. Buzzing sound in head, and in a few days left eye protruded. Well-marked exophthalmos, forward and downward. Pulsation of the eyeball and the mass at the upper and inner angle of orbit, with continuous bruit and systolic accentuation over brow and temple. Complained of noise, diplopia, and headache. Fundus negative.

Operation: Incision, eyebrow, angular. Superficial and temporal veins tied and superior ophthalmic ligated as far as possible in orbit. More edema at first, but no bruit, pulsation or fundus change. Exophthalmos gradually lessened. Vision, 20/20.

Also reports two other unrecorded cases. One, a double exophthalmos cured by ligation of common carotid. The other, unilateral, died after ligation of common carotid.

Halstead and Bender.

Man, aged twenty-four years. Wagon-wheel passed over his head just back of the eye, January 29, 1909. Unconscious three days. Left eye bulged more after accident than on entrance to hospital, when it was turned sharply toward nose and appeared paralyzed. Lids swollen and impossible to close upper lid, move the jaw or to swallow. Roaring noises synchronous with the heart beat could be heard from the time patient regained consciousness until he entered hospital. In bed two weeks after accident, during which sight in left eye became much impaired.

Examination August 27, 1909. Left eye turned in 45 degrees and very prominent, two-thirds in further forward than the right. Veins on upper lid very large and tortuous. Bloodvessels of sclera also dilated. Cornea vascular, and over a 4 mm. area in centre is a fairly dense cicatrix. Vision, right, 20/20; left, 20/30.

October 10. Pulsating tumor felt over lid and inner angle of orbit. Bruit heard over left temporal region and roaring noises complained of by patient, heard most distinctly over left ear.

October 14. Left internal carotid ligated near origin with chromic gut. At present left eye turns in and there is some exophthalmos but no bruit.

Lane.

Male, struck on head by brick, fracturing nose, three months ago. Twelve days later ectropion of lower lids, marked edema. Vision, 8/200, right eye; enormous dilation, retinal veins, small hemorrhages about disk. Pulsation, bruit, exophthalmos. Blowing sound in left ear. Pulsation continues over left temporal region with accentuated systolic murmur. Only general treatment and KI.

June 10. Patient sat up for first time, 5 A.M.

June 11. Became aphasic with right facial paralysis.

September 2. No pulsation; faint systolic murmur; vessels of conjunctiva bright red color. Vision left eye, 6/6.

Maher.

1. Man, aged thirty-five years, ten months ago, had had a blow on head with a stick. Was unconscious 30 hours and dazed a week. Three weeks after injury the right eye began to protrude and throb with marked pulsation, controlled by pressure on right common carotid. Bruit over eye and temporal region. Marked engorgement conjunctival vessels, edema of conjunctiva, pupil dilated, retinal veins dilated and tortuous, marked edema of optic disk and retina. Headache and whirring noise in head. Right internal carotid tied. Pulsation ceased at once. Exophthalmos diminished. Three years later no exophthalmos, slight pallor of disk, and only occasional headache.

2. Man, aged nineteen years, fell forty-five feet, fracturing base of the skull. Unconscious several days. Six weeks after injury left eye began to protrude and for some weeks progressed, then gradually subsided. The right eye became

more prominent. Pain and noises in head. Right eye proptosed and convergent, conjunctiva edematous, vessels full, limited motion of globe up and down, no motion outward, pupil normal, retinal vessels slightly tortuous and dilated. Vision, 5/18. Left eye not proptosed, movements up and down limited. Pupil dilated. Disk pale. Vision, 5/21. Loud bruit over right eye and temple. Left internal carotid tied. One month later marked subsidence; eye moved up and down but not out; headache better; but bruit persisted; vision same.

Weinkauff.

Widow, aged eighty-four years, with no known reason became sick April 16, 1908 with severe headaches, next day frequent vomiting appeared, and unconsciousness. Consciousness returned after a few days, but speech was still somewhat confused at first. It was noticed that the left eye was markedly pushed forward, and shortly afterward the right eye became affected in the same manner. The patient complained of serious disturbances of vision.

Patient was seen first on May 5, 1908. Consciousness normal. No headaches now and none present subsequently. Ringing in the ears exists unchanged since several years, deafness for a longer time. Old age pronounced. Arterial rigidity is not exceptionally pronounced, pulse irregular. Remained in about this condition for next six months, then died from sudden cardiac failure.

Examination. Slight facial edema, also edema of the overhanging upper lids. Globes directed downward, slightly divergent. Completely immovable and proptosed. They could not be pushed backward. The edematous bulbar conjunctiva pushed out between the lids. Media clear. Papillæ are cloudy and swollen. Numerous small hemorrhages of the retina. Retinal veins dilated only moderately and slightly tortuous. Sensibility of cornea gone. Fingers counted on both sides at ½ M.

In June the edema and exophthalmos began to go down

slowly. In the upper inner angle pulsation is clearly felt, deeply situated. Bruit heard synchronous with the arterial pulse over the upper part of the orbit, changing to a blowing murmur during diastole, heard loudest over nasal side. This murmur gradually increased in intensity in the next few days, "bau-sch, bau-sch." The patient did not notice this murmur, complaining only of the former continuous singing in the ears. Left vision now O.

July: Pulsating nodules began to form at inner and upper angle, which gradually became smaller.

August: Right side showed hardly any pulsation Compression of the right or left carotid produced no changes. Double carotid compression not tried. Pulsation of the bulb itself was not noticed, nor was pulsation of the retinal vessels seen.

October: Pulsation gone entirely.

November: Bruit completely disappeared. No exophthalmos. Right eye counted fingers at 2 M.; The papillary swelling had gone down. Left eye entirely amaurotic. Movability of the bulbs remained limited.

December: Patient died. No autopsy.

Hildebrand.

Young man, in 1893 fell from a ladder and broke his arm and sustained cerebral concussion. Blind in left eye on recovering consciousness. Four months later the left eye protruded slightly. Pupils dilated and motionless, optic nerve white and glistening.

Diagnosis. Laceration of optic nerve. One-half year later the globe was pushed very far out. Upper eyelid swollen, with marked enlarged vessels. Root of nose swollen and pulsation was felt there. Pulsating vessels ran backward from here. Globe could be easily and painlessly pushed back, and was directed inward and downward. Retinal veins dilated and tortuous. Arteries normal. Loud whistling sound heard over entire head with stethoscope, loudest between outer angle of left eye and left ear. Bruit disappears when

carotid in neck (left) is compressed. Patient complains of
the bruit, which he hears strongest in front of left ear.

Treatment. Carotid compression tried one year after
injury, for nine weeks for one hour a day, carrying out the
same treatment himself later at home. No result one-half
year later. Patient seen by Hildebrand seventeen years
after injury. Above condition. Globe shows slight pulsation
and hardly moves upward and outward. Lids are not swollen
or edematous. Vessels of forehead greatly distended and
tortuous. Right eye normal, veins slightly distended. Both
superior ophthalmic veins are involved. No operation.

Halstead.

Male, aged thirty-six years, was struck twice on the left
temporomalar region with a hard instrument, February 10,
1910. Unconscious a short time, then walked home. Blood
from nose and ears. Facial paralysis next day and roaring
in the ears. Two months later, when left eye was enucleated
for panophthamitis, the orbital contents prolapsed. Vision
20/40. Diagnosed as pulsating tumor of base of brain,
probably aneurysm.

October 5. 1910, stump of left eye removed. Right eye
signs of beginning venous stasis. Roaring in ears heard
in head; long, loud bruit over malar regions. Common
carotid and two divisions of superior thyroid ligated. Bruit
disappeared immediately. No brain symptoms.

Ransohoff.

Man, aged twenty-two years, received blow on right
temple during fight. No unconsciousness or dizziness,
October 18, 1905. On November 28, he suddenly noticed
that he could not see out of the right eye, which became
swollen and prominent; until within two weeks he could
not close the lid. Ringing and buzzing in the head, occasionally pain in forehead.

Examination. Man, aged twenty-two years, farmer;
healthy. Abducens paralysis. Pulsating exophthalmos.
Ocular media clear.

Operation. Common carotid, external carotid, and superior thyroid tied with catgut. Superior thyroid divided, common carotid divided. Abducens paralysis persists. Vision has improved much, subsequently the central scotoma disappeared, and neuritis cleared up. Cure.

Diagnosis. Arteriovenous aneurysm of internal carotid; rupture of abducens.

R. J. Schaefer.

Woman, aged seventy-four years, suddenly taken with vomiting and distress January 10, 1907. Went to bed. Soon after she felt severe headache, spreading to right eye. Next day noticed a brownish circle around the lids of right eye, and January 12, paralysis of upper lid occurred. No unconsciousness, but insomnia. Noises in head, and the previous deafness grew greater. Sees well. No previous serious illness.

Examination. Nothing in heart, lungs, or other organs. Several suffusions on right side of the face, especially around the right eye. Ptosis, exophthalmos, chemosis. Total ophthalmoplegia. Sensitiveness to pressure on the globe. Pulsation not present. Amaurosis. Retinal ischemia.

Operation: January 21. Protrusion now tremendous. Pulsation now evident. Bruit over right eye and side of head. Attempt made to ligate superior ophthalmic vein, according to Sattler's method. Great hemorrhage, and the vein could not be found. Tampon. Tried to find inferior ophthalmic vein. Could not. Had to tampon and give up operation.

Digital compression of common carotid tried at intervals. Suddenly, January 28, she could sleep and the bruit and noises no longer existed. Thrombosis of sinus thought to have occurred. The pulsating exophthalmos continued and the eye was nearly dislocated from the orbit. Enucleated January 30. Did not ligate common carotid at first (in disease), because he feared to do so on account of general arterial sclerosis. Died about February, 1910, from arterial disease.

Oppenheimer.

Had seen a case (erectile tumor) in which the common carotid was ligated. Secondary hemorrhage resulted fatally.

Kraupa.

Man, aged twenty years, jumped from a spring-board into a swimming pool. On coming to the surface he noticed a remarkable ringing in his left ear, which became more pronounced in the next few days. Also began a typical pulsating exophthalmos of left eye. Patient very alcoholic, otherwise sound. Short systolic bruit at apex. Hearing was slightly impaired in left ear. Typical pulsating exophthalmos in left eye. Media clear.

Digital compression carried out for a long time, and then Weil ligated the common carotid. Three months later high-grade exophthalmos still persisted, but the pulsation and the subjective symptoms have disappeared since ligating.

Five years later he came complaining of abdominal pain and examination showed very slight exophthalmos. He confessed having had syphilis one year before his eye trouble. Wassermann positive.

Cornea clear, movement normal. Pupils unequal, incomplete reflex. Thickening of walls of retinal veins, which was not altered by "606" and other treatment for two years. Increased blood-pressure in the veins assumed to be the cause. No exophthalmos or pulsation, but the retinal veins are still thickened.

C. S. Merrill (personal communication to Bedell).

Woman, aged fifty years, fell from a wagon, striking the back of her head, July 5, 1909. When seen had left-sided chemosis, external exophthalmos, and pulsation. Aneurysmal bruit. Compression of carotid stopped the bruit. Vision right normal, left nil. Dr. A. W. Elting ligated left external carotid. All symptoms relieved and eyeball returned to normal position. Some months later, vision in right eye 20/20, left eye, objects to outer side; optic atrophy.

Santos Fernandez dez Balbuena.

Man, aged forty-seven years Forty-two days before observation he was struck by a hammer; was unconscious for three days. On recovering consciousness he had noise in the head, with moderate exophthalmos and ptosis. Pupil normal. Conjunctiva congested. Compression of common carotid caused disappearance of symptoms. A week after observation gelatin injections were started (intravenous), 2 per cent., and 2 per cent. NaCl. One month later the condition was much better. Pulsation stopped and exophthalmos disappeared.

Lystad.

Boy, aged fifteen years, stoker on steamer, was wounded August, 1902, by a revolver in the right nasal aperture. Right-sided ptosis noticed on admission to hospital, besides a left spastic paralysis with incomplete anesthesia and much disturbance of hearing in left ear. Left hospital after three months and eight months later resumed his work.

About two years after his accident he gradually began to notice swelling over the right eye, and in the next year gradually increasing exophthalmos and bruit. Patient states that the swelling is greater just before a storm. "Barometer." Five years after trauma he received a blow with the fist over the right eye. Came to clinic for treatment July 27, 1907.

Typical pulsating exophthalmos. Movement of eyes normal. Stasis of retinal veins; no pulsation. Subjective and objective vessel bruits disappear almost entirely by compression of right carotid.

September 17, 1907. Right internal carotid was ligated. Not sufficient, so the external carotid and jugular vein (internal) were also ligated. Great improvement seen at first subsided during the next week, and in the beginning of 1908 the pulsation and exophthalmos were about as before ligation, and patient was unable to work.

January 24, 1908. Orbital operation performed (Prof. Schiotz): The pulsating mass in upper inner angle was ligated. There were a great number of very tortuous, thin-walled veins. Operation difficult. On removing dressings next day there was seen an enormous protrusion of the bulb and its surrounding structures. Intense headache and pain in eye. Subjective bruits unchanged, pulse slow, sensorium clear.

A slight swelling in the neighborhood of the left eye subsided after a few days. After three weeks the protrusion was distinctly smaller; pulsation and objective bruits disappeared. The subjective bruits were noticeably less, but severe headache and slow pulse persisted.

The exophthalmos slowly disappeared during the following weeks, the swelling over the eye grew less tense, and the pulse was normal.

Two months later he stood up. Slight posterior synechiæ; fundus not clear; hemorrhages. Tension increased 51 mm. (Schiotz). Fingers at 2 m. and field of vision concentrically greatly narrowed. After several months was able to work. Absolute glaucoma.

Eye enucleated at request of patient in December, 1908. No headaches subsequently. The subjective bruits come at times but very slightly. Otherwise normal.

Risley.

1. Knocked unconscious by fist blow on the ramus of right jaw. Four weeks later pain in head, diplopia, and confusion. Proptosis of right eyeball about 10 mm.; swelling of lid; conjunctiva chemotic, with full veins near inner canthus. Motion limited except downward. Systolic pulsation best heard over right eye. Vision 6/12. X-ray negative. Still under observation.

2. Man, aged thirty years. Three years before had had his head caught between a trolley car and an express wagon. Unconscious seven weeks. Abducens paralysis; slight prop-

tosis of right eye. Loud blowing systolic bruit heard over entire skull, but loudest over right eyeball and left frontal. Bruit lost on right carotid compression. X-ray negative. Still under observation

Haslam and Hird.

Woman, aged twenty-four years. Husband died of pulmonary tuberculosis. No history or signs of syphilis. Two days ago had pains around her right eye and noises in her head. Came on suddenly. Went to work next day and noises became louder then and the eye became prominent. No pain. Sight was bad but improved later. Went home to bed and was sick several times.

Examination. Proptosis (right). Subcutaneous and subconjunctival ecchymoses. Pulsation; eye pushed forward in systole. Double bruit heard over eyeball. Visible pulsation over right side of neck along the great vessels. Bruits could be heard over the whole of the skull. Pressure on the right common carotid stopped noises (subjectively), but they could still be heard by the stethoscope. Eyeball freely movable. Pupils equal and react normally. No signs of arterial disease. Six days later (after admission) she began to have paralysis of external rectus.

Six weeks after onset right common carotid was ligated at level of cricoid. Thyroid gland much enlarged. All symptoms improved except pulsation (very slight), and patient could still hear slight noise, and double bruit had become only systolic. Ten days later the noises and murmurs became worse, and next day the double murmur was present again. Abducens paralysis still persists.

Right internal angular vein was ligated one month later. Noises much less for three days afterward, and no thrill or pulsation was present. Not followed by thrombosis of cavernous sinus.

Eight months later patient has proptosis, pulsation, abducens paralysis, congestion of veins, bruit. Hearing on right side is defective. No visible change in optic disk. R. V. 6/24 (with glass). Right fundus shows congestion. Pulsation in arteries of neck above ligature.

Ginsburg.

Boy, aged eighteen years, was struck on the head with an iron object, August 26, 1910. Unconscious fifteen minutes. Hemorrhage from mouth and nose.

Personal History (three days later). Complains of headaches, very severe and worse at night. In the left eyebrow is a small skin wound. Bony rim is sensitive and swollen. Large ecchymosis under left lower eyelid. Left eye otherwise normal. Right eye: proptosis; immovable; lids congested. Pushing the globe backward causes pain. Bulbar conjunctiva is not sensitive in the nasal region, also on temporal side. Pupil medium wide; light reaction gone (direct and consensual). Disk cloudy; boundaries hazy. Fundus congested. No pulsation of vessels. Veins dilated and tortuous; arteries contracted. No hemorrhages. Amaurosis, V. zero.

Diagnosis. Fracture of the base and rupture of the optic nerve in optic canal.

September 4. Strong pulsation in retinal vessels noticed for first time. Pulsation of globe, synchronous with heart systole. Soft, blowing murmur heard over eye. Complains only of severe headaches.

Diagnosis. Pulsating exophthalmos.

September 10. Complains of noise in right half of head, disturbing sleep. Skin over temple, upper lid, forehead anesthetic. Cornea and conjunctiva insensitive. Compression of right common carotid causes subjective and objective bruits to disappear.

December 7. Ligation of common carotid below omohyoid.

December 8. Same bruit, but weaker.

December 9. Blowing bruit over forehead.

December 12. Proptosis unchanged, no infection in wound.

March 27, 1911. *Operation.* Ligation of vena angularis, frontalis, supra-orbitalis and palpebralis superior. All these veins divided. Could not see the superior ophthalmic vein on account of the thickening of other veins, especially the lacrimal. Ophthalmic vein grasped with Pean, also lacrimal. Levator palpebral superioris and tendon of the trochlearis divided to allow access to the ophthalmic vein. Peans left in place.

March 30. Bleeding from left ear. Proptosis greater than before operation.

St. Praes, April 17. Complete ptosis. Sensibility of skin and cornea slightly improved. Proptosis entirely gone. No ocular mobility. No pulsation. Vision O.

Microscopic examination of exsected veins shows thickening; three layers. Hypertrophic process is especially evident in middle layer, which consists of strong muscle fibers. Weigert's stain for elastic tissue demonstrated its presence.

Friedenwald.

R. S., colored, aged twenty years, applied for treatment November 11, 1909, because of pain in right eye, which she said had been bulging out of socket for eleven to twelve years. Pain had begun in the past year; condition otherwise unchanged. No history of trauma. For some months had heard a thumping noise in right ear, especially at night. Hearing perfect.

Present Condition. Right eye displaced forward and downward. It is very prominent and pulsates so markedly that pulsations can be seen many feet away. Easily palpable. Right eye about 12 mm. lower than left, and forced forward at least 5 to 6 mm. with each pulsation. Eyeball easily and painlessly pushed back into socket. Vision: Left, 16/15; right, 16/200. Ocular movements in right eye normal except upward. Diplopia. Pupils equal and react to light. Lids, conjunctiva, and anterior part of eyeball are normal. No tortuosity or congestion of retinal vessels. Right disk pàler than left. No bruit about the orbit. At the posterior margin of left sternomastoid is a short well-marked blowing sound systolic. At times a blowing sound is heard along the margin of right sternomastoid. X-ray shows enlargement of pituitary fossa, with irregularity. Right orbital cavity larger than left.

Reclus.

Woman, syphilitic, entered hospital July 18, 1906, for affection of the orbit. Treated for several months previously for syphilis. Five years ago began having rebellious headaches, especially at night.

February, 1906, was taken suddenly with fever and violent pains in the head, diagnosed as meningitis. Then the inner angle of the left eye began to be a little more prominent than the right, prominence consisting of pulsating vessels. One night later she was awakened by a sound like a locomotive blowing off steam.

Examination. Exophthalmos, swelling, and edema of upper lid, with a network of dilated vessels in it. Pulsation and thrill over these tissues and down the carotids on both sides. Bruit heard everywhere over the skull. It was a continuous whistle, with systolic accentuation. She complained besides of another bruit, like the chirping of a bird. Sugar and albumin in urine.

Digital compression of common carotid. Slight betterment, but later recurred. Gelatin injections. Lancereaux and Paulesco, following the first therepeutic suggestions of Carnot in the coagulating power of gelatin. Lancereaux cured a case by this method and presented him to the Academy.

Twenty-one injections given. One per cent. solution of gelatin in serum at first, then 2 per cent. as the 1 per cent. was found not active enough. Five per cent. is painful and causes a rise of temperature. Two per cent caused a slight rise. Injection into the muscles, not subcutaneous. Slight improvement was noted. Twenty-one more injections were given and the result was more encouraging. Altogether she was given 81 injections of 40 grams of solution, when she was taken with complete ophthalmoplegia (left) and ptosis. Regarded as specific and treated with gray oil injections. No improvement, and she is blind, with retinitis of that eye. Gelatin injections resumed, and after the fourth one she had acute swelling of upper lid with pain. Ice used locally. Pain disappeared and the vessels felt hard with no pulsation. Pulsating exophthalmos disappeared. No chemosis, or vascular tumor. The intracranial whistle and the attacks of headache persisted. Glaucoma of left eye.

Left common carotid ligated March 19, 1908. Intracranial bruit disappeared next day. Two months later well except for ptosis and ophthalmoplegia and blindness.

May, forty-four days after operation, she suffered an apoplectic stroke and died. Postmortem: Cavernous sinus full of hard clots and dilated to the size of a small nut, with the internal carotid ruptured 4 to 5 mm. Common carotid and internal carotid empty down to the place of ligature, where there is a clot about 2 cm. long. A second rupture of internal carotid into cavernous sinus existed on the other side, fresh. She had been having symptoms or right side for a short time, bruit, headache, and pain in right globe.

Wilder.

1. W. C., aged forty-two years, an American, was admitted October 31, 1910. Three weeks before was waylaid by a thug; struck over right eye. Unconscious. On recovering noticed lids of both eyes were swollen. Sight not impaired, but diplopia was present. Severe pain in right side of head, intermittent. These attacks became more frequent and severe and he came to hospital. Noticed roaring in ear on recovering consciousness, like a steam exhaust. Right eyeball began to protrude and swelling of lids did not diminish. The pain in the head became constant, radiating to back of the head and spine.

Examination. Right exophthalmos, conjunctiva swollen, and edematous. Conjunctiva veins engorged. Marked distention of angular vein at superior border of orbit. Cornea clear. Pupil dilated and inactive to light and accommodation. Mobiltiy of eyeball reduced to slight abduction only. Levator palpebralis also powerless. R. V., 20/60; L. V., 20/20. Fundus normal except for engorged veins. Optic disk redder than normal. Left eye normal. Hearing normal. Marked bruit, systolic accentuation, heard over right side of head and eye, most pronounced over zygomatic arch. At times faintly heard over left temple and eye. Bruit and subjective noises stopped on compression of common carotid. It was doubtful whether there was ever any pulsation of orbital contents, even when leaning over.

Operation November 10, 1911 (Dr. A. W. Bevan). Ligation of ' common carotid. Bruit stopped immediately. On recovery from anesthetic, noises were not heard. Pain in head persisted for a week and gradually subsided. Exophthalmos disappeared slowly. Swollen conjunctiva required massage and astringents. Mobility of eye slowly returned, pupil became normal. V., 20/30 at five weeks. Wilder thinks this was an aneurysm of the carotid (cavernous portion) not communicating with the sinus.

2. C. O., aged thirty-eight years, laborer, was admitted November 22, 1910. Struck on back of head by beer-bottle five or six months ago. Unconscious for some minutes. Again became unconscious; trephined. Regained consciousness after operation. Left hospital well after three weeks. Again struck on back of head with iron bar; unconscious. Scalp wound sewed; well. Two weeks later began to have headaches and noises in head and right ear. These continued steadily, and five weeks later noticed protrusion of right eye, later pain and lacrimation. Came to hospital.

Examination. Exophthalmos (about 10 mm.), directed downward and outward. Mobility of right eye limited to abduction and outward rotation. All muscles supplied by third nerve seemed to be paralyzed; fourth and sixth normal. No facial palsy. Pupil dilated. Ptosis. Chemosis of conjunctiva and fornix, with engorgement of veins. Angular vein not markedly distended. Fundus normal except for some engorgement of retinal veins. R. V., 20/40. L. V., 20/30. Tension of right slightly plus. High pitched bruit, synchronous with heart beat, heard over entire head, but loudest over temporal region of right side of right eye. Blowing bruit, accentuated in systole. Very slight pulsation of orbital contents seen and felt. Orbital pain and roaring in head, "like a waterfall." Hearing normal. Bruit and head noises ceased on compression of common carotid.

Diagnosis. Aneurysm of internal carotid in or near the cavernous sinus.

Operation. Ligation of common carotid. Dr. A. D. Bevan, December 12, 1910. Bruit stopped on ligation. Patient relieved of noises and pain at once. Exophthalmos gone in two weeks. Chemosis better. Partial recovery from the third nerve paralysis. Pupil still enlarged and immobile. Retinal veins still enlarged.

January 28, 1911. Hissing noises began occasionally, accompanied by exophthalmos, receding again. Some weeks later faint bruit heard over right mastoid and temple.

Internal carotid ligated April 5, 1911. When ligature was placed around vessel bruit ceased. (High bifurcation.) Found and ligated. Paralysis of muscles of left forearm and hand, difficulty in speech. No amnesia. Gradual return to normal. Exophthalmos still slightly present. Mobility good; right pupil 1 mm., larger than left, and mobile. R. V., 20/50; L. V., 20/20.

Ipsen.

Woman, aged forty-nine years, came to Rovsing's service June 1. Enlarged cervical glands of left side. Two miscarriages. Lately has had severe headaches back of the ear twice a year, causing shooting pains at the vertex of the head, and accompanied by vomiting. Normal in interval.

March, 1911. Fell against a tree and injured the left side of the head and neck, but there were no signs of basal fracture or unconsciousness.

May 7. Suddenly taken sick from no apparent cause. Intense pain in the right side of the head, with buzzing and sounds like machinery in operation heard. Vomiting.

Examination. Nothing abnormal seen, but next day the right globe was protruding, conjunctiva injected, and eyelids were swollen. These symptoms increased in intensity in next few days and the globe became immovable. Ten days later pulsation of globe and eyelids was noticed. This pulsation stopped upon compression of common carotid artery.

May 29. The left eye showed slight proptosis and pulsation, ceasing when right common carotid was compressed.

Examination, June 1. Same findings as above. Intraocular tension increased. Ophthalmoscope showed veins dilated to twice normal size; arteries normal. Total ophthalmoplegia. Vision of left eye was 5/12. Wassermann reaction was negative.

Operation (Dr. Theodore Rovsing). Ligation of right carotid. Immediate subsidence of objective symptoms. Discharged July 1, 1911. Recovered quickly, and now can read fingers at a meter's distance, but only on the temporal side. No headaches. Nevertheless, she feels a continual buzzing in the left ear, but this is checked by pressure on the left common carotid.

Silvan.

Boy, aged sixteen years, was sent to a specialist for a disturbance of the right eye.

October 20, 1913. While building a narrow bridge he was thrown out from the bridge against the right side of the head and neck; the left side of his head struck against a loaded wheelbarrow. He was rendered unconscious and remained comatose for an entire week. Immediately after trauma had hemorrhage from nose, ears, and mouth, and successively delirium and vomiting, without any general or circumconvulsive phenomena. On return to consciousness he remembered nothing of the accident, but psychic activity returned shortly, with no disturbance of speech or general motility or sensibility. From the beginning he notice a painful continuous blowing and rumbling noise in the head, more accentuated to the left in the neighborhood of the ear, like a jet of steam, with rhythmical accentuation with the radial pulse. This bruit was lessened without disappearing entirely, with little variation in time, when pressure was applied to the carotid area. At the same time the patient and family noticed that the right eye was made more bulging, and more inflamed than the other, and that pressure above this gave distinct pulsation with systole, and stopped the subjective systolic bruit. Facial paralysis of the left side from beginning. A month after injury the vision of the right eye began to fail. All the ocular muscles were intact; besides exophthalmos there was chemosis to a marked degree. Patient said the visual disturbance began with slight degree of pain, with the impression of confusion of near objects, without diplopia, or abnormal sensations nor painful phenomena of any kind. This progressed gradually and became worse, and at the end of four months after the accident vision was reduced to light perception

Examination. No visceral lesions; healthy; reflexes normal; intelligence and memory normal; motor and sensory perceptions normal; all reflexes normal; no headache or dizziness; no disturbance of walking or equilibrium; Exophthalmos directly forward; tension slightly increased; injection of bulbar and ocular conjunctiva, without chemosis or dilation of varicose veins; upper lid slightly succulent and thick; cornea not opaque; pupil dilated and did not react to light or accommodation; examination of fundus showed papilla inflamed greatly, edges sharply defined; central vein of retina congested, turgid, and tortuous; no hemorrhages; vision was reduced to simple perception of light, globe movable upward and downward and outward, but paralysis of internal rectus; pressure on the globe only moderatley reduced the protrusion, and produced an acute sensation of pain, and a light thrill was noticed synchronous with carotid pulse, which corresponded with the bruit, accentuated with each pulse beat, resembling blowing off of steam, incessant and disturbing, felt in skull, in temporo-auricular region. Stethoscope over the whole skull, but especially over orbit heard a bruit, soft, blowing, systolic accentuation slightly rough. This was heard along the course of the great vessels along the right side of the neck. Heart normal. The bruit, both subjective and objective, the thrill simultaneous with pulsation of the ocular glove when depressed, disappeared immediately and completely with compression of the right common carotid, but was unaffected by pressure on the left. V. R., 1/2; field of vision normally limited. Left normal. Olfactory nerve intact. Trigeminal normal. Vision in left eye paralyzed in all its branches. Ptosis. Eye closed. Palate (soft) half paralyzed and deviated. Other nerves normal.

April 28. Prof. Giordano ligated common carotid just below bifurcation. During the operation one could clearly demonstrate the stopping of the thrill and pulsation of ocular globe when it was depressed. The patient on recovery felt no longer the rumbling and whistling in the skull, and by the evening of the same day said that he could distinguish neighboring objects in a confused and uncertain way, which a week before he could not possibly discern. Vision progressed normally and rapidly, so that within one week from the operation the patient said that he could distinguish clearly objects near and far with precision, as before accident.

Examination, May 18, O. D. V., 2/3, em. O. S. V., 2/3, field of vision normal in both. Slight ptosis. Exophthalmos noticeably reduced. Conjunctival veins less injected. Eye could be pushed back without thrill or pain. Pupil moderately dilated and reacting well. Papilla less congested.

Retinal veins less tortuous and injected than before. Shining white spots with circinate arrangement near the papilla and macula, resembling the spots of albuminuric retinitis. Bruit and whistling in preorbital region disappeared shortly and definitely. Muscular exercise produced a very slight bruit over carotid region, not affected by posture of head, not subjectively noticed.

REFERENCES

Bodon. Deutsch. Zeitschr. f. Chir., vol. li, p. 605.

Ballin, M. Pulsating Exophthalmos with Successful Ligation of Carotid, Detroit Med. Jour., 1905–06, p. 20.

Barbieri. Exoftalmia pulsatil bilateral, Archivos de Oftalmologia Hispano-Americanos, 1909, p. 9.

Barlay, J. Exophthalmus Pulsans, Ungar. med. Presse., 1905, vol. x, p. 216.

Barrett and Orr. Case of Traumatic Pulsating Exophthalmos, Intercolonial Medical Journal of Australia, 1909, p. 492.

Beauvois, A. Traitement do l'exophthalmie pulsatile par la methode Lancereaux-Paulesco, Rec. d'opht., 1907, 3 s., vol. xix, p. 337–53.

Becker. Traumatic Aneurysm of Internal (Cerebral) Carotid with Pulsating Exophthalmos, Arch. of Ophth., 1908, p. 635.

Bedell, A. J. Traumatic Pulsating Exophthalmos, Arch. of ophth., 1915, vol. xliv, p. 139–53.

Buchtel, F. C. The Treatment of Pulsating Exophthalmos with Case Report, Ophth. Rec., 1913, vol. xxii, p. 75–79.

Bull, C. S. Pulsating Exophthalmos Traumatic, Tr. Am. Ophth. Soc., 1903.

Carreras-Arago. Exophthalmos from Traumatic Aneurysm of the Ophthalmic Artery Cured by Digital Compression of the Carotid, Rev. de cien. Med., 1887, vol. xiii, p. 97.

Clark, H. E. Case of Pulsating Exophthalmos, Glasgow Med. Jour., 1887, 4 s., vol. xxviii, p. 270.

Cunningham. Report of a Case of Gradual Occlusion of the Common Carotid Artery in the Treatment of Pulsating Exophthalmos, Jour. Am. Med. Assn., 1914, vol. lxii.

Despaquez. Bull. Soc. Franc. d'Ophth., N. S., xlx, 303–308.

Eliot. Ligation of Common Carotid for Pulsating Exophthalmos, Ann. Surg., 1912, vol. lv, p. 454.

Evans, J. Pulsating Exophthalmos, Brit. Med. Jour., 1906, pt. 2, p. 1305.

Eissen. Archiv. f. Augenheilkunde, 1890.

Eysen. Ueber die Behandlung des traumatischen pulsierenden Exophthalmus, Inaug. Diss., Berlin, 1908.

Ferandez des Balbuena, J. Tratamiento de la exofthalmia pulsátil par les inyecciones intravenosas, de suero gelatinizado, Arch. de ofthal., 1913, vol. xiii, p. 72–75.

Flemming, P. and Johnson, R. Traumatic Pulsating Exophthalmos Treated by Ligature of the Common Carotid Artery, Proc. Roy. Soc. Med., 1908–09, pt. 2, Clin. Sec., p. 14–16.

Friedenwald, H. A Case of Pulsating Exophthalmos without Bruit, Am. Jour. Ophth., 1911, vol. xx, p. 654.

Gibson, J. L. Pulsating Exophthalmos: postmortem, Australas. Med. Gaz., 1905, vol. xxiv, p. 107–09.

Gifford, H. Pulsating Exophthalmos Treated by Excision of a Dilated Orbital Vein, Ophthalmol., 1907–08, vol. iv, p. 20–25.

Ginsburg, J. Beitrag zur Behandlung des pulsierenden Exophthalmus, Klin. Monatsbl. f. Augenh., 1912, pt. 2, p. 698-712.

Golowin. Zeit. f. Augenheilkunde, 1890.

Halstead, A. E. Double Pulsating Exophthalmos; Report of a Case, Surg., Gynec. and Obst., 1911, vol. xii, p. 298.

Halstead, A. E., and Bender, A. J. Pulsating Exophthalmos; Ligation of the Internal Carotid, Surg., Gynec. and Obst., 1910, vol. x, p. 55.

Hansell, H. F. Pulsating Exophthalmos: Successful Ligation of both Common Carotid Arteries: Death, Jour. Am. Med. Assn., 1905, vol. xliv, p. 536.

Hasse, C. G. Pulsierender Exophthalmus des rechten Auges, Heilung durch Bindung der Arteria Carotis Communis, Arch. f. Augenh., 1886–87, vol. xvii, p. 25–30.

Hildebrand. Ein Fall von Exophthalmus pulsans nach verletzung, Aerztl. Sachverst-Ztg., 1912, vol. xviii, p. 10–12.

Hird, B., and Haslam, W. F. A Case of Spontaneous Pulsating Exophthalmos, Lancet, 1909, pt. 1, p. 462.

Ipsen, J. Et tilfælde of exophthalmus pulsans, Hosp.-Tid. Kbenh., 1912, 5 R., vol. v, p. 1009–17.

Jack, E. E. A Case of Pulsating Exophthalmos, Ligation of the Common Carotid; Death; Pathological Report by F. H. Verhoeff, Ophth. Rec., 1907, vol. xvi, p. 463–69.

Jacques. Exophthalmos pulsatile traumatique, avec epistaxis grave., guéri par la compression directe transsphenoidale du sinus caverneux, Revue heb. de laryn. d'otol. et de rhin., 1908, p. 72.

James, R. R., and Fadden, W. F. Two Cases of Pulsating Exophthalmos, in Which the Carotid Artery was Ligated, Lancet, 1912, pt. 2, p. 237.

Kennedy, R. Case of Traumatic Exophthalmos Pulsans; Ligature of Common Carotid; Cure, Glasgow Med. Jour., 1904, vol. lxii, p. 426–30.

Kraupa, E. Zur Kenntnis der Erkrankung der Netzhaut-Gefässe bei pulsierenden Exophthalmus, Klin. Monatsbl. f. Augenh., 1911, vol. xlix, pt. 2, p. 191–96.

Lane, F. Pulsation Exophthalmos, Ann. Ophth., 1911, vol. xx, p. 226.

Lewis, F. P. Pulsating Exophthalmos, Ligation of Orbital Artery; Recovery, Ophth. Rec., 1907, vol. xvi, p. 66–69.

Lystad, H. Traumatisk exophthalmus pulsans, Heibredet ved Orbital operation, Norsk Magazin for Loegevidenshaben, 1911, p. 416.

Lystad, H. Zur Behandlung des pulsierenden Exophthalmus, Klin. Monatsbl. f. Augenh., 1912, pt. 1, p. 88–92.

Lazarew. Ref. Jahres Ref. in Jahresbericht (Nagel-Michel), 1898.

McClennan. Pulsating Exophthalmos Due to Aneurysm of the Internal Carotid, Jour. Am. Med. Assn., 1911, p. 1552.

Maher, W. O. Notes on Two Unusual Cases of Pulsating Exophthalmos, Ophthalmol., 1914, vol. x, p. 407–09.

Mathewson, G. H. A Case of Pulsating Exophthalmos, Ophth. Rec., 1913, vol. xxii, p. 294–96.

Merrill, C. S. Unreported Case of Pulsating Exophthalmos, 1909.

Murray, F. W. The Treatment of Pulsating Exophthalmos, Ann. Surg., 1904, p. 421.

Noyes, H. D. Pulsating Exophthalmos, Tr. Am. Ophth. Assn., 1881, vol. iii, p. 308.

Orloff. Traitement de l'exophtalmie pulsatile traumatique, Annals d'oculistique, 1911, p. 40.

Ophthalmoscope. July, 1908.

Palen, G. J. A Case of Pulsating Exophthalmos, Jour. Ophth., Otol., and Laryngol., 1911, vol. xvii, p. 197–202.

Pincus, F. Spontanheilung eines traumatischen pulsierenden Exophthalmus, Zeitschr. f. Augenh., 1907, vol. xviii, p. 33–41.

Pooley. Arteria-venous Aneurysm (Pulsatory Exophthalmos), Arch. Ophth., 1908, p. 449.

Ransohoff, J. Pulsating Exophthalmos; Ligature of the Common Carotid, External Carotid and Superior Thyroid Arteries, Surg., Gynec. and Obst., 1906, pt. 3, p. 193–95.

Reclus. Sur une observation d'exophthalmos pulsatile, Gaz. des hôpitaux, 1908, p. 1001.

Risley. Traumatic Aneurysm of Cranial Artery, Annals Ophth., 1912, p. 375.

Rübel, E. Ophthalmoskopischer Befund bei pulsierendem Exophthalmus, Monatsbl. f. Augenh., 1913, N. F., vol. xvi, p. 62–65.

Santos Fernandez dez Palbuena. Exoftalmia pulsatil por aneurisma curado con las inyecciones de gelatina, Revista de Medicina Y Cirugia de la Habana Se Publica los Dias 10 y 25 de Cada Mes., 1907, p. 296.

Sattler, H. Ueber ein neues Verfahren bei der Behandlung des pulsierenden Exophthalmus, Klin. Monatsbl. f. Augenh., 1905, vol. xliii, p. 1–61.

Savariaud. Exophthalmus pulsatile, Bull. et mém. Soc. de Chir. de Paris, 1912, n. s., vol. xxxviii, p. 672.

Schaefer, R. J. Ein Fall von pulsierenden Exophthalmus, Deut. med. Wchnschr., 1910, vol. xxxvi, p. 124.

Schwalbach, G. Zur Behandlung des pulsierenden Exophthalmos, Klin. Monatsbl. f. Augenh., 1905, vol. xliii, pt. 2, p. 475–79.

de Schweinitz and Holloway. Pulsating Exophthalmos, Saunders, 1908.

Silvan, C. Sopra un caso di esofthalmo pulsante guarito in seguito alla legatura della carotide commune, Riv. veneta di sc. med. Venezia, 1914, vol. lxi, p. 51–64.

Slomann. Central. f. Chirurg., 1900, p. 182.

Sattler. Handbuch von Graefe-Saemisch, 1880. 1 Aufl.

Siegrist. Graefe's Archiv, 1900.

Wienkauff, K. Doppelseitiger idiopathischer Exophthalmus pulsans mit spontaner Ruckbildung, Arch. f. Ophth., 1910, vol. lxxiv, p. 352–56.

Wilder, W. H. Report of Two Cases of Pulsating Exophthalmos, Tr. Am. Ophth. Soc., 1909–11, vol. xii, p. 832–41.

Williams, G. Pulsating Exophthalmos, Proc. Roy. Soc. Med., London, 1910, pt. 3, Klin. Sect., p. 171.

Wing. Case of Pulsating Exophthalmos, Tr. Med. Soc., Washington, 1891, p. 123.

Wurdemann, H. V., and Placoe, N. M. Pulsating Exophthalmos, Ann. Ophth., 1904.

Wiesinger. München. med. Wchnschr., 1903.

Yvert. Cas remarquable d'exophthalmie pulsatile guérie des instillations d'adrenaline, Gazette des hôpitaux de Lyon, 1906–07, p. 89.

Zeller, O. Die chirurgische Behandlung der durch Aneurysma arterio-venosum der Carotis int. im Sin. cavernosus hervergerufenen pulsierenden Exophthalmus: ein neues Verfahren, Deutsche Zeitschr. f. Chir., 1911, vol. cx, p. 1–39.

DISCUSSION

DR. V. P. BLAIR, St. Louis, Missouri.—We are indebted to Dr. Rhodes for reviewing this subject. There is one point which was not brought out, and that is, the relation of the mortality as given to the ligature of the common carotid artery. Ligation of the common carotid in a young person is usually safe, but according to Kocher, ligation of the common carotid in an elderly man in whom there is arteriosclerosis is equivalent to a death-warrant. That is one of the greatest stumbling blocks in connection with operations on the posterior part of the jaw.

In a young person you may remove every structure on one side of the neck, except the internal or common carotid, with a fair chance of getting by with it; but in an old person the ligation of the artery is a very serious thing.

DR. ALEXIUS McGLANNAN, Baltimore, Maryland.—I cannot say anything definite with reference to the statistics regarding ligation of the common carotid in elderly people, but it is not necessarily a death-warrant. We have ligated the common carotid quite a number of times in connection with operations for extensive carcinoma of the jaw and mouth, for purposes of palliation, and the mortality has been *nil*. We have had no deaths as a direct result of ligation of the common carotid, so that I do not believe it is exactly a death-warrant as spoken of by Dr. Blair.

DR. GEORGE A. HENDON, Louisville, Kentucky.—I have ligated the common carotid in five old men over seventy years of age for cancer of the parotid gland without any bad effects; except in the majority of cases there was a recurrence of the malignant growth.

DR. J. M. T. FINNEY, Baltimore, Maryland.—There is one method of gradually cutting off the blood stream before ligation which was first suggested by my chief, Dr. Halsted, by means of metallic bands. Later that method has been developed by Dr. Matas and others in this country, who have thus succeeded in reducing the mortality of ligation of the common carotid very materially.

DR. GOODRICH V. RHODES, Cincinnati, Ohio (closing).—In regard to gradually shutting off the circulation, it has seemed to me the object of the operation of ligating any vessel or series of vessels is to reduce as much as possible the volume of blood flowing through the anastomosis. In other words, if we have a large amount of blood flowing through there it will blow out the clot. Gradually contracting the clamp may not do that primarily. It will only do it when the pressure of the clamp is such as to produce practical obliteration of the artery. That simply means that we are going to tie the artery anyway. If we practice in these cases compression of the artery for a definite time beforehand with digital compression, and study the effects upon the patient or even under local anesthesia practicing preliminary tying and watching the effect for a few moments, we could make our ligation immediately because these effects come on almost immediately with the exception of the ones that come from spreading of the clot later which cannot be avoided.

In regard to the operation on old people, the question comes up as to what condition we are operating for. A large proportion of these conditions in older people are from spontaneous rupture of the artery. They are not traumatic cases. These are more easily cured and present a more favorable prognosis than the traumatic cases, for the reason the thrombotic qualities of the blood are enhanced by the diseased condition of the intima of the vessel. If we can ligate in these cases we will get better results.

Dr. Blair mentioned the point that there was no question of the mortality being greater from ligation of the common carotid artery in older people than in younger people. I am not familiar with the figures on this point, but they can be deduced from my collected series of cases.

Dr. Blair.—That is Kocher's experience in surgery, and my experience has been the same.

Dr. Rhodes.—I do not remember offhand the percentage of fatalities following ligation of the common carotid artery in older people.

HIGH DEGREES OF HEAT VS. LOW DEGREES OF HEAT AS PALLIATIVE TREATMENT FOR ADVANCED CASES OF CANCER OF THE UTERUS

WITH AUTOPSY REPORT OF A CASE TREATED BY THE LONG APPLICATION OF LOW HEAT AS ADVOCATED BY DR. J. F. PERCY

BY H. J. BOLDT, M.D.
New York

DOUBTLESS all who have had experience in the treatment of cancer of the uterus, too far advanced for radical operation, will concede that the heat method, applied with the actual cautery, first brought to notice and strongly advocated by the late Dr. John Byrne, of Brooklyn, gives the most satisfactory results.

Radium and x-ray treatment, even with the newer methods, have not, so far as my observation goes, given better results—nay, nor as good results. Neither, in my experience, has intramuscular medication, with the various remedies used for experimentation from time to time, shown any noticeable improvement; although some observers have claimed not only improvement but absolute cures.

In this connection I wish to report the case of a patient sent to me from Mexico, who temporarily improved under radium therapy, to such a degree that the uterine bleeding and the pressure pain disappeared. The pain had necessitated the employment of narcotics by her home physician for some months previously. But after the first radium application no narcotics were necessary. The size of the cancerous mass, however, did not decrease, as was ascertained by rectovaginal examination. On the contrary it gradually increased. Seeing the publication of practically miraculous results emanating from European confrères, I advised the patient to seek *x*-ray treatment at Freiburg, where, I thought, the technic was better understood. It chanced though, that she was induced to remain at Paris, in the care of a physician generally considered as *the* expert in the use of radium—who assured her family that she could be cured. He retained her for four months, during which time the patient and family had been given repeated assurance of her gradual but steady improvement. Eventually she returned here to die, yet up to the last treatment, emphatic promises of final cure had been made. According to the nurse and the patient's family, the Parisian confrère asserted, that by his method of using radium success in such cases was invariable. While I do not doubt the intended correctness of published reports, I, nevertheless, must be convinced by personal observation before I ever again express faith in any remedy. No man is infallible and judgment and opinion will vary as long as the world stands.

Heat treatment, however, has stood the test of time, and clinical experience has shown that patients so treated live longer and are freer from the distressing symptoms than those under any other method of treatment. Indeed, Byrne assured us that a goodly number are cured completely of their disease by it.

Moreover, it is a comparatively safe therapeutic agent, if properly applied in selected cases; that is, where the disease has not already advanced so far that the bladder or rectum or both would probably be injured by a thorough application with the cautery.

Dr. Percy claims that his method of applying heat is more efficacious than that advocated by Byrne. Experiments; he asserts, have proved to him that low degrees of heat—

so low that the tissues are not charred—have a deeper destructive influence, if the heat application is made to cover a longer period of time. In order to get such low degrees he had a rheostat made which could be so regulated that only sufficient heat to obviate carbonization would pass to the electrode.

Charring should never be caused—only desiccation—according to Percy's theory. But, Byrne, too, said that heat must never be more than a dull cherry red. He used electrodes that were heated only by a battery, believing that there was more therapeutic value in the heat evolved from a battery than that from an electric current. Of course, comment on this is not necessary. But Byrne's reason for using low heat was also to prevent bleeding during the process of cauterizing which, he said, should a higher degree of heat be used than the dull cherry red, was likely to prove a very dangerous factor.

With the Byrne method and with my own, in which much higher degrees of heat are used, I have had extensive experience, covering many years; but with Percy's method my experience is comparatively limited, but theoretically, however, it impressed me so favorably that I have used it a number of times during the last two years.

Concerning Byrne's method and the still higher degree of heat method, I will not speak in detail, since I have, on former occasions, published my experience.

As said in the foregoing, the prognosis as to safety to life from operation is generally good—so good that a fatal result is a rarity. I have had but one fatal result from the high degree of heat, and that was after the patient had left the hospital, about two weeks subsequent to operation. Then, too, the circumstances were unfortunate in that the patient lived so far from my home that it required an hour to reach her. Moreover, the crisis occurred in the middle of the night, and I was not prepared to meet the condition with which I was confronted. The eschar was thrown off and bared the uterine artery which spouted in jets like a miniature fountain. The cavity was tightly packed with gauze, and I purposed to open the abdomen and tie the vessel if the bleeding did not cease by the time that I had prepared myself to do this. She died as the result of hemorrhage before I could do the operation.

The second death—which induced me to make this report —occurred after the application of the lower degree of heat, according to the Percy technic.

Mrs. D. F., the widow of a physician, aged sixty years. One pregnancy: twenty-eight years previously, was seen in February, 1915. She had a carcinoma of the cervix, too far advanced for radical operation. The palliative cautery operation was done with low heat. Time of cauterization, two hours. The immediate effect of the operation was good. The bleeding and the discharge ceased, and she left the hospital about the tenth day.

Reëxamination in April. The cauterized surface felt and looked smooth and was firm; no bleeding upon firm manipulation of the surface. But the rectal examination showed the tumor mass larger than before operation.

I felt that while the surface bleeding had ceased, yet the disease was active and had continued to progress. Therefore, I thought it best to make another application of heat to get a destruction of carcinoma cells farther distant. The cauterization was extended to a period covering two and one-half hours. At no time was the heat brought to a point to cause charring.

On the fourth day incontinence of urine commenced, due to separation of a slough, caused by the cautery.

The patient died of sepsis on the eighth day. The autopsy report is appended herewith.

But before including it, I want to say, that personally, I have never seen an instance in which slightly distant parametrial infiltration had become lessened after any cautery operation.

Percy says that a fixed uterus becomes movable under the application of low heat. This is true to a certain extent, but it seems to me that he makes an erroneous deduction. The mobility is brought about by the thickened paracervical tissue being dried out by the heat, and the cervix itself destroyed by the action of heat, so that it is natural that the uterus itself becomes more mobile, if previously fixed by the indurated base surrounding it. This is the case also with the use of high heat. The parametrial infiltration, however, a short distance from the uterus, does not become lessened. So that there is nothing new, nor an iota of superiority, much less peculiarity, in the lower heat degree method. On the contrary, it is inferior, if the time element be taken into consideration, since high heat will accomplish the same result in one-fourth the time.

PATHOLOGICAL REPORT FROM THE LABORATORY OF THE POST-GRADUATE MEDICAL SCHOOL AND HOSPITAL

Died 4.30 A.M., April 15, 1915.

Autopsy 1.15 P.M., April 15, 1915.

Clinical Diagnosis. Carcinoma of uterus.

General Inspection. The body is that of a well-developed and well-nourished adult female. The skin is white with a slight yellowish tinge. There is abundance of black hair intermingled with gray over the head. Pupils are equal, round and dilated, measuring 7 mm. in diameter. The teeth are in good condition. External orifices negative. There is a slight amount of purplish hypostasis over dependent parts; slight degree of body heat over chest; rigor mortis throughout. The chest is moderately full but the intercostal angle is less than a right angle. The upper part of the abdomen is on a level with the ensiform but the lower part is two finger breadths above ensiform.

Main Incision. There is 1 to 2 cm. of orange-yellow panniculus. Musculature deep red in color, moderate amount. The junctures of the costal cartilages and the ribs are well ossified.

Abdominal Cavity. The intestines are moderately distended with gas, bluish red in color, moist and glistening. There is no free abdominal fluid. In the pelvis the small intestines are matted together by recent fibrinous adhesions. On separating these adhesions an abundance of yellow purulent fluid escapes, estimated 80 c.c. This fluid is localized to the pelvis by adhesions between the intestines and a thin seminecrotic fibrinous membrane which extends backward over the uterus. The uterus is therefore within the pus cavity and has about it that purulent exudate. The liver is 1 cm. below costal margin. At the lower pole of the spleen and between it and the external abdominal wall is a recently formed abscess cavity measuring 5 cm. in diameter and filled with a yellowish creamy pus. The diaphragm on the left side is at the fifth interspace, on the right at the fifth rib.

Pleural Cavity. The lungs are moderately well collapsed and free. No increase of pleural fluid.

Pericardial Cavity. There is no increase of fluid and both the visceral and parietal pericardia are smooth and glistening.

Heart. Weight 340 grams. There is considerable amount of pericardial fat and the muscle is soft and flabby. Tricuspid valve admits two fingers; flaps negative. Pulmonary admits thumb with ease; flaps negative. Mitral admits two fingers; flaps negative. Aorta admits thumb with ease; flaps negative.

Lungs. Right lung—weight 270 grams. It varies from light to deep red in color; surface smooth; no areas of consolidation. On section bleeds freely and is aerated throughout. Left lung—weight 300 grams; similar in all respects to right except that it contains a few small calcified tubercles in apex.

Liver. Weight 1800 grams. It is dark, bluish red in color, smooth and firm. On section bleeds freely. Lobules stand out distinctly. There appears to be a moderate congestion.

Spleen. Weight 170 grams. The spleen is deep bluish red in color except for a yellowish area at one pole which forms border of abscess above described. On section the pulp is soft, deep red in color and the fibrous trabeculæ are quite prominent.

Kidneys. Right kidney—weight 350 grams. The surface is moderately smooth, dark red in color, but in places there are small yellowish white, slightly raised areas. The capsule strips with some difficulty, being moderately adherent in scattered areas, and exposes a mottled light to deep red surface with small yellow pin-point nodules distributed over it. The cut surface bleeds freely, is mottled light and deep red and has scattered throughout, but especially located in the cortical portion, yellowish areas varying from a few millimeters to 1 cm. in diameter, soft in consistency and outlined by a deep red border. The cortex is considerably thickened and poorly demarkated from the medullary portion. The ureter is congested, edematous and somewhat enlarged. Left kidney—weight 90 grams. The surface is indefinitely lobulated. The color is bright red and the consistency is very soft, almost cystic. The capsule strips with slight difficulty and exposes a light red, finely granular surface. On section the kidney substance is greatly thinned, due to the dilatation of the pelvis, and measures only 4 to 6 mm. in thickness. The cortical and medullary portions cannot be distinguished. The ureter is dilated and the walls greatly thinned in its upper two-thirds, but the lower third is constricted and near the bladder entrance is cord-like with no demonstrable lumen.

Genito-urinary Organs. The vagina contains gauze soaked in a yellowish-brown fluid. The vaginal walls are ragged and necrotic. The finger may be passed from the vagina directly into the bladder through an opening 3 cm. in diameter. By directing the finger posteriorly it may also be passed between the bladder and the uterus and directly into the peritoneal cavity. From this point the peritonitis apparently originated. The walls of the bladder are greatly thickened, measuring $1\frac{1}{2}$ cm., and the mucous lining is coated over with a foul-smelling brownish-red necrotic layer. The cervix has largely sloughed away and presents a ragged necrotic surface. A probe may be passed within the uterine cavity for a distance of $3\frac{1}{2}$ cm. The uterus measures $4\frac{1}{2}$ cm. in length, 7 cm. laterally and 5 cm. antero-posteriorly. The walls are $1\frac{1}{2}$ cm. in thickness. On section of the uterus and bladder a sharp line of demarcation exists between the necrotic tissue adjacent to the vagina and the living tissue above. Along the iliac vessels are numerous large and small indurated glands, some of them measuring $1\frac{1}{2}$ cm. in diameter.

Microscopic. Liver. The liver shows a condition of marked passive congestion and a mild chronic biliary cirrhosis as manifested by the presence of round cells and a moderate fibrosis about the bile ducts.

Spleen. There is some thickening of the capsule and a moderate increase in the fibrous trabeculæ, but the most striking feature is the intense congestion. The erythrocytes are in places so numerous as largely to obscure the normal pulp. The number of polynuclear leukocytes is considerably increased.

Right Kidney. The cortex is swollen and the glomeruli relatively diminished. The convoluted tubules are slightly dilated. The cells are swollen, finely granular and the nuclei stain poorly. Scattered throughout are small abscesses with hemorrhagic borders. The centres are filled with pus cells and numerous short gram negative bacilli. These abscesses are diffusely distributed throughout all parts of the kidney but are especially numerous in the cortex and apparently have had a hematogenous origin. There is marked general congestion and edema.

Left Kidney. The cortex is greatly thinned and the

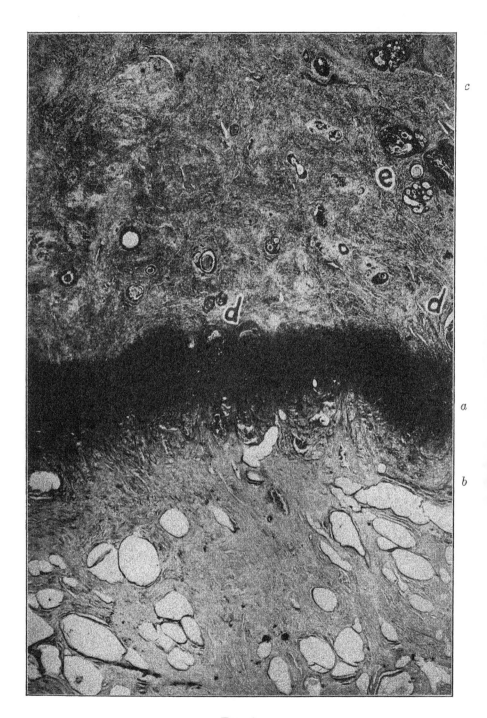

FIG. 1

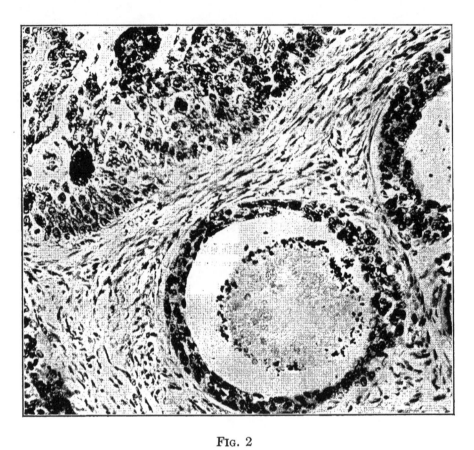

FIG. 2

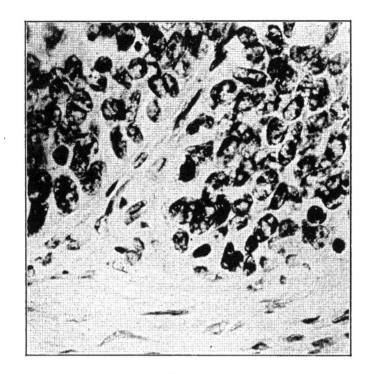

Fig. 3

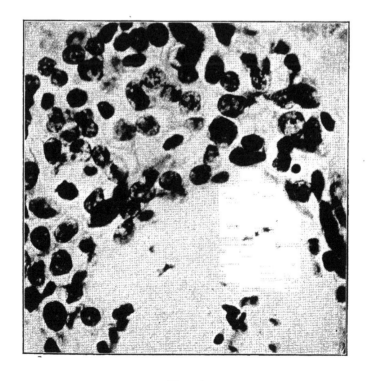

Fig. 4

glomeruli pressed together; many of them are hyaline. There is a diffuse fibrosis which increases as the pelvis is approached and encroaches extensively upon the tubules so that their number is greatly diminished. Lining the pelvis is a thick layer of old dense connective tissue through which very few if any collecting ducts pass. Scattered throughout are accumulations of round cells.

Bladder. A section passing upward from the vagina reveals a layer of necrotic tissue below, which is sharply demarkated from the living tissue above. Extending beyond this area of necrosis, however, is a diffuse fibrosis with numerous giant cells scattered through it, suggesting that a previous injury had produced such an effect. The epithelial lining has been largely denuded and there is in its stead a congested hemorrhagic granulation tissue. The submucosa is fibrosed and to a less extent the entire muscular wall. Smears and cultures from pus in the anterior cul-de-sac yields numerous colon bacilli.

Uterus. A section passing upward from the cervix reveals a necrotic layer which extends upward into the muscular walls of the uterus. Beyond this the tissue does not appear to be affected and well beyond the area of necrosis are nests of cancer cells, which, judging from the presence of mitotic figures, are still actively proliferating. There does not appear to have been any specific selective action upon the neoplastic growth.

Iliac Glands: Many of these glands are extensively invaded with cancer cells which present no evidence of degeneration.

ANATOMICAL AND MICROSCOPIC DIAGNOSIS

Immediate Cause of Death. Pelvic peritonitis, metastatic perisplenic abscess and multiple abscesses of right kidney.

Other and Contributing Factors. Carcinoma of uterus with extensive secondary metastasis of pelvic glands.

Sloughing of vaginal walls and subjacent portion of bladder and lower third of uterus.

Old calcified tubercles of apex of left lung.

Marked congestion and mild biliary cirrhosis of liver.

Marked congestion and leukocytic infiltration of spleen.

Hydronephrosis with atrophy of left kidney.

(Signed) R. M. TAYLOR.

Supplementary. Microscopic. The entire uterine wall with the exception of a small part of the fundus is invaded with carcinoma. This invasion is more extensive near the cervix and gradually becomes less as the fundus is approached. The process has evidently spread upward from below and has affected the entire thickness of the wall from the endometrium to the serosa. The neoplastic cells are irregularly arranged in large and small nests but sometimes occur singly or in rows. Some of the larger nests have broken down in the centre but the cells about the periphery appear to be living and actively proliferating. In some places there is a slight tendency toward a tubular or glandular arrangement, but for the most part this is not manifested. The general type of cell is large, though varying considerably in size, with a round or oval deeply staining nucleus and a relatively small amount of vacuolated cytoplasm. There is considerable fibrosis which bears a definite relation to the neoplastic invasion and has evidently resulted from the stimulus of the tumor cells. Bloodvessels are moderately numerous and are engorged with blood.

At the lower border of the uterus there is a distinct blue band passing across it (*a*, Fig. 1) which fades into the diffuse pink-staining necrotic tissue below (*b*). Above is a narrow hemorrhagic zone with numerous inflammatory, fragmenting and seminecrotic cells scattered through it. One may therefore start from below in the entirely necrotic tissue and by passing upward encounter cells in all degrees of degeneration until the apparently uninjured tissue (*c*) is reached.

The first intact cells to be met with are the mononuclear and polymorphonuclear inflammatory cells which undoubtedly have accumulated since the injury; the next are the connective-tissue cells. No tumor cells can be recognized in this seminecrotic zone. At several places (*d*) the zone passes directly through a nest of tumor cells; these cells appear to have been completely destroyed and only a mass of cellular detritus remains, while the connective tissue on either side and at the same level does not seem to be so severely affected as there still remain a few normal-appearing nuclei, yet the majority show evidence of fragmentation. A little farther inward this difference is entirely lost and the tumor cells show no morphological effect of injury and are evidently proliferating, as manifested by the presence of mitotic figures. Apparently unaffected cancer nests are found within 1 mm. of the necrotic portion.

In Fig. 2 is shown a higher magnification of some such nests, which are represented in Fig. 1 at (*e*) and are 3 mm. from the line of demarkation between the living and dead tissue. These cells present no morphological evidence of a degenerative change and many of them, especially those near the periphery of the nests, are in the process of division. Figs. 3 and 4 which are a higher mangification of selected fields from the same cell group show cells in the process of mitosis.

We come now to the practical part of the argument as revealed by the pathologic report. And in this instance the proverb that "one swallow does not make summer" does not hold good. Here we have one carefully studied case, with consideration of the therapeutic measures adopted, and it does show us definitely what we may expect. The results of Dr. Percy's experimentation fall to the ground, since his work was done on dead tissue (beef), and our deduction rests upon the action of heat on living tissue. We show with incontrovertible positiveness the fallacy of believing that the effect of heat applied in low degrees (so low that desiccation only takes place) and kept in contract with the tissue upon which its detrimental action on cell growth should be exerted over a long period of time extends for any considerable distance beyond the surface to which the cautery is applied; nor can it exert its destroying effect upon deeper seated cancer cells. This extensive action of heat, we must remember, was the belief that we entertained, and because of this some—particularly Byrne—held that cancer was actually cured by heat, even when past the stage of a radical operability (and this is the salient claim for Percy's technic). I too believed in the correctness of much deeper destruction of cancer cells than the vicinity of the cauterized surface, until this autopsy proved my misconception. I will say, however, that I at no time believed that any case of cancer of the uterus, if the disease had advanced a considerable distance into the parametria, or if the pelvic glands had become invaded by cancer cells, could be cured by heat treatment, despite the assertions of others of this possibility.

I did not believe it, because I have seen a large number of patients with advanced uterine cancer for whom I used the cautery treatment, and I have never seen a single instance actually cured. If this were possible, I should have seen, at least now and then, a cure. But they all died in the course of time, though they were made comparatively comfortable, and their life was, at least in my opinion, prolonged, particularly those in advanced years.

In the case of the patient whom I am considering, we had an instance in which a comparatively low degree of heat was used—at no time sufficiently intense to cause carbonization but just on the borderline—and its action was continued for two and one-half hours—a most trying procedure for the operator. And yet, directly beyond the "A" zone (see illustration) we meet with actively proliferating cancer cells. Only quite near, immediately in contact with the "A" zone, the cells appear destroyed. Particular attention is called to the unchanged condition of the carcinomatous iliac glands.

This one case alone gives us positive evidence that the actual cautery therapy has only superficial destructive ability on cancer cells, even when used as long as two and a half hours, and without carbonization. And on this the main stress is laid by Dr. Percy and others. It also verifies beyond a scintilla of doubt the statement made by me on several occasions that in my opinion the higher degree of heat will give precisely as satisfactory therapeutic results, despite the carbonization, as the lower degrees. In fact, one may destroy deeper and more rapidly with it; hence, it is superior to use for first cauterization.

The only valid objection to high degrees of heat that I can see is the smoke and the odor that occur during the operation. But this is of negligible significance. An essential advantage, nevertheless, is: One may finish a cautery operation in twenty minutes. But the greatest advantage is: One can practically strip the uterine and cervical structure so as to leave behind, as Byrne aptly called it, "only a shell of the uterus."

I had, before using the technic advocated by Percy, turned on enough current to bring the large dome platinum electrode up to white heat when taking off the tissue for the purpose of examining the parts before reapplying, and for the purpose of burning off the coating of carbon collected on the electrode. Practical experience has never shown any undesirable effect from this procedure. And after all, it is clinical experience that gives the decisive voice. But when applied to the tissues the electrode does not become so heated; the heat imparts then, as is evidenced by inspection, only a dark-to-light-red color to the electrode. But this does not become lessened so long as the current is kept on, and that is what I want for quick destructive work.

After the electrode has probably caused a fairly thick layer of carbonization structure, I raise the heat to a higher degree, so that it becomes a light red, the dark red having been used in the beginning.

Unquestionably this technic requires more skill and better judgment, but it is also more interesting and less monotonous than the slow desiccation process.

The making of manual examinations at intervals, to determine how much has been burnt out, are essential.

To Percy, however, much credit is due in connection with the cautery operation for uterine cancer—so much, indeed, that it cannot be overestimated—namely: To have the abdomen open during the operation, which is, from my point of view, more essential with the high heat advocated by me, than by his technic. Moreover, the necessity of having a thoroughly competent associate's hand in the abdomen, to control the vaginal operator's work. Because of the rapidity of the process, the abdominal assistant's work does not become monotonous either. He is constantly on the *qui vive*. I have occasionally controlled the electrode myself with my left hand, an assistant aiding my guidance from below. This is really the most satisfactory method, since an assistant's hand in the abdomen can never so accurately gauge what the operator wishes to accomplish, as can the operator's own hand.

The ligation of the internal iliac arteries is also a good intervention. This was first suggested and practised by the late Dr. Pryor, as a means of alleviating the bleeding and discharge as the result of advanced uterine cancer. It has been done a number of times by myself and others, particularly by Bainbridge in his blocking operation, for this purpose. The same is true for oöphorectomy. Dr. Percy did well to call attention to these procedures. And, then, too, the improvement that Percy made on the cooling specula devised by me is not to be underestimated. The speculum used by myself is illustrated as his No. 7, on page 305, *American Journal of Obstetrics*, August, 1, 1915. There are two lengths of my specula, and they have the advantage of a cock on the outflow tube, to regulate the rapidity of the flow of water, and always keeping the speculum vacuum filled.

While I would not like to work without my specula, the shorter and larger diameter specula of Percy are of great value in most cases (multipara, when the vagina is large and roomy). With cooling specula, there is not the slightest danger of ever injuring structures in the vagina or the vulva, not intended to be destroyed.

Danger of the structure being injured by high degrees of heat—as the bladder, rectum and ureters—is always present when the electrode is in the hands of one not accustomed to such work; but in the hands of a competent man, the risk is very slight, especially when the rule of removing the cautery-point for the making of examinations is followed and a competent observer has his hand in the abdomen. That the lower degrees of heat are likewise risky in this respect is shown by the result of our autopsy

It takes from one to two weeks for the separation and throwing off of the charred eschar. Then more or less bloody oozing begins to manifest itself from the raw surface. Acetone, applied as advised by Dr. George Gellhorn, overcomes this. Or one may use a strip of styptic gauze to pack the cavity.

But better still when the eschar has been separated completely—indeed, the ideal finishing treatment with heat is this: The desiccation of the cavity with low heat, without, however, the reopening of the abdomen, since the application of the low heat need not be employed longer than about twenty minutes, to bring about satisfactory desiccation. Although I have reopened the abdomen to do the secondary dessication, I do not find it imperative in the average case. One must not use force in applying the electrode then, because, if the main operation has been thoroughly done, the walls of the uterine shell are thin. I prefer this finishing operation to anything else and invariably employ it, if I may do so.

While the therapeutic value of radium in the treatment of cancer may be doubted by many, still there is so much evidence from men, both here and abroad whose judgment cannot be doubted, testifying to its curative effect, that it is my belief that more or less benefit may be obtained in some cases. Personally I have never seen more than temporary benefit. This, however, was in the instances in which I used radium alone.

It is for this reason that I would add the use of radium as an additional therapeutic agent after the final treatment— the dessication treatment—has been given. I commend it particularly since it can do no harm if properly used, and it may be of much benefit.

One may use 75 milligrams of radium, twenty-four successive hours through a filter, placed in a rubber capsule, the capsule being placed directly in the burnt-out cervico- uterine cavity, held in place by gauze packing, and left in twenty-four hours without seeing burns caused. I believe therefore that it is safe to leave it so long.

One word of precaution. Since my experience with a secondary fatal hemorrhage, I do not allow these patients to leave constant supervision until after the carbonized or charred eschar has been thrown off and when I feel confident that there is no further danger of secondary hemorrhage. They may be up and about as much and as soon as they wish after the operation. In fact, I encourage them to be out of bed to get fresh air, so as not to make them bed- invalids.

It must be obvious then that high heat and low heat should be used to bring about the best results obtainable from the heat treatment for uterine cancer that is too far advanced for radical operation.

To the late John Byrne, of Brooklyn, all credit is due for bringing the actual cautery treatment to our attention. To Percy is due the credit for enabling us to use heat more thoroughly and with greater safety, by calling our attention to the opening of the abdomen and having one competent to guide our work with his hand in the abdomen. And to

Pryor is due the credit of advising the ligation of the internal iliac arteries in cancer of the uterus to arrest hemorrhage and discharge, when too far advanced to do a hysterectomy.

DISCUSSION

DR. THOMAS S. CULLEN, Baltimore, Md.—Dr. Boldt has asked me to say a few words on this subject inasmuch as I had the opportunity of reading his paper before he presented it. He struck the key-note when he said that Dr. Percy had given us a good instrument, so that the chance of burning healthy tissue is reduced to the minimum; but he has shown us at the same time that he personally deserves priority for the adoption of this procedure which has been amplified by Dr. Percy.

Dr. Boldt has told us he has never seen thickening of the parametrial tissue diminish by heat. I have. In those cases where we used heat to get rid of the sloughing area of the growth we were amazed to see the apparently inoperable growth contract down until we could move it from side to side. This was not due entirely to diminution in the cancer but in a large measure to the getting rid of the suppurating area. The tissues assumed a more healthy character and the inflammation gradually drained out just as takes place where a carbuncle exists. We found after the use of acetone or the employing of formalin an edema of the broad ligament and the tissues became more friable.

Personally I do not know anything about radium from practical experience, and a good many practitioners are skeptical about its value; but there is no doubt that radium in inoperable cases of cancer does a lot of good. Both Dr. Kelly and Dr. Burnam have been devoting a great deal of attention to the treatment of cancer with radium and are most enthusiastic about what has been accomplished by it.

Sometime ago a case of far-advanced cancer of the cervix came under observation. The cervix was fixed on both sides and radical operation was out of the question. Dr. Burnam gave her two applications of radium and several months later I was able to satisfactorily remove this uterus which still presented a sloughing condition. I took sections from various portions of the cervix. The surface of the growth and the underlying tissue for at least 1 cm. showed coagulation necrosis. External to this there was some necrosis, but typical nests of squamous-cell carcinoma were still in evidence and in a fair state of preservation. The necrosis in the epithelium was noted farther out in the tissue than in the stroma; in other words the radium had affected the epithelium more than it had the stroma.

Dr. J. WESLEY BOVÉE, Washington, D. C.—I have been working for several years in galvanocauterization of the cervix for cancer, and, like Dr. Boldt, I devised a water-cooled speculum for this purpose, not as large and perhaps not as satisfactory as that of Dr. Percy.

I rise more particularly to speak of the fallacy connected with the suggestion of ligation of the internal iliacs in cutting off the blood supply. Since 1898, in my radical operations, I have been ligating the internal iliacs with the ovarian vessels, and I have never operated on a case yet in which I did not have to contend very vigorously with the bleeding which came from the branches of the inferior hemorrhoidals. If you cut off the internal iliacs, you still leave the ovarian vessels above which they connect with the hemorrhoidal vessels, and you get a blood supply as though you did not ligate the internal iliacs. One should be very particular to cut off the blood supply in various directions. I have felt I was not doing sufficient in cutting off the blood supply to these structures except by ligating the internal iliacs and the ovarians, and then, perhaps by galvano-cautery, cutting off the branches in the lateral walls of the vagina that came up from the inferior hemorrhoidal.

I am very much pleased with the work Dr. Boldt has been showing us, and particularly with what Dr. Cullen has been telling us about the failure of these agents reaching to any great depth; and I myself do not quite understand how we can expect to do away with cancer that surrounds the lower portion of the ureter by these methods without destroying the ureter and getting a ureterovaginal fistula. They speak of doing this work in such a way as not to injure the urinary or intestinal tract. An explanation of that would be very satisfactory to me.

Dr. CHARLES H. MAYO, Rochester, Minnesota.—Cancer of the uterus may be divided into cancer of the body of the uterus, which is the one for surgery without heat, and cancer of the neck of the uterus. The heat method now so much discussed can be applied to the treatment of cancer of the cervix. Our method for many years in the early cases of cancer of the cervix has been hysterectomy. For the late cases of fungating growths filling the upper vaginal vault and fixing the uterus we have resorted to the use of heat. The question is, how much heat does it take to destroy cancer cells—that is, if it is a cell—or some stimulus connected with the development of cancer, or if it is bacterial.

The experimental work on the transplantation of mouse cancer shows that much lower degrees of heat applied to the transplants when moved from mouse to mouse will absolutely prevent grafts from taking effect. This brings up the possibility that we may yet discover some bacterial cause for the development of cancer cells.

We have occasionally operated on a late case in which the upper vaginal vault was involved in the fungating mass, with advanced pelvic involvement, and after using the cautery have written the family physician that the case was too far advanced for hysterectomy. But we dealt with the local condition and have advised (after Findley) the local use of acetone to stop hemorrhage.

We have operated on 70 patients with the Percy method. In 20 the uterus was removed later. A number were palliative operations. In 20 patients who were later subjected to hysterectomy a specimen was secured from the cervix, for the laboratory, and then the slow burning was continued. In 16 of these no trace of the disease was found in the uterus after the hysterectomy. With rapid application of heat, such as with a hot knife or wire, we do not seemingly get as good results. Carbon is the best non-conductor we can get. It must be scraped from the heater often. If enough heat is applied good results will be obtained. What one wants is a broiling penetration. To avoid secondary hemorrhages, ligate the internal iliacs as Clark has done and one or both ovarian arteries. In the first six cases we applied heat for thirty-nine minutes, then brought it up to forty-eight minutes as an average, and now it is sixty minutes. It is the slow application of heat to the uterus held in the gloved hand that produces the results. If you keep up this broiling penetration the same as is experimentally shown in the transplantation of mouse cancer one will get results. If it is done too rapidly one may as well use some other method. In two of our cases treated by the Percy method a violent spreading caused cracks in the vagina which became inoculated with cancer. This is preventable.

Dr. J. SHELTON HORSLEY, Richmond, Virginia.—With the possible benefits which may be derived from the Percy cauterization method the possibility of vaccination may come in with some of the cures by the Percy cautery method. The results of the biological treatment of cancer are certainly not brilliant. Serums have failed, but there have been a few cases quoted in the literature, as adenocarcinoma of the uterus, that have been apparently cured after vaccine treatment. In this zone in which all tissues are not entirely destroyed, but in which cancer cells are attenuated, it is quite possible that in this zone the attenuated cancer cells may act as an autogenous vaccine and be of some benefit, independent of the tissues that have been entirely destroyed.

Dr. ALEXIUS McGLANNAN, Baltimore.—The most important lesson to be drawn from this paper and discussion is that we should be very careful in drawing conclusions as to the methods of curing cancer. As far as our knowledge at the present time goes, we believe that a wide operation in early cases brings about a cure in most instances, and all the palliative methods, those other than a wide operation in the early stage, are likely to end in failure. The occasional cures reported are either accidents or are cases in which the end-results have not been followed or in which the patients have not lived long enough to show the ordinary final results.

Dr. HENRY T. BYFORD, Chicago.—Dr. Mayo has clinched the question by saying heat will cure cancer. It depends, however, upon two things: whether cancer is due to the cell action or to germs. Cancer cells can be destroyed by low degrees of heat. It is probable that the germs can stand as much heat as the tissues in which they develop. It is also probable that the germs get beyond these so-called cancer cells that are already deficient in vitality, and one has to destroy the normal tissue about them.

Another thing is, in different parts of the tissues there are variations in the circulation. In the more vascular areas heat does not penetrate quite the same as in the less vascular areas, and it is impossible to depend upon its action beyond the necrotic zone. Hence, I do not think we are going to be able with the heat method to develop an actual cure of cancer. It remains a cautery.

Dr. CHARLES R. ROBINS. Richmond, Virginia.—I got the Percy habit at the Mayos, and I must say that the idea of thorough action by the Percy cautery appealed to me very strongly, and after I began to use it I adopted the procedure of removing a piece of tissue and having a microscopic examination made before the operation, and then having a microscopic examination made after the application of the cautery; and in those cases that have not been too far advanced the report has come back that there was an absence of cancer cells in the uterus after the application of the heat. For that reason I have adopted the use of the Percy cautery as a routine measure in all cases of cancer, whether they are primarily operable or not, because I believe that the destruction of the cancer cell before a radical operation would be a safeguard to the patient.

I do not recall how many Wertheims I have done in the last two years—it is probably eight— but of the cases that were cauterized, I have not at the present time had any evidences of any recurrence whatsoever. Some of the cases were what we call border-line cases where there was a slight infiltration of the broad ligament.

One of the greatest fields of usefulness for the Percy cautery is to cauterize the cases we expect to operate on anyway.

The microscopic examination was made by a competent man in each of my cases, and there were no cancer cells remaining in the uterus.

Dr. J. Wesley Bovée, Washington, D. C.—There has been a great deal of stress laid in this discussion on the presence or absence of cancer cells in the uterus. They do not give us trouble. It is the cells outside of the uterus that cause trouble. If cancer cells in the uterus alone should bother us, we would have only to do a hysterectomy. Therefore, it is the cancer cells in the higher lymphatic chains that give us the trouble, and demand the radical procedures in vogue.

Dr. C. Jeff. Miller, New Orleans, Louisiana.—I have used the cautery in a large number of cases of cancer of the uterus and have observed a number of cases in which the Percy cauterization method has been applied, and during the past nineteen months I have used radium in advanced cases of cancer of the cervix, and can speak for my results in 26 cases of inoperable carcinoma treated up to the first day of December, 1915. I believe that radium offers the best results in advanced carcinoma of the cervix than any other method I have heretofore used. If the ultimate results of radium should ever prove to be as good as the primary results, then radium offers the best treatment for advanced carcinoma.

Of 26 cases, 6 are apparently well. All were advanced to such an extent that operation was out of the question. These patients are free from pain and the parametrium appears to be free from any disease. A large number of the rest of the series were markedly improved from four to eight and twelve months, but several of them now show evidence of returning trouble.

Hemorrhage is a very common and troublesome accompaniment of advanced carcinoma. The effect of radium in these cases is uniformly good. In only one instance have I failed to check bleeding. Moreover, sepsis promptly subsides and the vaginal vault appears to heal without contraction or marked evidence of scar tissue.

Three patients died within three months after treatment. The longest time that has elapsed in the favorable cases was eighteen months. The first case treated is still well and enjoying good health.

If cancer could be confined to the uterus, I believe radium would cure the majority of them, but, unfortunately, radium may not reach cancer nests far out in the parametrium or in the iliac glands, and these patients after improving for months or years will show a recurrence. As Dr. Bovée has said: "It is not the cancer cell in the uterus that gives trouble, but the metastases to remote areas." Within the radius of the uterus and the parametrium, radium exerts an immediate effect which is decidedly better than cautery or hysterectomy in advanced cases, and I believe the permanent effect will prove to be as good as from Percy cautery or hysterectomy in so-called borderline cases. It can be used without causing pain, there is no necessity for an anesthetic, and the sepsis is as promptly controlled as hemorrhage.

I may mention one case that entered the hospital with a hemoglobin percentage as low as 16 per cent. and had been having a temperature ranging from 99° to 101° F. for six weeks. I do not believe that even an anesthetic would be safe in this case, to say nothing of the effects of cautery. The patient gained 19 pounds in two months, is free from pain, and there is no evidence of the cancer mass left about the cervix.

If radium produces such marked changes in the hopeless cases, it shows that it has a wide field of usefulness in cancer of the cervix.

DR. W. P. CARR, Washington, D. C.—I want to call attention to the fact that there is a very great difference in cancers.

Some of them are very much more amenable to heat, to radium, and the *x*-ray than others.

I have, for instance, sent two cases to Dr. Burnam for treatment of inoperable cancer of the uterus. One of them was apparently cured and has been well for four years. The other one was not benefited in the slightest degree, although she had just as much treatment, and was apparently a similar case.

While the average penetration of radium is only 1 or 2 or 3 mm., there are cases in which it penetrates much deeper, and in some cases of sarcoma of bone it will penetrate very large tumors and cure them absolutely. The same variations follow *x*-ray treatment of cancers.

I had occasion to remove both breasts for cancer not long ago in a case that had been thoroughly treated with the Coolidge tube, and sections of the tumor showed that nearly every cell in both breasts had been destroyed. Cells in the breast were in a state of coagulation necrosis, clear through the thickness of three inches. In some cases the radium or *x*-ray does penetrate very much more than in others. The same thing may apply to heat, and from the varied experience and conflicting testimony we get from men who use it, that must be the case. In some cases it is more effective than in others.

Dr. HERMAN J. BOLDT, New York City (closing).—I am very grateful for the free and liberal discussion that my paper has received. It shows that this subject is still of interest to everybody. I regret very much that Dr. Percy was not here to take part in this discussion. I had requested him to do so, and sent him a copy of my paper which would enable him to know exactly what was going to be said by myself.

I think this work should be carried on further, if there is anyone intersted in the treatment of cancer, by heat by animal experimentation.

I am sorry Dr. Cullen left the hall, because he misunderstood me if he was under the impression I said that the parametria did not become diminished in thickening. The thickening of the parametrium close to the uterus does become diminished, but the infiltrated parametria do not become diminished appreciably much beyond the area where the heat is applied. The thickening becomes lessened only to the extent that we can reduce the edema by the penetration of heat.

Dr. CULLEN.—That is, you have fixation, you have plenty of room all around afterward?

DR. BOLDT.—Any kind of heat will do that, slight or low degrees of heat.

DR. CULLEN.—By the treatment you have gotten rid of the sloughing area; you have diminished the amount of absorption, and you have relieved the indurated and inflammatory area.

DR. BOLDT.—I think I mentioned that in my paper.

Dr. Bovée is perfectly right in saying that ligation of the internal iliac arteries is not sufficient. Dr. Bainbridge brought that out in connection with blocking in ligating the internal iliacs and ovarian vessels. It is a good preliminary measure if there is going to be an extensive operation.

With regard to what Dr. Mayo said about cancer being cured by heat, I grant that if the carcinomatous elements are superficial, so far as the effect of the nearby action of the heat will affect them, we may bring about a cure, but it is incomprehensible that we can possibly get heat to kill carcinoma cells when in one instance it was proved that at a distance of 3 mm. away from where the cautery was placed we had still living carcinoma cells. Can we not expect them in the parametria? It is a physical impossibility to determine why we have them in one case and why we do not have them in another case.

Dr. Mayo has told us that in some 16 cases there were no evidences of carcinoma cells present after the cauterization treatment. There is only one conclusion to be drawn from that statement, namely, that the *carcinoma* cells were superficial. It could not be in one class of cases that cancer cells were destroyed, whereas in the other class they were not destroyed. A good deal depends upon the depth of penetration and the invasion of the carcinoma cells. The subject requires much more study.

What we have tried to do is to get at the truth; I do not care whose method it is or who is entitled to priority. However, I maintain that great credit is due to Dr. Byrne, of Brooklyn, who first called attention to the method some thirty-five or forty years ago.

Dr. Robins said he always uses heat as a method preliminary to performing a radical operation. It does not seem to me that is exactly the point. If a case is suitable for a radical operation, why not go ahead and do it. I admit it is hard to decide when to do a radical operation in the case of a uterus that is not freely movable and when we have other methods of treatment at our command, such as radium and the x-ray. If the doctor can assure us that the uterus will become movable later as a result of preliminary treatment, I say go ahead, then, and do a radical operation.

I fully coincide with what Dr. Miller has said regarding the use of radium, and from the limited experience I have had with it, I will say that radium certainly does give decided temporary relief, so far as bleeding and pain are concerned; but in my experience that relief has not been permanent and that, sooner or later, patients are just in as serious a condition as they were before, or as though we had never used anything.

IMPLANTATION OF THE TRIGONUM INTO THE SEGREGATED LOWER END OF THE ILEUM

By Vilray P. Blair, A.M., M.D.

St. Louis, Missouri

THIS single case is reported partly because the operation proved a failure, in that the patient died, and partly because it was designed with the hope of overcoming two of the obstacles that have been encountered in the attempt to form a visceral receptacle for the urine in exstrophy of the bladder. The difficulties lie in preserving the blood supply to the trigonum and in protecting the kidneys. In regard to the former it succeeded but presumably failed in the latter.

The patient was a girl, aged six years. At examination the labia majora were found well formed posteriorly and separated widely anteriorly. There were two small "dog ears" on the anterior median part of the labia majora which somewhat resembled and were taken for the labia minora. Between the posterior parts of the labia majora was a transverse slit three millimeters wide with a somewhat fluted mucous lining. This was taken for the external opening of the vagina. The umbilicus was low. Below the umbilicus the recti muscles seemed to separate, leaving a hernial protrusion which extended from the umbilicus to the pubis and when the child cried, stood up about five centimeters. Most of this protrusion was covered with skin but its extreme lower part was red and apparently covered by mucous membrane; this patch was about two centimeters across. In this there were two small vertical slit openings, one millimeter long from which urine came in jets alternately. The left slit was at a higher level than the right. The diagnosis was exstrophy of the urinary bladder, complete absence of all bladder wall except the trigonum, deformity of the external genitals and absence of the lower end of the vagina.

The operation was done in two steps. The first consisted in dividing the ileum ten inches from the cecum, the cut end of the distal segment being closed by suture; the proximal part being implanted into the ascending colon. The idea was to use the ten-inch segment of the ileum for the urinary receptacle in the hope that the ileocaecal valve would protect the ureters from ascending infection. At the second operation this segment was found to be free from feces. There was some discussion at the time as to the propriety of turning the urine into the right half, the absorbing part of the colon, but there seemed to be no evil result from this.

The second stage of the operation was done three months later, when the trigone was free from the abdominal wall and left attached to a triangular flap of peritoneum attached below and containing a ureter at each border. The blood supply was so free that many ligatures had to be applied after the trigone was freely mobilized. No difficulty was encountered in making a lateral implantation into the lower segment of the ileum. It was also possible to cover the site of implantation and the raw surface of the peritoneal flap, carrying the ureters, with parietal peritoneum even down to the triangular ligament which was developed into a thick ligamentous band that replaced the symphisis pubis. There was no subsequent urinary leakage.

A third operation, viz., the strengthening of the wall at the site of the hernia by the transplantation of fascia lata had been contemplated for a later date.

The child apparently did well for a year, holding its urine all night and during the day passing it about each two hours with plenty of warning. They lived at a distance and only one specimen of urine was obtained, which was six months after the implantation. Examination showed a specific gravity of 1016, alkaline, some albumin, no sugar and no casts. The child at this time was in excellent health. About one year after the second operation the child became sick, lost weight, and had a waxy color. When seen two months later she looked bad and complained of a great deal of cramping pain in the lower abdomen, which suggested that a urinary calculi might have formed in the new urinary bladder. An x-ray picture could not be made without an anesthetic, and a request to come to the hospital was deferred. The blood at this time showed a slight leukocytosis and 77 per cent. polymorphonuclear cells. About one month later the child died; no autopsy was performed, but the attending physician reported death due to uremia.

REPORT OF A CASE OF EXSTROPHY OF THE BLADDER OPERATED ON NEARLY THIRTY YEARS AGO; WITH SUBSEQUENT HISTORY

By Randolph Winslow, M.D.
Baltimore, Maryland

In May, 1886, Georgie T., a white female child, aged six years, was brought to the Hospital of the Good Samaritan, Baltimore, by Dr. Samuel T. Earle, who placed her under my care. She was a small, but well nourished and very intelligent child, who was in a deplorable condition. In addition to a large congenital prolapse of the rectum, she was suffering from exstrophy of the bladder, the opening being 2½ x 2 inches in diameter and trefoil in shape. The exposed mucous membrane was red, vascular, and bleeding; covered with mucus, ammoniacal and offensive in odor. There was constant dribbling of urine and her skin and clothing were always wet. The pelvic bones were widely separated and her gait was awkward and waddling. No hernia was present in either groin. There was no urethra but only a shallow groove where the urethra should have been. The labia were separated from each other and the clitoris was not seen. The vagina was apparently present but nothing was determined in regard to the uterus and ovaries. The umbilicus was absent. Her appetite was good. Dr. Earle operated on the prolapsed rectum with the thermocautery, and subsequently he narrowed the anal orifice, eventually curing her of this malady.

On June 1, 1886, I performed a modified Wood's plastic operation for the relief of the exstrophy. An umbilical flap was turned down with its raw surface outward and two small flaps were turned up from the vulva and sutured to the lower edge of the umbilical flap, leaving a small opening at the lower margin for the escape of urine. Two lateral abdominal flaps of considerable size were raised and twisted with their raw surfaces inward so as to cover the other flaps, and their margins were sutured in the middle line. Catgut sutures were used for holding the raw surfaces together and sublimated silk for the external wounds. A large portion of the extensive raw surface of the abdomen was closed with sutures, leaving only a narrow uncovered strip to be healed by granulation. The umbilical flap consisted of very thin skin and but little subcutaneous tissue, while the lateral flaps were pretty thick and vascular. The surfaces were dusted with iodoform and covered with gauze and absorbent cotton. The patient was considerably shocked but rallied easily and she suffered little or no pain subsequently. The urine escaped freely from the small opening between the flaps. For several days her temperature remained nearly normal but on the third day febrile symptoms began to set in and an examination showed the wound to be in good condition, but an erysipelas ambulans was discovered traveling upward from the buttocks toward the flaps. On the fifth day the erysipelas reached the flaps but was fortunately very superficial in character and did not cause much disaster. A strip of the left flap about one-half to three-quarters of an inch in width along its middle and lower edges sloughed and left a gap to be healed by granulation. This gap was materially lessened by the use of deep silver wire sutures shotted on lead plates. Healing of all wound surfaces was accomplished in about six weeks.

The condition of the child was vastly improved but there was, of course, no continence of urine. It was possible, however, to keep her drier, more comfortable and less offensive to her neighbors. This was about as good a result as was attainable at that time; indeed, any other operation would have been well-nigh impossible on account of the marked prolapse of the rectum that was present. At the present day I think some other procedure should be employed in cases of exstrophy of the bladder, and I personally favor the implantation of the ureters with the trigone of the bladder into the sigmoid or rectum, the extirpation of the remainder of the bladder and the closure of the gap in the abdominal wall with sutures.

I have not though this case worthy of publication on account of the method of procedure employed or by reason of the success of the operation, but because of her subsequent history, of which I have only recently become cognizant. After remaining six months in the Samaritan Hospital, she was removed to Bay View Asylum, where I subsequently saw her upon several occasions; the last time probably in 1890, when she was ten years of age.

In Howard A. Kelly's *Operative Gynecology*, 1898, Vol. 1, p. 319, I find the following account evidently referring to the same girl. "In a case of a girl of fifteen (G. T., No. 3869, October 14, 1895), the pubic bones were separated 4 cm. with a thin sharp-edged fibrous band between them; above this there had been a total defect of the anterior bladder wall, covered by inverted flaps of skin taken from the sides and so adapted as to leave only a small orifice open just above the fibrous band, through which the urine escaped. By rectal examination, I found an infantile uterus and ovaries, and on making a cystoscopic examination between the flaps two little oval openings representing a double hymen were discovered on the posterior wall of the bladder; a sound passed them led up to the cervix uteri."

I lost sight of the girl and did not know what had become of her until January, 1914, when I received a letter from Dr. Charles B. Reynolds of Philadelphia in regard to her. She had been married some years and had been delivered of a child by Dr. Reynolds a short time previous to the date of his letter to me. This was her third child; the first having been born in November, 1901 following an instrumental delivery, according to her statement. The second child was delivered by podalic version in July, 1903, and was born dead. The mother was badly lacerated and had her injuries repaired at the Cambridge, Maryland, Hospital.

During the third labor in December, 1913, Dr. Reynolds saw her in consultation and finding her condition serious had her removed to the Medico-Chirurgical Hospital, where she was etherized and delivered of a large dead baby that presented by the breech. While she was in the hospital a skiagraph was taken of her pelvis which showed an absence of the symphisis pubis and a gap of three inches between the pubic bones. In commenting on her condition, Dr. Reynolds says, "She appears to be a strong and otherwise well developed woman and quite intelligent." She was sensitive about her malformation and disinclined to allow any examination of her genitalia.

In January, 1915, she was delivered by Dr. Reynolds of a fourth child, a girl weighing nine pounds, which was born alive. This was a shoulder presentation which was delivered by podalic version. Exstrophy occurs much less frequently in females than in males but the condition is none the less deplorable. In many cases both the external and internal organs of generation are malformed or undeveloped and the woman, if she lives to adult life, is usually incapable of bearing children.

The first fact, therefore, that makes this case noteworthy is that she has come to term four times within a few years. Secondly, the labors were all dystociæ; one child having been delivered with forceps and the others either by podalic version or by breech extraction.

When we consider the absence of the symphisis pubis and the wide separation of the pelvic girdle; the diastasis of the recti muscles and the weak condition of the lower abdominal

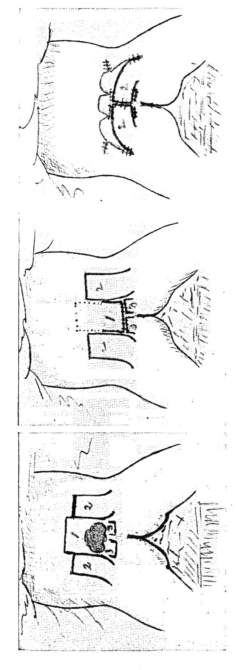

FIG. 1   FIG. 2   FIG. 3

FIG. 1.—Exstrophy of the bladder. Flaps outlined. 1, Umbilical flap; 2, lateral flaps; 3, labial flaps.

FIG. 2.—1, Umbilical flap reversed and united to reversed labial flaps 3, 3. The shaded portion indicates the raw surfaces of these flaps.

FIG. 3.—2, 2, Lateral flaps placed over the other flaps and united in the middle line. All the portions sutured. Shaded portion indicates the extent of denuded surface which could not be sutured and which healed by granulation in a few weeks.

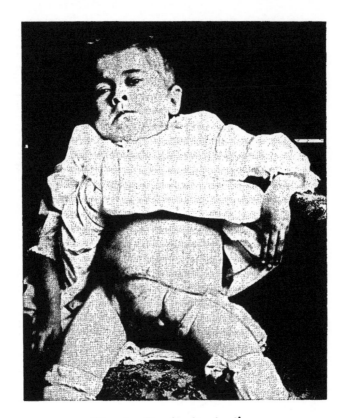

FIG. 4.—Result after healing.

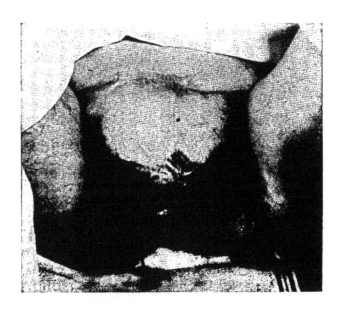

FIG. 5.—Condition of parts in December, 1915.

wall, it is not remarkable that she was unable to give birth to a child in the normal manner and that the deliveries were all abnormal.

I find it stated by Da Costa that only 30 per cent. of the victims of this malformation live beyond the twentieth year; it is therefore very gratifying to me to know that this woman, upon whom I operated twenty-nine and a half years ago, is still alive and in reasonably good health.

In a letter received from Dr. Reynolds on December 10, 1915, he says: "The woman is well nourished, intelligent, and is enjoying good health, though she has prolapsus uteri. She is able to perform her regular household duties satisfactorily."

DISCUSSION ON THE PAPERS OF DRS. BLAIR AND WINSLOW

Dr. Ernst Jonas, St. Louis, Missouri.—So far as the flap formation is concerned as recommended by Dr. Winslow, it is the usual flap formation which was done until recently in a great many cases of epispadias. I should like to ask Dr. Winslow if there was continuation of the growth of hair on the flap turned in with the skin surface toward the bladder. If I am informed correctly, that was one of the reasons why these operations for epispadias were given up. We used to read in the text-books that when the skin surface is turned toward the bladder, no hair formation takes place in later life, but that does not seem to be true in those cases that we have observed and on which we have operated.

Dr. William D. Haggard, Nashville, Tennessee.—I would like to relate a case of exstrophy of the bladder occurring in a woman, twenty-nine years of age, in whom I transferred the base of the bladder according to the Maydl method into the sigmoid, and at the end of a year the woman was quite well. She retained her urine three hours during the day and from four to six hours at night. She had absence of the vagina. The cervix-uteri presented between the gap of symphysis pubis two and a half or three inches apart, and looked exactly like a urethra. She also had no umbilicus. The Maydl operation, while tedious, was not as difficult as I anticipated, and the result was very satisfactory.

DR. RANDOLPH WINSLOW, Baltimore (closing).—I have not seen this woman for twenty-five years. I am under the impression that Dr. Cullen repaired her perineal injuries at the Cambridge (Maryland) Hospital, and I have been told, he said, there was hair growing in the bladder, but as to the accuracy of that statement I do not know. Do you remember that?

DR. CULLEN.—I did not operate on her. In the first place, I have never seen hair on the inside of the bladder, which proves conclusively there was no hair in that case, if I did do it. In the second place, I have never operated on a case with complete incontinence.

DR. WINSLOW.—Didn't you see this case?

DR. CULLEN.—I did not.

DR. WINSLOW.—In the first place, a woman is not likely to have hair on the skin of the epigastrium from which the large flap was made. The small flaps from the labia majora were sutured to the lower edge of other flaps; they did not go into her bladder. I do not believe she has had any stone in the bladder.

RESULTS OF OPERATIONS FOR EXOPHTHALMIC GOITRE

By E. S. JUDD, M.D.

AND

J. D. PEMBERTON, M.D.
Rochester, Minnesota

IN this review of cases of exophthalmic goitre, we have endeavored to ascertain as nearly as possible the results of operation for the condition. As is well known, it is difficult to determine when a condition of this kind is cured, and that some of the patients who are apparently cured may ultimately have relapses. In order that a sufficient length of time should have passed since operation, only the patients operated on in 1909 and in whom a definite diagnosis had been made were selected for this study.

In these cases the diagnosis of exophthalmic goitre was based on the clinical history and the histologic changes in the tissues when a part of the thyroid was removed. In a certain number no tissue was removed, ligation of the thyroid vessels only being done. In most instances, however, the thyroid was resected. The cases were all in the hyperplastic, toxic group, as described by Plummer and Wilson. (There was a definite so-called hypertrophy in all of the thyroids removed which was diagnosed by the clinician as exophthalmic goitre and by the pathologist as hyperplastic thyroid.)

Of the 176 patients in the series (operated on in 1909) we have been able to trace 121 by correspondence and subsequent examinations. A number of these have returned several times for examination, and many of them have reported by letter several times.

It has been our custom to ligate the superior thyroid vessels in two types of exophthalmic goitre cases. In one type the disease was mild and we hoped the procedure might be sufficient to effect a cure. In the other type the disease was severe and one or more ligations were done as a preliminary to resection. These patients were advised to return in three months for the removal of a part of the gland, but some of them were so greatly improved by the ligations that they did not return. Of the 121 patients that were traced, 56 were ligated; 36 had primary resections of the thyroid; 20 had preliminary ligations followed later by resections. Nine of these patients were operated on for recurrence at which time either one of the vessels was ligated or a part of the remaining piece of the thyroid was resected. The patients have been classified in five groups.

Group I. In this group there were 55 (45.4 per cent.) patients cured; *i. e.*, those who had been well for some time and as far as they knew, or as we could judge, were completely relieved of all their former symptoms. In 16 of the 55, primary resections had been done; in 11 resections following ligations, in 24 ligations alone; and in 4 secondary ligations or resections following resections. We believe that the preliminary ligations should nearly always be followed by thyroidectomy, and that when ligations alone are done, late recurrences are much more common. On a number of occasions we have done thyroidectomies for the recurrence of symptoms after patients had been well for more than five years following ligation. One patient in this group was well for more than five years after the ligation of both superior thyroid vessels; then all the symptoms of hyperthyroidism gradually returned and the gland was resected. The following histories are illustrative of the cases in this group:

A30233.—Mrs. A. M. B., aged twenty-seven years. Examination October 18, 1909. Acute symptoms of hyperthyroidism began about five and a half years before. Enlargement of the thyroid first noticed five years before. Six months before the appearance of the goitre she began to lose weight, was restless, irritable, and had slight tremor and general nervousness. Pulse, 60. Two weeks after the goitre appeared, there was a rather sudden onset of tachycardia with diarrhea. Pulse, 170. There had been nausea and vomiting and edema of the feet for six weeks. All the symptoms, except gastro-intestinal, had continued for two years. She was exhausted, unable to work and lost twenty pounds during this time. During the last three years there had been gradual improvement. At the time of examination the pulse was 130; there was dyspnea, exhaustion on exertion, and restlessness. Very little change in the size of the goitre, if anything a little smaller. She had some difficulty in swallowing. Electrical treatments had been given. The thyroid was firm, the right lobe larger than the left. Heart regular and not enlarged. Strength fair, and nutrition good. The exophthalmos which had existed for five years was quite marked, uneven, more noticeable on the right side.

On October 20, 1909, the right lobe and isthmus were extirpated. The pathologist reported hyperplastic thyroid. The patient had a normal convalescence and left the hospital in a few days. She was the wife of a physician and we were thus able to follow her condition accurately. One year after the operation only a slight trace of trouble remained. Four years later her husband reported that she was entirely well though the right eye was still a little more prominent than the left. At the present time she is entirely recovered and there is no evidence of her old trouble. In a letter she stated that it was about two years after the operation before she considered herself well. She now works with perfect ease. Her pulse is about 80. She has gained about ten pounds in weight. Her voice is clear. She is in fact in splendid health.

A29110.—Male, aged twenty-seven years. Dr. N. B. examined September 17, 1909. The goitre was first noticed two years before. Hyperthyroidism probably started at about the same time. A small nodule in the right lobe of the thyroid was first noted, since then, tachycardia and some loss in weight and strength. From that time palpitation, tachycardia, loss of weight has been variable. He had spells of diarrhea for two or three days at a time, sweating profusely. First noticed exophthalmos about six months before. Tremor was not noted until a few months before, since then symptoms gradually became more severe. The thyroid was rather soft, and the right lobe somewhat larger than the left. There was slight enlargement throughout the gland. Heart normal in size. Pulse 120, soft and slightly irregular. White blood count, 6320; total lymphocytes, 49 per cent. Operation September 20, 1909. Extirpation of the right lobe and isthmus. Pathologic report: Hyperplastic thyroid.

One year after the operation this patient reported that he was much improved, though there was still slight evidence of the old trouble. Six months after the operation he had had a relapse of the tachycardia, but this cleared up in a few months. He can now do as much work as he could before the beginning of his trouble. The exophthalmos has entirely disappeared. Present average pulse rate 85; normal weight before his trouble began was 150 pounds, present weight is 165 pounds. His voice was not affected by the condition.

A20797.—F. E. K., male, aged forty years. Examination March 2, 1909. The goitre was noticed nine months before, though there may have been some evidence of hyperthyroidism for two years. He had acute illness two years before which was called grip. He has been a little nervous for years, and thinks that his present trouble has been coming on gradually for several years. He had lost thirty pounds in weight and complained of weakness, nervousness, and dyspnea on exertion. There had been no vomiting nor diarrhea. Examination showed a hard gland, generally enlarged. No dilatation of the heart and no evidence of myocarditis. Pulse 120 to 130. Exophthalmos regular and quite marked. The first operation was done March 6, 1909, when the right lobe and isthmus were extirpated. After this he felt fairly well when resting. He grew stronger, less nervous, and gained ten pounds in weight immediately after the operation, but lost it after working two weeks. When he returned for examination October 22, 1909, his pulse was 120. During August and September he had about ten attacks of biliary colic, with diaphragmatic spasms, and was obliged to take morphin several times on account of pain. October 29, 1909, the left lobe was resected. The pathologic report on both pieces of tissue was hyperplastic thyroid.

This man reports that about eight months elapsed after his second operation before he considered himself entirely well, but he is as well as before he began to have the trouble. He can now do his work with ease. The prominence of his eyes has disappeared. He regained the thirty pounds in weight and now weighs 150 pounds. This patient has recently undergone a successful operation for gall-stones.

A26401.—A. M., female, aged sixteen years. Examination July 17, 1909. Goitre first noticed one and a half years before. She had been nervous for several years and had noticed tremor. There had been a gradual onset of symptoms of hyperthyroidism, tachycardia, dyspnea, palpitation, loss in weight, etc. Ten months before the symptoms had been severe and for several weeks she had been unable to be on her feet for any length of time. She had spells of diarrhea lasting three or four days at a time and several spells of nausea and vomiting. Exophthalmos for eleven months. The thyroid was enlarged; thrills distinct; the left lobe larger than the right. Heart dilated one and one-fourth inches to the left. Systolic murmur at the apex. Pulse rate 150 and full. White blood count, 8000; total lymphocytes, 42 per cent. Operation July 29, 1909; ligation of both superior thyroid arteries.

This patient writes that she is much stronger than at any time before she had the trouble. There has been no recurrence of symptoms and she can do more work than before. The prominence of her eyes has gradually diminished; the appearance of her neck is normal. Pulse 80; hands steady. She has not taken medicine since her operation. She thinks that about six months elapsed before she was entirely well.

A27574.—Mrs. A. O. M., aged thirty-four years. Examination August 1, 1909. This patient had a goitre at the age of eighteen which disappeared. Her mother had one at twenty and it disappeared. The second goitre was first noticed about a year ago. Symptoms of hyperthyroidism, tachycardia, nervousness, and enlargement of the thyroid, had persisted for about five months. There was an irregular nodular enlargement of the gland. Heart not dilated; pulse, 110 to 120. Some prominence of the eyes. White blood count, 9200; total lymphocytes, 47 per cent. Operation, August 18, 1909; ligation of the superior thyroid vessels. For more than two years after this, during which time she gave birth to a child, she felt well. In January, 1911, she returned, stating that for two months she had been having palpitation, dyspnea and nervousness, though not nearly as severe as before the ligation. She had lost seventeen pounds in these two months. On January 10, 1911, the right lobe and isthmus were removed. Pathologic report: hyperplastic thyroid.

She now reports that she is well. She thinks it was about six months after the second operation before she was entirely well. She had a few slight temporary attacks of palpitation and nervousness. The prominence of her eyes has diminished. Pulse 68. Normal weight before her first symptoms was 110; just previous to the thyroidectomy, 98; present weight, 124. She had no trouble with her voice. Her husband, who is a physician, writes that in his opinion she is as well now as before the beginning of her illness.

Group II. In this group of 22 patients (18.1 per cent.), all were practically cured of their symptoms but still at times had slight evidence of the disease. Many of these are entirely well, though occasionally under sudden nervous strain they show that they are not entirely normal. In this group there were 11 primary resections, 4 resections following ligations, 6 ligations and 1 secondary resection. Some of the case histories are given as typical of results in the group.

A27928.—Mrs. A. A., aged twenty-eight years. Examination, August 19, 1909. The goitre was first noticed two years before; the hyperthyroidism probably started five months before when the goitre rapidly increased in size. There was a sudden onset of typical hyperthyroidism, profuse sweating, rapid loss in weight, etc. Examination showed the thyroid generally enlarged, bruit and thrill marked over arteries. Pulse, 160. Exophthalmos marked. Long, harsh systolic murmur. On May 24, 1909, both superior thyroid arteries were ligated.

One year after the operation the patient wrote that she was apparently entirely well. She now writes that she is not quite so well; is nervous at times, but does not think there is any evidence of her old illness. Her general strength is improved, but she tires more easily than before she had the trouble. A slight enlargement in the region of the thyroid can be felt. Pulse, 85; weight about normal. No tremor.

A30012.—Mrs. J. M., aged fifty-four years. Examination October 11, 1909. This patient noticed the goitre four months before. Hyperthyroidism had probably lasted about eight months. She was weak and unable to do her housework. She lost about fifty pounds in weight. Tremor gradually became worse, now affecting her entire body. She was nervous and irritable and perspired easily. The thyroid was found generally enlarged, the right lobe larger than the left. It was firm, rounded and regular in outline. Heart slightly enlarged; heart sounds slightly deficient, regular at apex. Systolic murmur. Pulse 120, regular and of good quality. White blood count, 9900; total lymphocytes, 35 per cent. Operation October 19, 1909: thyroidectomy; extirpation of the right lobe and isthums. Pathologic report: Hyperplastic thyroid.

This patient has written that all of three years elapsed before she considered herself well, and at present her nervous condition is not good. However, there has been no recurrence and no evidence of the old trouble. Her strength has improved; she is able to do her housework. No exophthalmos. No tremor. Weight before the appearance of symptoms was 180; previous to the operation 140; at present, 200 pounds. Her voice has not been affected.

A26468.—D. B., woman, aged forty-three years; schoolteacher. Examination July 19, 1909. The goitre was first noticed four months before at which time symptoms of hyperthyroidism developed; palpitation, tachycardia, dyspnea, sweating. She complained of being hot; gradually developed tremor and diarrhea. There was no vomiting. The symptoms were progressive until May or the first of June, when they reached their height. For some six weeks she could hardly get about. She was treated by rest and gradually grew better. Exophthalmos was present. The thyroid was hard with areas that felt cystic. The right lobe was considerably larger than the rest of the gland. Heart dilated one-half inch to the left; mitral systolic murmur. Pulse 140, but tension good. White blood count, 10,000; total lymphocytes, 30 per cent. On July 30, 1909, both superior thyroid arteries were ligated. She returned in May, 1911, stating that after the ligations she was in bed most of the time for three months because of palpitation and irregular heart action; since then she has been weak and unable to do much work. Palpitation occurs on excitement or exercise. Pulse from 80 to 90. Prominence of the eyes less. Operation May 15, 1911. Thyroidectomy; extirpation of the right lobe and isthmus.

This patient reports that her nerves are not so strong as they were before her illness. She is troubled more or less with sleeplessness, but her general health has improved and she can work with more ease. The prominence of her eyes has disappeared; there is no enlargement of the neck. Average pulse, 80. No tremor. Normal weight, 100; previous to operation, 75; present weight, 100. She cannot use her voice as well as before.

Group III. In this group of 7 patients were those who reported that they were markedly improved but most of the time there was some evidence of the old trouble and those who retained a little exophthalmos or nervousness. Most of them had entirely regained their normal weight and physical strength; 3 of the 7 had been simply ligated. In all probability if these 3 patients and the 6 in Group II who had simply been ligated would have resections now the few remaining evidences of the disease might entirely disappear. One of the patients in Group III had a primary resection; 1 had a resection following ligation; and 2 had secondary resections. A typical case is as follows:

A28982.—N. M., female, aged twenty-four years. Examination September 14, 1909. There had been gradual onset of nervousness, tachycardia, dyspnea, sweating, etc., several years before, and the patient had stayed in bed the greater part of a year. She then improved until within the last three months when she became gradually worse. There was a firm prominence of the right and left lobes of the thyroid. Marked bruit of the upper poles. Heart regular; not dilated. Pulse, 140. Marked systolic murmur at the apex. Exophthalmos quite marked. White blood count, 6000; total lymphocytes, 33 per cent. Operation September 22, 1909. Ligation of both superior thyroid arteries.

Recent report states that she has never considered herself entirely well, though her strength has gradually improved. Pulse, 92. There is some tremor; shortness of breath. Normal weight before her first symptoms, 151 pounds; present weight, 112. She has had an attack of jaundice, with rheumatism and gastric disturbance, since her operation.

Group IV. In this group we have placed 5 patients in whom there was slight improvement. In 1 a simple ligation had been done and this patient might now receive considerable benefit from a resection. As a rule, marked benefit follows ligation; if not, cure should not be expected in case the patient should have a thyroidectomy. Three of these 5 patients had primary resections, and 1 was operated on a second time with little or no improvement. The following case represents this group:

A23024.—Mrs. A. G., aged forty-three years. Examination April 30, 1909. Hyperthyroidism had existed for five years. She visited our clinic in 1904, when the diagnosis of Graves's disease was made. She was weak at that time and did not stay for treatment. She improved following this attack and her condition continued to be nearly normal for about a year. One year prior to her second examination she began to lose weight rapidly (fifteen pounds). After three or four months she again improved and was fairly well until April of the following year when she had a spell almost as serious as the first one. Exophthalmos at that time was quite marked. There was considerable enlargement of the right lobe of the thyroid, and slight enlargement on the left side. Heart irregular in rhythm and force. Dilated one and one-fourth inches to the left. Pulse regular, 114. White blood count, 5700; total lymphocytes, 36.6 per cent. August 5, 1909, double ligation of the superior thyroid vessels was done. August 26, 1909, the right lobe was extirpated.

This patient writes that she is not as well as she was before her original attack; her strength has improved, but her general health is not good. Pulse, 80. No tremor.

Group V. The 8 patients in this group derived little or no benefit from the operation. One had a primary resection, 1 a secondary resection and 6 were simply ligated. The following history is representative of this group:

A27142.—Female, aged nineteen years. Examination August 3, 1909. This patient had noted nervousness, not marked, for about three years. For the past nine months she had been easily exhausted. There were increased dyspnea, nervousness and difficulty in getting up stairs. She had two or three spells of vomiting; was frequently nauseated; her feet were swollen. The thyroid was found moderately hard and nodular. There were thrills over the superior thyroids. Heart slightly dilated. Pulse, 144; some exophthalmos. White blood count, 6200; total lymphocytes, 34.9 per cent. Operation August 5, 1909: ligation of the superior thyroid vessels. May 9, 1910: thyroidectomy; extirpation of the right lobe and isthmus.

This patient has not been as well as she was before the beginning of her illness. Her general health improved for a time, but there has been a recurrence of the former symptoms. The eye prominence diminished for a time and again returned. Pulse 118, and irregular. There was tremor and some hoarseness.

In addition to the 121 patients, 3 others were traced, but sufficient data to classify them were not obtained. Patients who are benefited, but not cured, by the removal of a part of the thyroid will in many instances improve greatly with a resection of the remaining part of the gland. This point has been demonstrated in 9 of our patients in whom the symptoms recurred and the second operation was done;

4 of these 9 patients were cured by the secondary resection; 1 was practically cured, though slight evidence of the disease remained; 2 were greatly improved. These results tend to bear out the impression that if the patients are not cured it is because enough of the gland has not been removed.

An effort has been made to determine the factors pertaining to exophthalmic goitre which would indicate the results from operative treatment that might be promised patients. In this, however, we have been only partially successful. In 8 of a group of 13 unsuccessful cases there was considerable dilatation of the heart at the time of operation, and several of the patients had developed edema. A complete cure could not be expected in this type of case; nevertheless, in several instances great benefit was derived from the operation. Twenty-five of the 55 patients who were cured had some dilatation of the heart at the time of operation.

The oldest patient operated on (fifty-seven years of age) and the youngest (four years and two months) were cured. The average age of the patients cured was 30.7 years; the average age of patients deriving little or no benefit was 29.1 years.

In the series of 120 patients traced, there were 107 females and 14 males. All but 2 of the males were benefited. The average length of time in which these patients had had symptoms before coming for treatment was about the same in the group of cured (19.3 months) as in the group receiving no benefit (22.2 months). The average length of time required to effect a cure was 17.9 months. In the second and third groups, in which were included the patients who were better but not cured, the average length of symptoms was longer; in Group II, 31.6 months; in Group III, 49.2 months. Despite the fact that the statistics do not emphasize this point, we believe that more cures and better results will be obtained in patients having symptoms for short periods than in those having symptoms for a number of years. The average duration of symptoms in patients who were cured was 19.3 months. It would seem reasonable to assume that if patients could have been treated within the first year a larger percentage would have been cured.

All these patients had some degree of exophthalmos (Stellwag or von Graefe) before operation; many of them complained of pain and tension of the eyes which usually disappeared soon after operation. Often they stated that their eyes felt much better even before there was any appreciable change in the degree of prominence. From our observations it would seem that the exophthalmos is one of the last symptoms to subside; sometimes it persists long after all other evidence of the disease has cleared up. Seventy-five patients reported that all prominence of the eyes had disappeared or was greatly diminished.

The functional results in our cases have been very satisfactory. A low collar incision just above the clavicle reflecting the superficial tissue flaps, severing the muscles just below their upper attachment on either side, if necessary, is inconspicuous. This incision heals quickly and normal motion of the head and neck returns in a few weeks. In a small number of patients there has been some disturbance in the voice, though this has been temporary. It is apt to be most marked about the fourth or fifth day when the edema is greatest. In one instance there was total loss of the voice for two months, when it rapidly returned to normal. The characteristic squeaky goitre voice so often heard in exophthalmic patients before operation usually completely changes to normal by the time the wound has healed. Some of our patients who speak with the normal motion of the vocal cords have complained of the voice being weak or tiring easily. At times it is husky, and there is difficulty in singing. All these symptoms usually subside in a very short time.

Of the 176 patients operated on in 1909 (some had three operations), 21 died, 7 in the hospital. All were females; the oldest forty-six years of age, the youngest fifteen. In 5 a single ligation only was done; in 2 there were resections. The average length of time symptoms had existed prior to operation was 29.5 months. One of the patients who died following resection had had a ligation and seemed entirely well. About five years after the ligation in our clinic, she had a hysterectomy performed elsewhere. The goitre symptoms recurred, growing gradually worse, and she returned to us for resection.

The histories of the patients who died show that they were all operated on at the time of the maximum severity of the disease. If we had realized then as we do now the danger of operative interference at the height of any attack of hyperthyroidism, the patients might have been carried past the period of maximum severity before operating. In all these patients hyperthyroidism was the clinical diagnosis of the cause of death; 4 showed dilated hearts and edema. The average loss of weight of the 7 patients at the time of operation was forty-two pounds. The average white blood count was 7800, and the average lymphocyte count 49.3 per cent.

Fourteen patients have died since leaving the hospital; 1 ten months after a double ligation. This patient had a recurrence of the trouble; was operated on elsewhere and died. The average length of time between operation and death in these 14 patients was 14.1 months. In 11, ligations were done; in 2, resections; and in 1 there was a recurrence. The average age was 34.1 years. Eleven had dilated hearts; 4 systolic murmurs. There was edema in 6 and evidence of nephritis in 4. From this review of the histories of patients who have died it seems evident that the condition was extremely toxic. It is quite probable that most of them died because of continued intoxication which had produced irreparable damage, usually in the heart, liver, and kidneys.

Better judgment as to what should be done and when to do it has lowered the mortality considerably in the past five years. In the series of letters received from exophthalmic goitre patients during the past few months, 11 mention having borne healthy children since operation. One woman had had three children. In two pregnancies 1 patient had had a recurrence of all the symptoms of hyperthyroidism and, because of this, abortions had been performed. This patient's report did not make clear that she was really suffering from hyperthyroidism when pregnant. Her chief symptom was vomiting and this, of course, may have been the pernicious vomiting of pregnancy; however, she had had one normal pregnancy without serious vomiting, before her attack of hyperthyroidism. Eight of the women who have had children since operation have been classified in Group I as cured; 2 of them in Group II as improved, and 1 in Group III in which no benefit has been derived from operation.

Judging the results in this series of 121 patients, a cure may be expected in about 45 per cent. In addition to this, about 23 per cent. will be practically cured, although a slight trace of the old trouble may persist. Our statistics show that an additional 4 per cent. obtained some benefit. About 5 per cent. reported that they had received no benefit.

UNILATERAL HEMATURIA ASSOCIATED WITH FIBROSIS AND MULTIPLE MICROSCOPIC CALCULI OF THE RENAL PAPILLÆ

By R. L. PAYNE, JR., M.D., F.A.C.S.
Norfolk, Va.

DURING the past decade there have been many articles written on unilateral hematuria and like all other unsolved pathological problems, there have been quite a diversity of opinions expressed.

At the meeting of this Society in 1912 the writer presented a paper (*Surgery, Gynecology and Obstetrics*, July, 1913) setting forth a resumé of the various pathological interpretations published up to that date and related a series of experiments which helped to eliminate the acutely developing vascular lesions as a causative factor of unilateral renal hemorrhage.

A large number of careful observers have reported the evidence of chronic inflammation in sections of kidney tissue removed from the type of case under consideration and our studies of personal cases before and since 1912 have confirmed the belief that chronic inflammatory changes are the principle factor in the production of unilateral hematuria.

We also advanced the theory, in the paper above mentioned that chronic inflammatory changes raise the local vascular tension to the point where rupture of the capillaries occurs with a resulting hemorrhage.

The following case is presented, not with the idea of drawing therefrom any definite deductions but for the purpose of explaining and defining our interpretation of the pathology present in this particular case.

C. H. J., male, aged twenty-seven years; occupation, school teacher; family, past and social history negative.

Present History. Seven years ago first observed the presence of blood in urine. This occurred at varying intervals of time until three years ago since which time there has been blood continuously present in the urine.

The patient has never suffered a particle of colic or pain, nor has there been associated any spells of fever. The amount of urine passed has always been plentiful but the patient gives the history of persistent constipation. There had been a perceptible loss of weight and the patient looked very anemic.

Physical Examination. On physical examination neither kidney was palpable and there was no tenderness over either loin space. X-ray examination was negative for stone and the microscope revealed an abundance of blood in the urine but no pus, no crystals and no casts.

Cystoscopic examination showed a normal bladder with bloody urine spurting from the right ureter and clear urine from the left side. No resistance was met with either ureteral catheter but the separate specimens showed with the microscope clear urine from the left kidney and bloody urine from the right side. Functional phthalein tests showed a normal output from the left side and a marked reduction from the right kidney. Bacteriological studies of the separate specimens was negative from the left kidney but showed a few colon bacilli from the right kindey.

Bacteriological study of the bladder specimen also showed the presence of colon bacilli.

Operation was decided upon because the writer has observed several of these cases relieved by section of the kidney from pole to pole and down to the pelvis in the absence of any demonstrable lesion to the naked eye.

At operation the kidney seemed normal in appearance and

size and no stone or new growth could be demonstrated. Upon bisection the cortex and parenchyma showed nothing definite but every single papillæ was intensely congested and the tip of every papillæ presented a cherry-red appearance which coincided macroscopically with the classical description of an angioma.

The writer had never before done a nephrectomy for this condition but it did not seem reasonable that bisection with suture could relieve this particular case, not did it seem possible that the experience of Fenwick (*British Medical Journal*, 1900, No. L, p. 248) could be applied to multiple angiomata of every papillæ.

Bearing in mind the normal functional test of the left kidney, nephrectomy was accordingly done, and herewith is appended the pathological report by Dr. Wm. De B. Mac-Nider, of the University of North Carolina.

Gross Appearance. "Kidney in 10 per cent. formalin $4\frac{1}{2}$ x 3 x $1\frac{1}{2}$ inches. Capsule easily removed, not adherent and surface smooth and normal in color. Cut surface shows a normal relation of cortex and medulla.

"The cortex is uniformly pale. All of the pyramids appear congested. This congestion macroscopically takes the form of streaks running in the long axis of the pyramids. In several instances these streaks lead to areas of congestion, reddish brown in color which surround or cap the apices of the pyramids. All of the renal papillæ show marked congestion.

"*Microscopic Pathology.* There is no increase in inter-tubular connective tissue and no sclerosis of the vessels. The glomeruli do not show any increase in capsular connective tissue. There is, however, quite an uniform increase in connective-tissue cells between the capillary loops of the glomeruli. This connective-tissue change is likely of recent development because connective-tissue fibers have not been laid down.

"The capillaries in this area are intact, hence, there is no evidence of the hematuria having originated from a ruptured

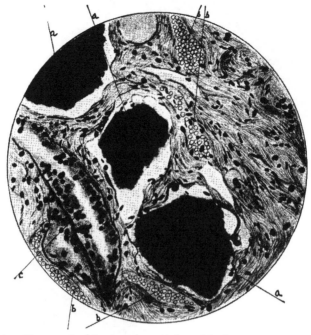

FIG. 1.—Camera lucida drawing, *Leitz* obj. $\frac{1}{6}$ oc. 2. Three calculi are shown at *a* surrounded by a proliferation of connective tissue. At *b* are seen dilated capillaries packed with blood cells. *c*, a papillary duct cut in its long axis.

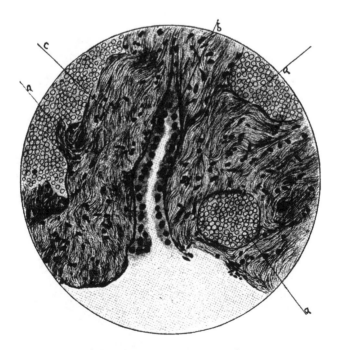

FIG. 2.—Camera lucida drawing, *Leitz* obj. $\frac{1}{6}$ oc. 2. Taken from a section through the apex of a renal pyramid. At *a* the enormously dilated venous spaces are seen. The connective-tissue overgrowth at *c* is marked. At *b* is seen a papillary duct cut in its long axis.

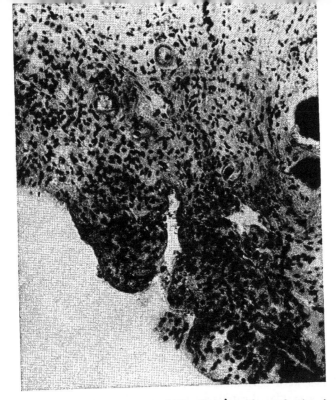

FIG. 3.—Microphotograph, × 188. Section through tip of papilla. On free surface is seen a ruptured capillary which still contains some blood cells. Two calculi are also shown.

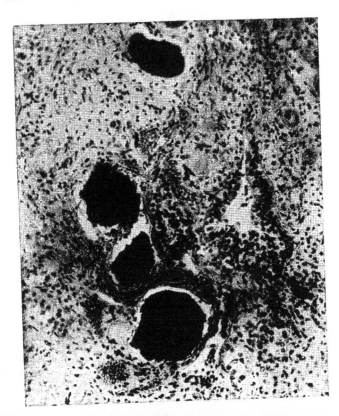

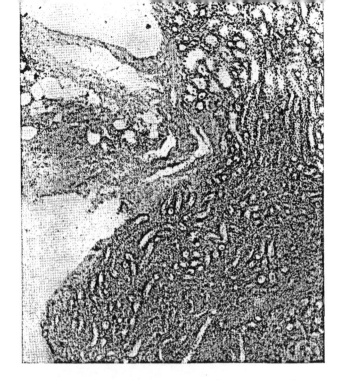

FIG. 5.—Microphotograph, × 55, showing large section of papilla
with ruptured capillary and much hemorrhage on free surface. Also
large number of dilated sinuses scattered throughout section.

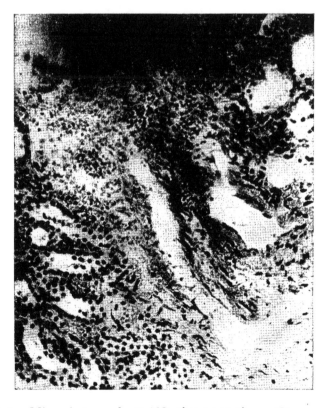

FIG. 6.—Micro h t   n h × 182 of same section as Fig.

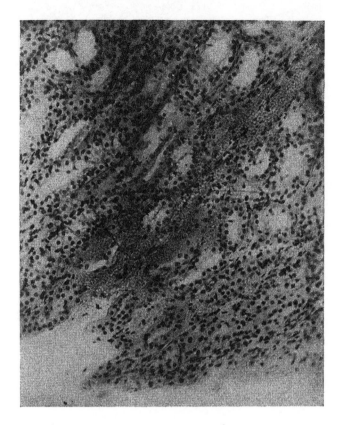

Fig. 7.—Microphotograph, × 152. Section through tip of papilla showing a dilated capillary cut in its long axis. It is still filled with blood but ruptured on the free border of the papilla.

capillary loop or loops. The epithelium of the cortex appears normal. The tubules in the cortex occasionally contain granular material which shows an absence of red blood cells.

"Sections were made passing through the papillæ and pyramids both in the long axis of the pyramids and at right angles to the axis. Such sections show the epithelium of the tubules in this zone of the kidney to be fairly normal. In the region of the papillæ there is a distinct increase in intertubular connective tissue. This increase is not uniform in its distribution.

"Located in the region of the papillæ and principally between the tubules but rarely inside a tubule are numerous calculi which are microscopic in size. Surrounding and in the region of such concretions there is an unusual overgrowth of connective tissue. In this connective tissue, usually between the tubules, the small veins and capillaries are hugely dilated into venous sinuses.

"Many of the small calculi lie in close apposition to these vascular sinuses. Such sinuses are well filled with blood. In such areas the tubules may be compressed by either the dilated capillaries or the intertubular calculi.

"All of the papillæ show dilated capillaries in a net-work on the surface, many of which were ruptured with free blood escaping. These numerous but small varices were evidently the source of the hemorrhage.

"The origin of these varicosities is not clear. It would seem, however, that the numerous though small calculi, aided by the connective tissue they had originated, succeeded in causing an obstruction to the venous return and a subsequent dilatation of the capillaries with resulting varicosities."

The writer does not believe that deductions can be drawn from one case. The facts here presented would, however, lend weight to the theory of those who believe chronic inflammation to be the cause of unilateral renal hemorrhage.

Briefly, to summarize, we have a case of so-called essential hematuria which shows in the kidney removed that macroscopically the only part of the organ involved in a pathological process is the papillary area.

Microscopically the cortex and medullary portion is pathologically negative, while the papillæ show definite lesions as follows: (1) Numerous microscopic calculi; (2) overgrowth of connective tissue; (3) hugely dilated capillaries; (4) calculi lying in close apposition to dilated capillaries; (5) dilated capillaries in a net-work on the free surface of papillæ, many of which are ruptured with free blood escaping.

It is not the part of this paper to discuss the question of infection, hematogenous or otherwise, whether the stones were the beginning of the process, whether the connective-tissue overgrowth was the cause of the varicosities, or in any way to theorize concerning the causative factors involved, but to report accurately our findings and partly show them in the accompanying illustrations.

Finally, after five years of study of so-called essential unilateral hematuria, both clinical and experimental, together with an intimate knowledge of the literature, this is the first instance, known to us, where the definite source of the hemorrhage and the probable cause thereof in a case of symptomless unilateral renal hemorrhage is shown.

PANCREATIC CYST AS A CAUSE OF UNILATERAL HEMATURIA, WITH REPORT OF A CASE

By JOSEPH RANSOHOFF, M.D., F.R.C.S. (ENG.)

Cincinnati, Ohio

THE report of a single case before a body, singly and collectively, as experienced as the Southern Surgical Association requires some justification. This I believe I can claim for the following report, because of an error in diagnosis, largely attributed to a symptom hitherto undescribed in connection with an abdominal growth, which in itself is rare. For cystic tumors of the pancreas are surely not common.

So far as I can now recall, I have had an opportunity of operating on only 6 cases. From the enormous material of the Mayo Hospital for the last two years one must conclude that pancreatic cysts are rare. Of a little over 5000 abdominal operations performed in 1914, only two were for pancreatic cysts. Among 4764 sections in 1913 there were none for pancreatic cysts, although in that year 6 cases were so diagnosticated. Whether these cases were, at operation, found to be something else, or the carriers of the supposed cysts developed a chilliness of the pedal extremities (rarer even than pancreatic cysts at Rochester) the reporter sayeth not.

In a very extensive review of the literature I have found no other case in which, as the one to be presented, profuse hematuria was a cardinal symptom and led to an error in diagnosis.

W. L., aged sixty-one years, farmer, referred by Dr. Conard, of Blanchester, O., to whom I am indebted for the history previous to the patient's admittance to the hospital. The father died at seventy of mastoid disease; mother at sixty of tuberculosis. One sister died of tuberculosis at thirty and one of pneumonia. One brother is living, aged fifty years. The patient was always strong and well until three years ago. Habits excellent. The present illness began three years ago with violent abdominal pains in the region of the umbilicus. The pains lasted for five or six days and disappeared after free catharsis. Their exact nature could not be determined. There was no elevation of temperature, no tenderness that could be particularly localized. During convalescence there was severe pain in the left arm and shoulder, which lasted for several days, but could not be explained.

A year ago the patient had a similar attack, from which he did not recover as promptly as from the first. He could not walk erect, there was tenderness on pressure in the left hypochondriac region and in the region of the left kidney, but no tumor mass could be felt at the time.

In June, Dr. Briggs recognized a tumor in the left upper quadrant. The patient has not been well since, but did not present himself for examination again until September 6, when he came on account of passing large quantities of blood with the urine. At this time he stated that he had for a number of years pain on the left side, under the ribs, and this was at times followed by the passing of bloody urine. During the last year the patient has lost over thirty pounds. He has coughed a great deal, and a single examination of the sputum showed the presence of tubercle bacilli.

Condition on admission to the Jewish Hospital, September 14, 1915: well-developed male, weighing 190 pounds, but evidently much reduced from his normal weight. Facial expression that of prolonged suffering. Pulse about 90. Systolic blood-pressure, 110; temperature normal; hemoglobin, 90 per cent.; red-blood count, 4,200,000; white-blood count, 8700. Polymorphonuclears, 74; mononuclears, 3; large lymphocytes, 7.4; small lymphocytes, 15; eosino-philes, 1.4. Urine dark in color, almost chocolate and contains a large amount of blood intimately mixed with the urine. No clots. Negative for bacilli. Stools normal in color and consistency. Negative for occult blood.

Physical Examination. Percussion negative. Auscultation reveals coarse moist rales over the greater part of the left lung, which accounts for the profuse expectoration. The sputum repeatedly examined for tubercle bacilli was negative, although the report of Prof. Wooley states that pretty nearly everything else, streptococci and staphylococci, diplococci and sarcinæ, were present. It is probable that the tubercle bacilli found on one previous examination before the patient's admission to the hospital came from the mouth or gums, which were in bad order, the latter being very much retracted. The x-ray of the chest was negative.

Abdomen. In the upper left quadrant, a tumor nearly as large as an adult head is palpable. Viewed from the foot of the bed the upper half of the abdomen showed the tumor projecting in a graceful curve, the highest point of which is fully two inches above the general level of the integumen. The lower abdomen shows nothing abnormal. Percussion over the growth elicits a flat note, which extends over the axillary line, and continues to the spine, except for a tympanitic band, descending from above and to the left of the median line, and evidently produced by the colon. There is a fulness in the left costol iliac space. The tumor is distinctly fluctuating. The x-ray examination shows a normal shadow of the lower half of the right kidney. In the upper part of the abdomen there is a tumor shadow, which extends to the right of the median line and lifts the left half of the diaphragm. The colon filled with barium bovilac shows no distention.

Cystoscopic examination, bladder and ureteral orifices

normal. From the left ureter there is a rhythmic expulsion of a bloody stream. On account of the exhausted condition of the patient ureteral catheterization was refrained from, and the injection of indigo-carmin used. Within five minutes a nearly black stream was belched from the right ureter and one almost as dark from the left.

Clinical Diagnosis. Cystic sarcoma of the left kidney without any question mark. Operation September 17, 1915, gas ether anesthesia, left lumbar incision through costo-iliac interval, with easy exposure of the left kidney. When this was brought into the wound no trace of the tumor was found, although the kidney looked somewhat larger than normal, and rather darker in color; An incision through the peritoneum to the inner side of the colon permitted the palpation of a large retroperitoneal growth, which could be best reached from in front. The kidney being anchored, the incision over it was closed with layer sutures. Median incision first disclosed the spleen, which projected below the lower border of the ribs, and measured approximately eight inches in both surface diameters. Its surface was dark purple. The sharp anterior edge overlapped the cystic growth, which it was now evident projected between the transverse colon and the greater curvature of the stomach. The diagnosis of pancreatic cyst was of course easily made, and after tapping and excision of a portion of the cyst wall, the remainder was attached to the abdominal wall. The operation was completed in the usual way of draining cysts of the pancreas. There were over 1000 c.c. of the fluid removed. This was rather viscid, blood stained and contained a large numer of little yellowish masses, globular in shape, eaily crushed, and looking not unlike miniature butter-balls. A few of these were adherent to the cyst walls. They consisted in fact of saponified fat.

The analysis of the fluid made by Prof. Reemelin, showed positive evidence of (1) alkaline protease, (2) amylase, and (3) lipase. Evidently, therefore, the digestive ferments found were of pancreatic origin. The cyst wall, according to the report of Prof. Wooley, contained no pancreatic tissue. It is composed of a typical granulation tissue, of which there are very many polymorphous leukocytes, indicating that the cyst was of a chronic inflammatory character.

Subsequent History. The error in diagnosis evidently did not influence the postoperative course. The wound in the kidney healed by first intention. From the third day on the urine became less and less bloody, and after the end of the week had become clear, and remained so to the end. The abdominal incision did not do so well, but for a period of three weeks gave us much concern on account of the irritation of the skin from the discharge, which is common after pancreatic drainage. Unfortunately the pulmonary condition recognized before the operation was aggravated, and pneumonic patches developed first in the lower part of the right lung, and gradually extended upward. The profuseness of the expectoration suggested the possibility of a pulmonary abscess, although x-ray examination and very careful physical examination made by Dr. Rachford demonstrated only a progressing bronchial pneumonia. To this the patient succumbed nearly seven weeks after the operation. The abdominal wall was almost completely closed and drainage so slight as to require dressing only ever three or four days.

REMARKS. So far as my knowledge goes from a rather extensive study of relevant literature the case presented is unique in that renal hematuria was caused by a pancreatic cyst. It doubtless was the result of pressure on the left renal vein. A like pressure on the splenic vein, caused the enlargement of the spleen to four or five times its natural size.

With the proverbial superiority of hind sight, it is clear to me now that an error in diagnosis might have been avoided by two methods of examination which were not practiced, because in my judgment there was a limit to the amount of investigation which the exhausted patient would tolerate.

Had we resorted to an x-ray plate of the stomach and colon simultaneously filled with barium the relation of the tumor to the stomach and colon would certainly have been demonstrated. Again, an injection of collargol into the pelvis of the kidney would likewise in all probability have shown a normal renal pelvis, which does not go with tumors of the kidney, since it is quite certain that almost every growth of the kidney associated with hematuria can be recognized by the deformity which the collargol distended pelvis reveals upon the radiogram.

Furthermore, the hematuria in the total absence of clots looked clinically more like that which attends an inflammatory condition than that associated with tumor of the kidney. It would have been possible perhaps to drain the cyst from the wound in the loin, as has been done by Pierce Gould and Johnston, but by the time the nature of the growth was made certain by the abdominal incision the posterior one had been definitely closed.

Since there is said to be more rejoicing in heaven at the return of one repentant sinner than at that of ninety and nine of the righteous, I venture to hope that the report of an error in diagnosis, and that in a case finally ending in death, will prove at least as welcome as that of ninety-nine successful cases, to my as yet uncrowned and wingless colleagues of the Southern Surgical and Gynecological Association.

DISCUSSION ON THE PAPERS OF DRS. PAYNE AND RANSOHOFF

DR. FRANCIS R. HAGNER, Washington, D. C.—The paper read by Dr. Payne is certainly a very instructive one. Recently an article was published by Dr. Bassett, of Denver, in which he mentioned infection as a cause of the majority of the cases of hemorrhage from the kidney. Anything we can find which will enable us to clear up these so-called symptomless hematurias is certainly a great help to us, and the case cited by Dr. Payne bears this out. I understood him to say the patient had a colon infection. It seems to me that was a coincidence; that as a result of this inflammatory condition in the papillæ the calculi found at this point is an interesting observation. So far, I have not seen any mention of this before.

Many of us do not realize that we are doing a partial nephrectomy when we split a kidney from pole to pole. I have operated on three patients who have had this done some years before, and the destruction of the kidney from the incision is really remarkable. I am sure, that possibly one-quarter or even more of the secreting structure of the kidney was destroyed by that incision and the consequent scar-tissue formation.

With reference to the case reported by Dr. Ransohoff, I believe in his case the hemorrhage was probably due to pressure on the renal vein. Quite recently I had a case upon whom a prostatectomy was done some three years ago, and this gentleman came back to me with a hemorrhage from the left ureter. I catheterized this and found a stricture just at the entrance of the ureteral orifice, and on the other side the urine was clear. A catheter was finally introduced, the stricture was dilated, and the catheter passed up to the kidney. The urine was very bloody. Next day the hemorrhage stopped, The patient had had three recurrences of hemorrhage in that way, and after simply dilating the ureter the hemorrhage stopped immediately. It may have been pressure on the renal vein of the dilated pelvis that caused the hemorrhage. The phthalein output in this patient with hemorrhage is the same in the two kidneys.

DR. THOMAS S. CULLEN, Baltimore, Maryland.—I have been much interested in Dr. Payne's paper. When working in Professor Orth's laboratory in Göttingen in 1893 I saw many kidneys with small round whitish-yellow or yellow spots on the surface or in the cortex. These were calcified glomeruli. The water in the small river passing through Göttingen contains much lime and it is possible that this was responsible for the calcification of so many glomeruli.

In Dr. Payne's case there was no calcification in the glomeruli. I would like to ask him whether in his case the calcification was in the connective tissue or in the collecting tubules themselves.

Dr. Hagner has spoken of the injury inflicted in the kidney by the cutting. Max Brödel has given us many valuable surgical hints by his wonderful injections of the kidney, thus clearly showing us where incisions can be made with the minimum danger to the kidney.

The silver wire method of opening the kidney as employed by my brother, Dr. Ernest K. Cullen and by Dr. Dergee is fraught with little danger to the kidney and with an astonishingly small amount of bleeding. In a case of one-sided hematuria I exposed the kidney and found the surface covered with many small abscesses. These I opened with the point of a knife. I then split the kidney, using the silver wire method. Many more miliary abscesses were opened in the cortex. The kidney wound was now approximated by matress sutures of catgut, and the kidney surrounded by iodoform drains. The patient promptly recovered, had no more hematuria and subsequently passed through two normal labors.

In connection with Dr. Ransohoff's report, I would like to mention the case of a woman, slightly past middle life, who was suffering from gall-stones. On opening the gall-bladder I found some discrete stones and a putty-like material lined the gall-bladder. Shortly after she returned to her home she complained of severe abdominal pain in the epigastric region, and in a few months the upper abdomen was markedly enlarged. I made a median incision above the umbilicus and found a pancreatic cyst containing several liters of fluid. The cyst was drained and the patient speedily recovered.

Dr. FRED. W. BAILEY, St. Louis, Missouri.—I wish to report a case similar in clinical appearance to the case related by Dr. Payne. A boy, about eight years of age was suffering with constant hematuria which had been increasing for about six months. He had been under the care of a very competent internist without any particular improvement, long-continued bed rest, dietetic and medicinal attention being ineffective. Tests at intervals showed but little reduction in kidney function, the patient being too young to successfully undergo ureteral cauterization. The x-ray showed the kidney on the right side to be twice as large as the left. Pain was constant in right lumbar region. He was going down hill so rapidly that we determined to make an exploration.

Through a median incision, the patient's abdominal cavity was explored. I found the left kidney normal in size for his age. The right kidney was greatly enlarged, of soft resistance and irregular in its outline. I immediately closed the incision and through an oblique posterior incision, delivered the right kidney. It proved to be twice the normal size with a double ureter joining about two inches below the lower pole. The kidney was incised from end to end, and the macroscopical picture of the pelvis and pyramids was almost identical with that described by Dr. Payne. There were two pelves, the upper one twice as large as the lower and the opening between the two was almost closed. Each pelvis had its individual ureter.

The kidney was removed and the progress of the case watched with great interest for a few days. The boy made a complete recovery. The urine did not entirely clear up for ten days. It is now about four months since the operation. Unfortunately the specimen was lost in the laboratory and the microscopical picture therefore, cannot be recorded. It would be interesting to know how much the congenital condition had to do with the hematuria, acting, I should judge, as a predisposing factor encouraging infection or irritation because of deficient drainage. Clinically, the surgical act was justified by the constant pain, x-ray findings and rapid decline.

I would like to ask Dr. Payne in closing the discussion to tell us if there are any steps in the technic by which we can determine with more accuracy, the functionating power of the kidney in a boy of that age.

Dr. Bransford Lewis, St. Louis, Missouri.—These two papers are very interesting contributions to the etiology of hematuria as well as to other phases of the subject.

With reference to the subject of infections in causing hematuria, we know that infections will cause unilateral hematuria and to such a serious degree that one has to take out the kidney to save life once in a while. Also, you can resort to ureteral catheterization and inject medicated fluid up into the kidney pelvis, relieve the patient, and thus avoid the necessity of a nephrectomy.

Another interesting point is, whence comes the infection which gives rise to the interesting sequelæ? Late studies seem to indicate that focal infections in various parts of the body play an important part. Instead of there being simply an ascending infection from an infected bladder, we may have a focal infection giving rise to hematogenous kidney infection and hematuria, and that is a more interesting phase of the subject, it seems to me, than even some of these others.

A professional friend of mine of Chicago recently told me

he had a brother who had an infective nephritis with hematuria, and he was treated locally in several different ways without any success. Finally, they found he had an infected tonsil, which was removed, with benefit to the kidney. There was a definite improvement in the kidney condition after the removal of the tonsil, but after some weeks there was a relapse. They looked after the tonsil again and found a little tab still remaining from the incomplete removal of the tonsil, and when they removed this tab they found an abscess cavity underneath it. This was completely removed and the kidney condition cleared up without recurrence.

We all know the vast influence of focal infections coming from the tonsil, and it is well to keep this in view in connection with hematurias and with infections of the kidney.

Dr. John T. Moore, Houston, Texas.—I desire to report a case of cyst of the pancreas about the size of one's head that gave rise to no hematuria. I was called to see the case in consultation with Dr. R. H. Moers of Houston. The patient was a woman, aged forty-nine years, referred to him by a doctor in the country who said she had a tumor. When she came into the hospital she had a consolidated left lung due to pneumonia. We thought probably this was a tuberculous pneumonia, but failed to find tubercle bacilli, and after keeping her under observation for a little while the pneumonia cleared up. The woman's history was that of a tuberculous patient we think. We thought she might have a tumor of the kidney. This we excluded by catheterization of the ureters, finding the urine normal from each kidney. By exclusion, we came to the conclusion she had a cyst of the pancreas. At operation Dr. Moers made a median line incision and found the diagnosis to be correct, and at my suggestion he drained under the ribs on the left side. This woman had a very precarious time for three or four weeks. The cyst discharged quite a good deal, but finally closed. She at last improved, but is now dying, I understand, from tuberculosis. It was proved before she left Houston that she had a tuberculous lung. Although there was a good deal of pressure upon the left kidney, there was no hemorrhage from that side at any time.

Dr. R. L. Payne, Jr., Norfolk, Virginia (closing).—I am very grateful to the gentlemen for their remarks addressed to my part of the two papers.

To be coherent in my reply, I will first say to Dr. Bailey that it is a difficult problem to determine the functional test in a young child. You can with the smallest Nitze cystoscope under general anesthesia sometimes do it.

In reply to Dr. Cullen's question as to stones in the tubules, the majority of stones were between the tubules and a few in the tubules. For reasons which I did not explain in my paper we naturally leaned to the infectious theory in this case, and possibly some focus, such as Dr. Bransford Lewis mentioned, was at the bottom of it. It must have been a hematogenous infection, and the chronic constipation and the presence of colon bacilli in the bladder possibly had something to do with it.

Directing my remarks to the question brought up by Dr. Hagner relative to bisection of the kidney, we have found in our experimental studies on dogs' and rabbits' kidneys subsequently removed, that over one-third of the kidney structure was destroyed by scar tissue.

I was much interested in Dr. Ransohoff's case. It is an instructive one and brought to my mind the first experiments we did in trying to produce the condition of unilateral hematuria. Unquestionably this thing is due to congestion, and there are three ways of producing congestion of the kidney, first by slow occlusion of the renal artery; second, by ligation of the renal vein, and third, by division of the nerves going into the kidney, removing the vasomotors and getting chronic dilatation. In our experiments none of them resulted in a unilateral hematuria. Therefore, we were able to conclude that the acutely developing vascular lesions had nothing to do with the clinical condition. It must be a chronic inflammatory condition, and that brings us down to the salient point where the pathologic problem has never been solved, and that is because our interpretation of nephritis is so distinctly at variance. There are two factors at work in nephritis, one of vascular changes and the other of epithelial changes, and some men call a nephritis such when they find only epithelial changes, while others interpret the vascular changes alone. Both should exist to have a true nephritis, and I think a better term in these cases seeking to explain the condition is a chronic inflammatory change.

CAUDAL ANESTHESIA IN GENITO-URINARY SURGERY

By Bransford Lewis, B.S., M.D., F.A.C.S.

AND

Leo Bartels, M.D., F.A.C.S.
St. Louis, Missouri

History. In 1901–1903 Cathlin[1] proposed the use of normal saline injections into the sacral canal for the purpose of allaying certain nervous manifestations connected with the urinary tract—enuresis in boys and girls, tabetic crises, etc. Encouraged by some success in this endeavor, the same author later tried to induce anesthesia by injecting in a similar manner, but this proved unsuccessful with him and with other French experimenters of that period.

It was not until 1910 that material success was reported in this regard. Then Läwen[2] described his use of 1 or 2 per cent. solutions of novocain in normal saline solution used in this way and the anesthetic effect he secured therefrom.

Gros[3] advised an alkaline base for the solution as promoting the intensity of anesthetic effect, and made use of novocain bicarbonate, together with a small addition of adrenalin.

Läwen made use of the sitting posture for the patient until the anesthesia was well under way, and began with 20 or 25 c.c. While he mentioned that the anesthetic effect was somewhat variable, he claimed that very satisfactory

---

[1] Les *I*njections epidurales, *P*aris, 1903, p. 89.
[2] Centrbl. f. Chir. 1910, No. 20.
[3] Arch f. exper. Path. und Pharmacie, p. 708.

results were obtained in many instances. Analgesia had been noted in the gluteal region, rectum and anus, skin of the scrotum and penis, and of the upper and inner parts of the thigh; and in women, the vulva and vagina. Läwen thought that probably the prostate, also, would be found to be analgesic through the same agency, though he had up to the time of his report had no opportunity of confirming this belief.

In reviewing the subject of nerve-blocking for local anesthesia, Harris[1] mentioned the sacral method and reported having used it with good effects. This was our first introduction to the method. While we then had little to go on, the method seemed logical; and we had had experience with Cathlin saline injection in certain cases with varying success but no bad effects.

To date we have essayed caudal anesthesia in some eighty odd cases, with results so favorable that we feel justified in making the report herewith presented.

ANATOMY. Thirty-one pairs of nerves branch off from the spinal cord, emerge through the foramina and are distributed to the several parts of the body which they innervate. They are divided into five groups—the cervical, dorsal, lumbar, sacral, and coccygeal.

SACRUM. Although originally composed of separate segments, the sacrum in adult life is blended into one bone. For present consideration its most interesting features are its *central canal* and its *foramina*. The canal is a continuation downward of the spinal canal, but at the second sacral segment communication between these two parts is cut off by the closure of the dura mater around the nerve branches. This is not only demonstrable anatomically, but Läwen[2] found that colored fluids injected into the sacral canal never appeared in the spinal canal or colored the upper part of the cord, showing the complete isolation of these two parts

[1] Surgery, Gynecology and *Obstetrics, F*ebruary, 1915.
[2] Deutsch. Ztschr. f. Chir., 1911, p. 300.

of the canal from one another by closure of the dura mater. So that although the nerves are transmitted from the spinal canal down into the sacral canal, there is no other communication between the two. This fact marks the distinction between this method of securing anesthesia and that termed spinal anesthesia, in which the fluid is injected directly into the spinal canal. It likewise indicates that the two methods should not be confused with one another.

The nerve branches that descend thus from the spinal into the sacral canal are called the sacral nerves. From the sacral canal they pass through the sacral foramina out into the pelvis, forming then the *sacral plexus*, one of the most important of whose branches is the pudic, distributed to the genito-uninary organs.

The sacral canal is enclosed in bony walls except at its lower end; here through non-development of the spinous processes the posterior bony wall is lacking and is replaced by a ligamentous membrane or covering. This opening is called the *sacral hiatus*.

It is through this hiatus that the needle is directed for delivery of the fluid for anesthesia. The opening is variable in size in different individuals (Fig. 1), but is practically always large enough to permit the introduction of a needle.

The sacral canal is flattened from before backward, and its caliber grows smaller as it curves downward toward the coccyx (Fig. 2). In the male the curve of the sacrum is fairly evenly distributed over the whole length of the bone, but in the female the upper part or base of the sacrum is projected more sharply backward for the increase of pelvic capacity pertaining to that sex. These variations have an influence on the ease or difficulty of introducing the long hollow needle through which the injection is made. The axis of the canal must be threaded by compensating movements while advancing the needle.

DISTRIBUTION OF NERVES FROM THE SACRAL PLEXUS.—The chief divisions of the sacral plexus are the sciatic and pudic nerves. The pudic terminates in three branches, namely, (1) the dorsal nerve of the penis; (2) the perineal nerve; and (3) the hemorrhoidal. These supply the skin and the structures of the penis, scrotum, perineum, prostate and bladder; and the inner surface of the thighs, posteriorly. A structure *exclusively* supplied by a certain nerve may be anesthetized by deadening that nerve; but when the structure is supplied by another nerve, also, the deadening of one nerve only does not suffice for anesthesia; the collateral nerve holds the tissues in a sensitive condition. This accounts for the fact that the lower extremities are not made analgesic by anesthetizing the sciatic nerve. Collateral innervation maintains sensibility.

PREPARATION OF SOLUTION.—Various drugs have been added to the novocain solution to make its effect more efficient and enduring, but our experience has led us to believe that the two most useful adjuvants in this respect are potassium sulphate and adrenalin. The addition of these drugs permits the use of novocain in much weaker solution while still retaining its effectiveness.

Chloretone, although a local anesthetic and antiseptic, has been discontinued by us because of its irritating effects and also because analgesia has seemed just as good without it. The following solutions are freshly prepared before using:

A. 1 per cent. solution of novocain.

B. 1 per cent. solution of potassium sulphate.

When ready for use these two solutions are combined in a sterile glass, and two drops of adrenalin solution (1 to 1000) are added for each 30 c.c. of the combined solution. Freshly distilled sterile water should be used for making the solutions.

DOSAGE. From 40 to 90 c.c. of the combined solution is injected, according to each individual case—the more sensitive individuals and the major operative procedures requiring the larger amount.

Prostatectomies demand larger quantities and more complete anesthesia. If one injection does not produce sufficient anesthesia, an additional amount may be used. For this reason the needle may be allowed to remain in the canal for fifteen or twenty minutes, providing for the additional amount if it is found necessary.

TESTS FOR INSENSIBILITY. It is not advisable to apply tests before fifteen minutes following the giving of the injection. They are liable to lessen the confidence of a nervous patient in the success of the method. At twenty minutes the effect should be manifest or at its best. In prostatectomies or vesical operations, a part of this time is occupied in making the prevesical incision under ordinary infiltration anesthesia (Fig. 9). When the operator arrives at the bladder wall he finds it insensitive and ready for incision. Previous to this, if desired, a test may be made by sounding the prostatic urethra and bladder, both of which should be influenced by the caudal anesthesia.

SUCCESS AND FAILURE. Just as with the use of drugs for any purpose and by any method, so there is a certain variability in the effectiveness of this method for producing anesthesia. Aside from individual susceptibility, there may be other reasons explanatory of this. The capacity of the sacral canal may be large or small, requiring a greater or lesser amount of fluid to fill it and exercise the pressure-effect on the nerves that is so essential.

We have found it serviceable to use a larger quantity of the more dilute solution than was formerly employed. Eighty or ninety c.c. of the $\frac{1}{2}$ per cent. solutions seems preferable to half that quantity of 1 per cent. solutions.

Läwen reported 15 per cent. failure in 47 cases, using 20 to 30 c.c. of 1 to 2 per cent. solutions. Our earlier experience gave about the same percentage of success (85), which seems likely to be improved under further study and use of the method. Its newness to us, together with the paucity of literature regarding it, led us to feel our way in increasing the quantity of fluid injected rather than striving too ardently for uniform success.

But lately we have used 80 or 90 c.c. of anesthetic fluid in a number of cases, without observing that it induced any more disturbance than the lesser quantities had given. The hypodermic administration of morphine or pantopon, given shortly beforehand, contributes to the effectiveness of the result.

Harris says that so far the nerve-blocking methods have been accompanied by no mortality. With two possible sources of danger eliminated, the sacral method of nerve-blocking would seem capable of maintaining that enviable reputation. These possible dangers are: injection of the fluid into a vein (Fig. 8) and injection into the spinal canal. They are obviated by definite maneuvers related in the description of Technique.

It is difficult to anticipate any other cause for anxiety in this respect.

The difficult cases for caudal anesthesia are the obese, the very nervous, the hysterical, and children. Läwen has advised against its use in the aged, but we have found that these are the very cases in which it is especially advantageous. It has made operation possible in a number of cases debilitated and decrepit from advanced age and the ravages of urinary obstruction and sepsis, its freedom from shock and other depressing influences making it particularly desirable for this class of cases.

TECHNIC OF ADMINISTRATION. The patient is placed on his right side, with his head slightly elevated, and is instructed to bow his back strongly, bringing his knees and chin as near together as possible.

The area over the sacrum and the immediate neighborhood is cleaned with benzine, dried and painted with iodine.

The sacral hiatus is sought for and is found just below the spinous process and above the coccyx (Figs. 5 and 6). The rudimentary sacral spinous processes lead down to it.

Having infiltrated the skin and deeper soft tissues over the hiatus with the same anesthetic fluid as is to be used for the sacral canal, a little massage serving to diffuse the solution to better advantage, the long needle fitted with a trocar wire is inserted into the sacral hiatus (Fig. 7), passing through the membrane that covers the hiatus. The needle in being introduced is at first held at an angle of 45 degrees with the skin surface, but as soon as the operator feels the penetration of the membrane by the needle, the syringe is depressed almost to a level with the body-plane at that point.

The needle is made to follow the axis of the canal, which it penetrates for a distance of one and a half or two inches. When placed, the trocar wire is withdrawn and opportunity is given for avoiding the two dangers previously alluded to. If the needle has gone up too far and passed through the guarding dura mater into the spinal canal, evidence will be given in the escape of numerous drops of spinal fluid through the needle. In this case the needle must be withdrawn until its point rests in the sacral canal and no more spinal fluid flows. If there is bleeding, indicating that a vein has been punctured, the position of the needle is changed so that an inadvertent intravenous injection be not given. In case there is no bleeding it is well to make assurance doubly sure before injecting the anesthetic fluid. To that end a few drops of normal saline solution are first injected and permitted to return through the needle, thus removing a possible clot or shred in the needle. Blood will assuredly flow at this point if a vein be the resting place of the needle.

If not and all things seem satisfactory, the injection is proceeded with—20 c.c. at a time being sent slowly and steadily through the needle by the Record syringe, repeated until the desired quantity is reached.

Some patients indicate the blocking effect on the nerves by complaining of pains or peculiar sensations down the

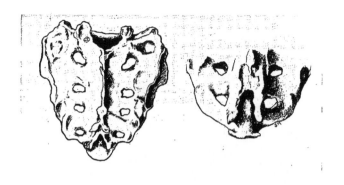

Fig. 1.—Sacra, and varying forms of sacral hiatus. (P. Bull.)

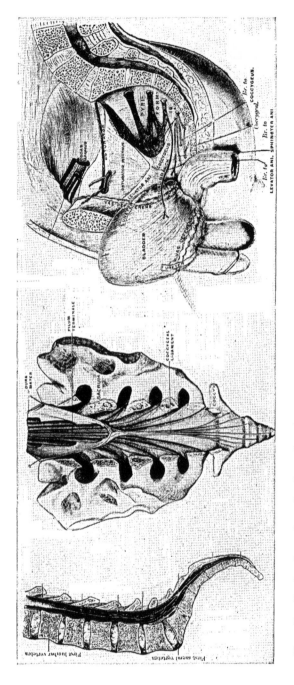

Fig. 2   Fig. 3   Fig. 4

Fig. 2.—Sagittal section of spine, showing spinal and sacral canals (Cunningham).

Fig. 3.—Showing separation of spinal and sacral canals by closure of dura mater. Sacral nerves exposed (Gray-Spitzka).

Fig. 4.—Sacral plexus of nerves and distribution (Gray-Spitzka).

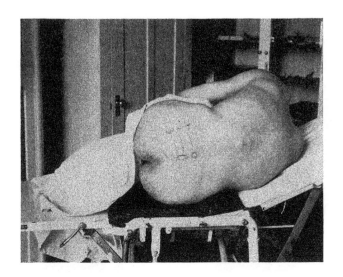

FIG. 5.—Landmarks for caudal anesthesia.

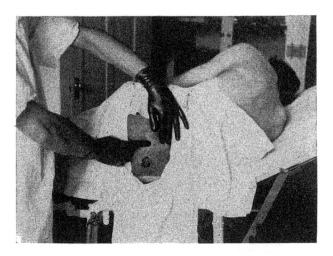

FIG. 6.—Finger covering the hiatus.

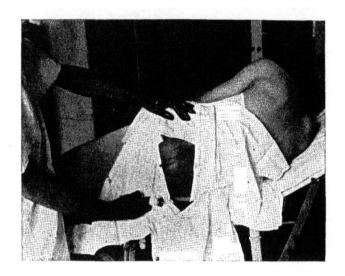

FIG. 7.—Needle inserted into sacral hiatus.

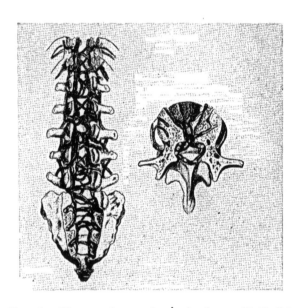

FIG. 8.—Venous plexus of spinal column (P. Bull.)

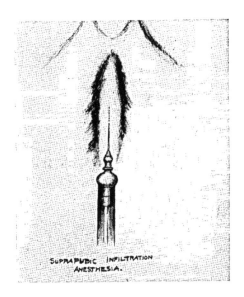

FIG. 9.—Infiltration of suprapubic tissues.

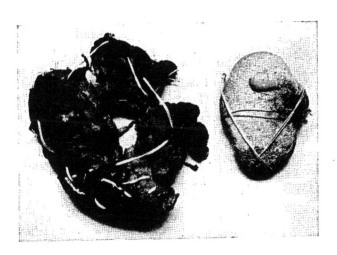

FIG. 10.—Prostate and vesical stone removed under caudal and
infiltration anesthesia.

thighs and legs. It has seemed to us that anesthesia portended better when such complaints are made.

Occasionally it is found that a curved needle is more favorable for threading the canal than a straight one—conforming to a more sharply curved canal or a smaller hiatus.

UNTOWARD EFFECTS. On one occasion, before the technic described was adopted, the beginning of the injection was marked by emphatic complaints by the patient of severe pain in the head and chest, weakness, with undue frequency and irregularity of the pulse. It was recognized at once that the injection was *intravenous* and it was promptly discontinued. The symptoms passed off shortly afterward and there was no objectionable after-effect.

At other times we have noted transient indications of weakness, moisture of the skin, frequent pulse, etc., but whether these were due to the effects of the injection or to nervousness and apprehension on the part of the patient, it has been difficult to say. We have had patients that fainted incidental to a rectal palpation of the prostate, from the strangeness of the situation and nervousness of the patient. So that it is not always easy to differentiate between nervousness and toxicity. However, the effects have never proved serious in any case as yet. Harris says that nerve blocking methods have as yet no mortality. We hope that they may continue to occupy that enviable position.

If less than a toxic amount of novocain be used, and it is used under the plans and precautions described, we can see no reason why it should prove dangerous or show a mortality.

TOXICITY. In referring to the toxicity of novocain, Braun[1] says that while he had never noticed any disturbance following the subcutaneous injection of 2 per cent. solutions, Läwen had observed typical poison symptoms following the injection of 25 c.c. of 2 per cent. solution into

[1]Local Anesthesia, translated by Shields, 1914, p. 124.

the sacral canal. The symptoms consisted of nausea, sweating, anemia, rapid pulse, frequent respiration, feeling of oppression and haze in front of the eyes. The authors had noted that these symptoms could be avoided by making the injection slowly. In experience on the nerve trunks of the lower extremities, Läwen had used as much as 2.1 grams of novocain without toxic effect. In one case the patient had received 20 c.c. of 4 per cent. solution (15 grains of novocain); in another 30 c.c. of 2 per cent. solution. He has injected 50 c.c. of 1 per cent. solution and larger quantities of 0.5 per cent. solution. In only a few of the cases were toxic symptoms noticed. Finally,[1] Braun remarks that, "Since Läwen has shown that the 4 per cent. novocain-suprarenin solution is harmless, even in large quantities, the author has been using this solution." And he further remarks, "The toxic action of this drug is less than that of any hitherto known anesthetic substance."

ADVANTAGES OF SACRAL ANESTHESIA. The preëminent advantages of this method do not appear in ordinary routine surgical cases. These can be anesthetized with ether or gas-oxygen with little risk, if administered by an expert. But when an aged individual, so reduced by pain and toxemia, and by back-pressure in his urinary tract that he is utterly miserable and decrepit; so debilitated that he has no resisting powers to stand further depletion; and seems both ripe and ready for dissolution; and so old that there is no promise of restoration from this source—then we have the patient for whom this mode of anesthetic is appropriate and most advantageous. It is a question then of safety first, of life and death, not simply a choice between several equally safe methods of anesthesia.

Anesthetized by this method, we have seen just such cases undergo various operative measures connected with the bladder and prostate, who both during and after such

---

[1] Local Anesthesia, translated by Shields, 1914, p. 180.

operations were serene and comfortable, free from cardiac, pulmonary or gastric disturbances, and ready at once to take liquids and light nourishment.

ILLUSTRATIVE CASES. CASE I.—P. K., aged sixty-three years; laborer; poorly nourished; chronic rheumatic and inebriate; poor risk from every standpoint. Arteriosclerosis and myocardial degeneration present. Urinary tract septic; urine loaded with pus and bacteria; urination every five to forty minutes. Repeated septic chills and fever. Cystoscopy showed large intravesical prostatic hypertrophy, together with a stone almost as large as a hen's egg. After five days' preparatory treatment the patient was operated on by the suprapubic route, under caudal and infiltration anesthesia, as described, the specimens shown in Fig. 10 being removed. The patient suffered none at all, either from pain or shock, and expressed himself as more comfortable after operation than before it. Recovery was uneventful and the patient was ready to leave the hospital in three weeks.

CASE II.—Wm. McG., aged seventy-six years. Very feeble; ill nourished; emaciated and cachectic. First essay at cystoscopy under ordinary methods of local anesthesia was a complete failure, the patient squirming and resisting to a degree that prevented even the introduction of the instrument into the bladder. With this experience in mind, and with memories of previous attempts at instrumentation by other surgeons, the patient very impressively informed us that he would submit to operation or anything we wished to do, *only on condition that it was done under ether anesthesia*. In this stand he was backed up by his family. His enfeebled condition made it highly desirable that he be operated on without the addition of any factors of shock or disturbance. Bronchitis present forbade the use of ether.

A little diplomacy paved the way to the use of caudal anesthesia for a second attempt at cystoscopy, five days after the first one. The effect was all that could be desired. The patient was comfortable throughout; relaxation permitted the introduction and complete manipulation of the cystoscope, and from this very satisfactory examination there was confirmation of a previous suspicion of prostatic carcinoma. This diagnosis explained the hyperesthetic condition prevailing locally as well as the unpromising condition generally. Nevertheless, it was still considered advisable to operate to relieve the obstruction and sepsis present.

The caudal anesthesia had been so eminently pleasing to the patient that he made no further objection to its use in the subsequent major operation; and it was applied with equally as much satisfaction. After suprapubic opening of the bladder, the larger proportion of the growth, hard, dense and resistant, was removed by digging, tearing and morcellement, leaving at least a good channel for the escape of urine, if not preventing the future return of the growth. The latter had involved adjacent structures to a degree that made radical removal out of the question.

But the caudal anesthesia was both effective and innocuous; the patient was in as good condition after the operation as before, and his progress since then has shown that neither operation nor anesthetic added to his disability or distress and it is expected that the remaining tenure of life may at least be more comfortable.

Other, simpler cases might be related in which everything has gone more evenly than in these, but it must be remembered that it is solving the difficult and unpromising cases that makes the method attractive or worthy.

Summary

Prostatectomies	13
Cystoscopies	68
Cystotomies	2
External perineal urethrotomy	1
Rectal carcinoma	1
Total number of cases	85

RESULTS.   10 of the 13 prostatectomies needed no other anesthesia.

2 required a small amount of ether.

1 required complete ether anesthesia, there being no effect from caudal injection.

46 of the 68 cystoscopies gave excellent analgesia.

13 gave partial analgesia

5 gave no analgesia; 3 of these 5 failures we believe due to faulty technic.

1 of the cystotomies (for calculus) gave good analgesia, and the prostate could have been enucleated.

1 required a small amount of ether, as curettement of a carcinomatous mass was done.

The one case of external urethrotomy (perineal) gave complete analgesia.

The one rectal case (carcinoma) was a failure.

SOME OBSERVATIONS ON LOCAL ANESTHESIA

By Herbert P. Cole, M.D., F.A.C.S.
Mobile, Alabama

An examination of the records in my service shows that within the past twenty-four months we have performed an increasing percentage of our general surgery under local anesthesia.

Many of the major cases were selected for local anesthesia, as they offered grave operative risk under a general anesthetic.

The following is a partial list of the operations performed:

Appendectomy, acute and chronic 25
Appendicular abscess, drainage of 2
General peritonitis, drainage 4
Abdominal drainage and repair of old appendix sinus . 1
Abdominal adhesions, separation of 2
Laparatomy for removal of towel present in abdomen for
    six months 1
Exploratory laparotomy 13
Enterostomy 1
Gastro-enterostomy for ulcer or carcinoma 8
Abdomen, gunshot wound of 2
Cholecystotomy 8
Herniotomy 17
*O*variotomy, removal of 43 pounds ovarian cyst . . . 1
Nephrectomy 1
Thyroidectomy. 5
Uterus, suspension of 1
Ectopic gestation, salpingectomy 1

Breast, radical amputation of, for carcinoma 3
Skull, large osteochondroma of, decompression . . . 1
Skull, elevation for depressed fracture of 1
Skull, decompression of, for epilepsy 1
Orbit, exenteration of, for sarcoma 1
Superior maxilla, resection of 1
Gland of the neck, extensive resection of 1
Foot, amputation of 2
Os calcis, resection of 1
Shoulder, repair of gunshot sinus of 1
Internal cuneiform, resection of right 1
Hypospadias, extensive operation for 2
Prostatic abscess, drainage of 1
Vesical drainage, perineal 1
Suprapubic fistula, repair of 2
Cystotomy, suprapubic 1
Prolapse of the rectum, radical cure of 1
Hemangioma of anus, removal of large 1

Seven operations were performed during pregnancy, with no maternal mortality and with a loss of one fetus, as follows:

Appendectomy (chronic interval cases 3, appendix abscess
    drainage, 1) 4
Herniotomy, inguinal 1
Uterus, postoperative adhesions 2

In the first decade there were seven major operations under two years of age, as follows:

Artificial anus for anorectal imperforation, third day of
    life (death in twelve days from bronchopneumonia) . 1
Herniotomy, bilateral, for incarceration (age three weeks) 1
Herniotomy, left, incarceration (age three weeks) . . 1
Thoracotomy, empyema (under two years of age) . . 4

Forty-seven cases were operated on between the ages of fifty and eighty-seven and were almost exclusively selected for local anesthesia because of cardiovascular or renal contra-

indications to general anesthesia. The following is a partial
list of the graver cases:

Extensive operation for carcinoma of the sternum, eighty-
seven years of age   1
Exenteration of the orbit for sarcoma, eighty-one years
of age   1
Herniotomy for large strangulated hernia, seventy-eight
years of age   1
Amputation of the foot for gangrene, seventy-one years of
age   1
Gastro-enterostomy for inoperable carcinoma of the
pyloris (age seventy-one and fifty-nine)   2
Posterior gastro-enterostomy for ulcer of the duodenum,
fifty-six years of age   1
Cholecystotomy, rupture of the gall-bladder, third day,
fifty-two years of age   1
Cholecystotomy for gall-stones, age sixty-two and fifty-
two   2
Cholecystotomy (for gall-stones) age fifty-two (in addition
through the same incision, appendectomy for cystic
appendix and posterior gastro-enterostomy for ulcer of
of the duodenum)   1
Gangrenous appendix, ruptured (patient sixty years of
age with active pulmonary tuberculosis and a patient
sixty-six years of age with extensive peritonitis) . .   2
Appendectomy, chronic appendicitis (fifty years of age)   1
Nephrectomy for adenoma of the kidney, patient fifty-two
years of age   1
Radical amputation of the breast for carcinoma, sixty
years of age   1
Perineal drainage of prostatic abscess, sixty-two years of
age   1
Radical cure for prolapse of the rectum, sixty-nine years of
age   1
Enterostomy on the fifth day for ileus and peritonitis,
sixty-five years of age (death on the eighth day) . .   1
Peritoneal drainage for peritonitis of unknown origin on
the sixth day, patient sixty-eight years of age (death on
the fourth day)   1

We note a mortality rate of $4\frac{2}{10}$ per cent. in 47 cases
in the fifth to ninth decade. Cases selected for local anesthesia as being grave operative risks. Of the two deaths,

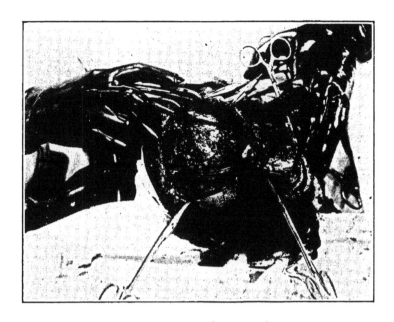

*F*IG. 1.—Decompression for epilepsy.

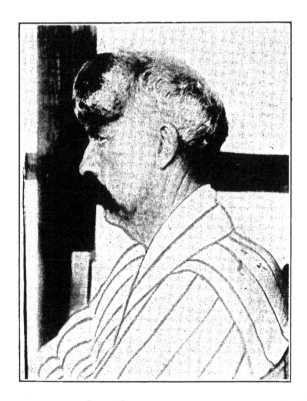

*F*IG. 2.—Decompression with removal of large osteochondroma
of the frontal region.

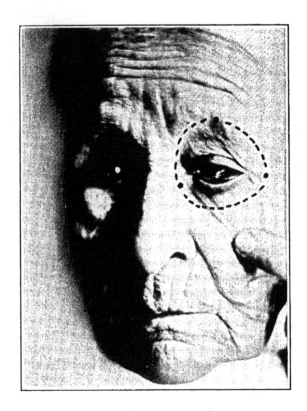

Fig. 3.—Exenteration of the orbit for sarcoma.

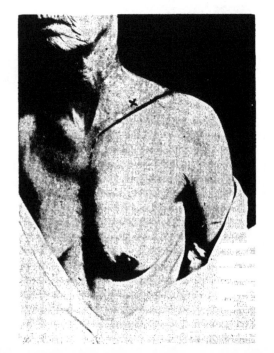

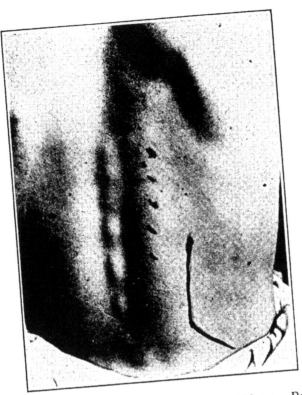

FIG. 5.—Nephrectomy for adenoma of the kidney. Points of intercostal infiltration and injection.

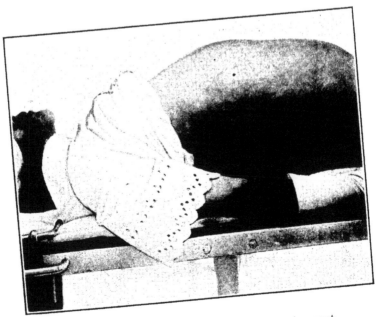

FIG. 6.—Ovariotomy for 43-pound ovarian cyst.

neither can be considered primarily a result either of the anesthesia or the operation.

We note one death in seven major operations on infants under two years of age. We note a mortality rate of 14 per cent. in these infants offering a grave mortality rate from any procedure. The single death from bronchopneumonia twelve days after operation cannot be primarily considered death from anesthesia.

IN CONCLUSION: The selection of local anesthesia, as the anesthetic of choice, in cases offering grave mortality risks, is a factor of safety too potent to be neglected.

Utilization of local anesthesia methods permits of extensive surgical procedure in cases otherwise inoperable.

DISCUSSION ON THE PAPERS OF DRS. LEWIS AND BARTELS AND DR. COLE

DR. J. A. CRISLER, Memphis, Tennessee.—I have been very much interested in these two papers, especially since we have done a considerable amount of work under local anesthesia. We have reported 172 major operations, including practically all ordinary surgical operations, done under local anesthesia with the aid of one tablet of morphin, one-quarter of a grain, and hyoscin, one-hundredth of a grain. This number included also 13 cases of operations done upon the Gasserian ganglion by my associate, as I do not do that work. All manner of goitres and all hernias and some gall-bladder cases and many other major cases, have been operated under local anesthesia. The aged stand it better than young and nervous people.

There is one point I want to ask Dr. Cole to explain, and also to accentuate the value of the method described by Dr. Lewis. We have had three epileptiform convulsions to occur in women while on the operating table who apparently were in perfect health insofar as these symptoms were concerned. They gave no history of epileptiform attacks, yet while undergoing operations in the neighborhood of the uterus, bladder, and ovaries, developed hard convulsions, so that we have abandoned the use of local anesthesia in operations around the bladder and uterus.

Dr. James E. Moore, Minneapolis, Minnesota.—When we first began to use local anesthesia I was considerably prejudiced against it because the only drug we had at our disposal then was cocain, which we all know is dangerous; but it has gradually grown upon me until I have arrived at the point where I think its use is indicated in a great many cases. The idea of its use was impressed upon me the moment a patient was admitted to the University Hospital, Minneapolis, on the medical side, who had a bad heart lesion; her kidneys were badly diseased; she had a large fibroid tumor of the uterus; the abdomen was greatly distended, and, generally speaking, the woman was in a very bad condition. Giving her a general anesthetic was of course out of the question. A medical man asked me to come in to see if we would admit her to the surgical side. He did not expect we would. I talked with Dr. Strauchaur, who is an expert in the use of local anesthesia. I said, "I throw up my hands; I cannot do anything for this woman in her condition." The doctor said, "With you permission, I will operate on this woman under local anesthesia." I said to him, "go to it." To make a long story short, he did a complete abdominal hysterectomy under novocain anesthesia. The woman did not suffer pain or did not suffer shock, and three days after operation, the day before I left home, she was as comfortable as any hysterectomy patients I have ever seen.

It was not intraspinal injection, but local anesthesia alone.

Dr. C. E. Caldwell, Cincinnati, Ohio.—I hesitate to say anything on this subject of local anesthesia, although I have been particularly interested in it, having recently done quite a number of operations under local anesthesia, particularly herniotomies, and just recently I had a case which proved to me the value of local anesthesia in conditions where general anesthesia would be out of the question.

This man was sixty-seven years of age, a chronic alcoholic, with very bad kidneys, casts in his urine, albuminuria, very low hemoglobin content, and a myocarditis, with a very irregular, intermittent pulse, and he came to the hospital after a severe attack of cholecystitis, and remained there for nearly six weeks, getting him into a condition where operation would be advisable. At the time he was ready to leave the hospital, and feeling it would be fatal if he had another attack, I suggested that an operation be carried on under local anesthesia. This was done under the infiltration method with novocain,

1.5 per cent., waiting a sufficiently long time for the anesthetic to have a full effect, and that is the principal thing. My idea is the patient must not suffer the first pain. If you start by causing the patient a little pain, he is put in a psychic condition where he anticipates more; but if you can succeed in opening the abdomen without pain, one will succeed in doing what he wants to do with comparatively little disturbance. In this case there were extensive omental adhesions to the abdominal wall and under surface of the liver; these adhesions were so dense around the gall-bladder that it was with considerable difficulty I broke them up, and the gall-bladder of the *en retrait* type could not be delivered, but I succeeded in opening it, and in delivering a single stone, and draining successfully the submerged gall-bladder. From the time of the operation, two weeks ago tomorrow up to the present time, the man has had absolutely no postoperative symptoms. He has had no pain, no distress of any kind. He asked for a high-ball while he was on the table, and we got it for him before he left the operating room. The only pain he suffered was in closing the abdominal wall when there was traction upon the parietal wall, the anesthetic effect having worn off. I injected a little more novocain to relieve the suffering, and the closure was made with comparative comfort. The patient said he would not care to go through the closure very often, but the operation was entirely successful under local anesthesia. It is the first cholecystostomy I have done under local anesthesia, and I am encouraged to feel that perhaps in some cases it may be advisable to resort to it.

Dr. WILLIAM R. JACKSON, Mobile, Alabama.—I would like to ask Dr. Lewis how long the effect upon the anesthetized area lasted, and did these patients have any inability with reference to their locomotion? In other words, were any of these patients ataxic after operation under local anesthesia?

Dr. A. C. STOKES, Omaha, Nebraska (by invitation).—I wish to thank the members of the Association for the privilege of taking part in this discussion. I have listened with great interest to the papers which have been read at this meeting, and I appreciate this opportunity of saying a few words.

Local anesthesia is a very interesting subject to me although the technic of it has not been well worked out. There are, however, certain principles which we are coming to. First, I believe that morphin and hyoscin and drugs of that kind should be gotten away from as far as possible, as their use in a great many cases is not valuable, and in some cases their use is detrimental. Take old men upon whom we operate for the removal of the prostate, and old women upon whom we operate, and they do not tolerate morphin well at all.

A second point I would make is that the local anesthetic effect should be, if possible, in the neighborhood of operation, as the infiltration of large nerves distant from the field of operation is more or less dangerous and difficult. We should not get too far away from the place on which we intend to operate.

In the third place, almost any operation that has been done under general anesthesia can be performed under local anesthesia, but that does not mean that most of the operations should be done under local anesthesia. There are certain operations which of necessity should always be done under local anesthesia, while other operations should be done under a general anesthetic. It seems to me, minor operations upon the extremities, operations upon the fingers, operations upon the scrotum and penis and lower limbs, can be performed better under local anesthesia than by general anesthesia, and the results be equally as good. Operations for complicated hernia, operations upon the scalp, the abdominal wall or a simple gall-bladder or appendix can be done as successfully with local as with general anesthesia.

DR. BRANSFORD LEWIS, St. Louis, Missouri (closing the discussion on his part).—A well-defined mortality attends various methods of anesthesia, the largest of all pertaining to spinal anesthesia. The question in many of these old prostatic cases is whether they can undergo operation at all or not. We have operated with success on one patient under caudal anesthesia, who had complete retention and had used a catheter for six months. Phthalein was given forty minutes before the color showed up in the urine. The specific gravity was 1004. The phthalein test in the first two hours gave 8 per cent. We rejected the man for operation. We told him he would have to continue using the catheter and sent him back home. Under the continued use of the retained catheter he came back and the phthalein output was 12 per cent. in two hours. We sent him back home again and after two months we received a report to the effect that the phthalein output was 14 per cent. That shows how the phthalein output came up under the influence of complete drainage. The patient subsequently came back for further examination and we found he had 14 per cent. phthalein in the first two hours, and his urine was in much better condition. He was a bad risk for any kind of operation with general anesthesia, so we put him under caudal anesthesia, operated on him without any depression at all.

This case illustrates in a very striking way our favorable experience with caudal anesthesia. It does not produce any shock.

Comparing caudal anesthesia with the infiltration method of anesthesia in cases of prostatectomy, I will say that I have never been able to do prostatectomy with comfort to the patient and with satisfaction to myself under the method of direct injection into the prostate. Dr. Allen, of New Orleans, tells us he does it, but I have not been able to do it. With caudal anesthesia we get regional anesthesia through anesthetizing the sacral plexus. You do not have to go into the prostate, and under difficult conditions make an injection that has limitations from the standpoint of capability. So I think in certain of these urinary operations preference is definitely in favor of the caudal method. The anesthesia will last for two or three hours. The patient can take fluids immediately after the operation. The advantages of caudal anesthesia are greatly in its favor in a large proportion of cases.

DR. H. P. CÓLE, Mobile, Alabama (closing).—In reply to the question of Dr. Crisler, I have not seen epileptic convulsions following local anesthesia except in one case, that of a man who had from four to twenty epileptic convulsions a day, so it was not a surprise to me for him to have a convulsion while on the operating table. His pulse increased to 140 while I was operating on him. I have not seen epileptic convulsions in the other cases.

As Dr. Stokes remarks about scopolamin and morphin, there are undoubtedly cases where the use of scopolamin and morphin is a serious detriment to the individual. I think the majority of cases should be under some form of preoperative sedative and careful preoperative control by the operating staff if you do major surgery under local anesthesia.

One of the main points of failure of successful local anesthesia is in not accurately controlling the surroundings under which you do the operation.

As to the field of local anesthesia in abdominal surgery, it is more difficult to do successful abdominal surgery under local anesthesia than under general anesthesia. Increasing experience gives one a little education in the factors which produce shock and more successsful work is now being done in the abdomen than in the beginning.

Closing the gall-bladder cases is difficult and painful, and where extensive work is required to be done on the gall-bladder it cannot be done with any great comfort.

There is one factor I would call attention to and that is, where extensive operations are done wounds do not heal as readily under local as they do under general anesthesia.

INTUSSUSCEPTION IN INFANTS

By Lewis S. McMurtry, M.D.

Louisville, Kentucky

INTUSSUSCEPTION is essentially an accident of infancy, since three-fourths of the cases obtain in children under two years of age. In a series of three hundred (300) cases collected by Grisel, two hundred and four (204), that is 68 per cent., occurred in breast-fed infants under one year of age. Universal clinical experience confirms these observations, showing that intestinal invagination is an affection of the first period of childhood and particularly is observed in breast-fed infants. Another fact equally well established is that this accident occurs most frequently in vigorous children, and consequently is more common in males than in females.

Of all the varieties of intestinal invagination the ileocecal is by far the most common, and almost invariably is found in cases of infants and young children. Grisel concludes that in infancy 82 per cent. at least are of this variety. The anatomical explanation of this fact doubtless is that the normal ileocecal junction is in the form of an invagination. In infants the cecum is provided with a long mesentery, permitting wide excursions of that viscus; with advancing age the cecum becomes more and more fixed to the posterior abdominal wall, while the small bowel retains its mesentery and consequently its extensive mobility.

The intensity of reflex action is very great in infancy and childhood. Intestinal irritation and muscular spasm beget contraction of the bowel, and peristaltic contracture, aided by straining, drives the contracted bowel into the segment below. The mechanism is the same as that by which a portion of intestine forces its way into a hernial sac. A moment's consideration of the anatomical relations of the ileum and cecum at the point of junction will show how readily the smaller tube may be telescoped into the larger tube as a receptacle. The mesentery is carried in with the attached segment of invaginated bowel, increasing its bulk and adding to the obstruction, forming a vascular and constricted pedicle; venous congestion begets swelling and bleeding, and later follows arterial constriction and gangrene. Under continued peristalsis aided by straining, the invaginated bowel may involve the entire colon and present at the rectum. The tumor of intussusception consists of a mass of invaginated ileum, cecum, colon and mesentery, varying in size with the extent to which the entering segment has advanced in the lumen of the colon. The functional result of this departure from normal anatomical relations is partial or complete obstruction. The mobility of the intussusception is in proportion to the length of the mesentery, and rotating on this as an axis may be carried into the pelvis, up beneath the liver, or to the opposite side of the abdomen.

The onset of this affection is marked by sudden, violent, acute pain. As already stated, the child is vigorous and breast-fed, with good digestion and corresponding disposition perhaps while asleep it is awakened by pain and cries piteously. The pain continues with increasing severity, and the face becomes pale and features pinched. The temperature is low, perhaps subnormal, and vomiting occurs. These symptoms are coincident with the accident. The vomit consists at first of recently ingested food, later of bile; it rarely becomes feculent. Vomiting is due to pain and shock, and the arrest of the fecal current. Usually the vomiting is intermittent, ceasing for an hour or two and then returning. This symptom is rarely absent and is aggravated by food and medicines, especially laxatives which are so frequently given in the initial stage of the disease.

After a few hours the symptoms may spontaneously abate and reaction takes place. This is due to edema and does not indicate release of the invaginated bowel. This temporary relief from pain and shock often proves fatal by obscuring the diagnosis.

Obstruction is not an early symptom of intussusception; it comes on secondarily. Hence at first the child expels gas and fecal matter, but very soon—within a few hours—blood and mucus appear in the stools. Blood and mucus exude from the mucous surface of the invaginated intestine, and pass from the bowel. After the first few stools the discharges from the bowel consist altogether of bloody mucus. As a rule the child will cry and strain and this characteristic bloody stool will be expelled. This symptom is almost pathognomonic. When a healthy infant cries with sudden violent abdominal pain, exhibits the symptoms of shock, vomits, and has frequent stools of blood and mucus, a diagnosis of intussusception, even though no tumor may be found, is practically justified.

As the edema of the invaginated intestine increases the obstruction becomes complete, and as a rule the abdomen becomes tympanitic. If the obstruction is not relieved the patient will succumb to exhaustion and the toxemia resulting from the devitalized intestine. The duration of the disease if left to nature is from two to seven days. In very rare instances, spontaneous sloughing and expulsion of the intussusception, with recovery, have occurred, but this is a rare termination of this affection. It may be laid down as practically an established fact that if an invaginated intestine in infancy is not released within twenty-four hours, the child will die. Exceptions to this will be few and infrequent.

The diagnosis of intestinal invagination during the first

year of life can usually be readily established by the observance of the symptoms described. The sudden onset of violent pain, with shock, vomiting, bloody stools and perhaps an abdominal tumor are as a rule sufficient. The tumor is a variable symptom. In sixteen cases reported by Elliot a tumor was found in ten cases; in six cases no tumor could be felt. While the tumor is most frequently found in the right iliac fossa, it may follow the course of the large intestine and be found under the liver, or may reach the left side of the abdomen and be palpated by the finger in the rectum. In all cases a rectal examination should be made. The bloody mucus which soils the examining finger is significant. It has been suggested that a roentgenogram of the intestine after an injection of bismuth be made, and this procedure has been utilized as a diagnostic aid. Such investigation should be made in every case when practicable, and will often establish a positive diagnosis in doubtful cases.

The most frequent error in diagnosis is to take the beginning of invagination for an attack of enterocolitis. The sudden onset of pain, the frequent bloody stools so characteristic, and without the profuse diarrhea of enterocolitis, together with the rapid alteration of the patient's condition, should suffice to make the distinction.

This condition might readily be confused with acute appendicitis. The tumor of invagination is usually sausage-shaped and mobile; while in appendicitis the swelling is diffuse and immovable. Moreover, appendicitis is marked in the beginning by fever: this does not obtain in intussusception.

In dealing with a case of suspected intussusception in a baby the physician should if possible decide the diagnosis before leaving the house. He should study the case closely, give it immediate attention and weigh each symptom carefully. The fate of the patient depends on early diagnosis.

The excessively high mortality following the treatment of intestinal invagination in infants, even in the most skilled hands, invites attention to this subject and has impelled the writer to offer this paper. One cannot but be impressed with the analogy between intussusception and strangulated hernia; indeed, intussusception is of itself a hernia. The infant at the breast is a very uncertain quantity in surgery, and, moreover, the fact that the hernia involves visceral structures exclusively and is wholly within the abdomen conduce to a more mortal condition than a superficial hernia.

Cathartics and opium for obvious reasons have no place in the treatment of intussusception. Attempts at reduction by means of distention, either with gas or fluids, with inversion of the patient, bear the same relation to this lesion as taxis in strangulated hernia.

In all cases in which the diagnosis is made within a few hours after the telescoping has occurred immediate operation should be done. In that very large proportion of cases in which the surgeon is not called until twenty-four hours have elapsed since the invagination occurred, swelling has taken place to such an extent that very seldom will distention by air or water succeed. There is reliable testimony that in some instances it has succeeded, and hence it should be given a trial in all cases where the disease has advanced beyond the period of operative treatment. The patient should preferably be anesthetized and the body inverted, while by the aid of a soft-rubber catheter and funnel placed above the patient warm saline solution is introduced into the bowel. Gentle palpation along the course of the colon should be applied by the surgeon while the water flows into the bowel. Unless the diagnosis was erroneous, this treatment did succeed in case No. 4 in the appendix to this article.

When abdominal section is done success will depend more upon the operator's expedition and skill, with refinement of manipulation, than in perhaps any other abdominal operations. The young infant is easily shocked. It is very important that the invagination should be reduced by pressure from the apex of the intussusception so that it is pushed out from within instead of being pulled out. The appendix should not be removed unless absolutely necessary, and every effort made to abbreviate the operative procedure. In my own experience I have found chloroform preferable for anesthesia.

It is well known that after release of the invaginated intestine there is a tendency for recurrence of the invagination. To prevent this several operative procedures have been utilized. One is to shorten the mesentery by securing it in a position parallel to the intestine. Elliot adopted the method of attaching the disinvaginated intestine to the parietal peritoneum by a few sutures of catgut. This last method proved satisfactory in his cases. Every addition to the operation that is not absolutely necessary should be omitted, and every moment of time should be conserved in the patient's interest. Even with the best judgment and skill, the mortality of the operations done the first twenty-four hours stands at 40 per cent.

When an irreducible invagination is found, the best procedure perhaps is to establish an artificial opening in the intestine and wait until a later date for the resection of of the invaginated bowel. There is, however, but little choice between this and resection of the intestine at the time, since both procedures are followed by an extremely high mortality. Special methods of resection have been devised by Maunsell, Barker, and others, but unfortunately all methods of resection have yielded poor results. Indeed, a resection of the invaginated intestine in infancy is almost invariably fatal.

I append herewith four illustrative cases of intussusception in infants under one year of age. Two late cases were not operated upon and both died. One was recognized early, operation done and recovered; another came late, and unless there is an error of diagnosis, recovered without operation.

CASE I.—Helm S., male, aged eleven months. Seen with Dr. Sidney J. Meyers. The patient, a vigorous breast-fed child, had been well until three days before, when seized with acute abdominal pain, and shortly afterward had repeated attacks of vomiting. In the evening of the day of attack the child strained and passed blood and mucus from the bowel. This child had suffered with diarrhea some months before, and at first this attack was regarded as a renewal of the previous illness. On the following two days the vomiting was repeated and the mucus and bloody stools persisted, and the child was prostrated and was growing weaker. On examination at my first visit, the temperature was 101° F., pulse 160, respiration 34. The abdomen was prominent and slightly distended, and an oblong tumor, somewhat tender, was felt above and to the right of the umbilicus. Castor oil had been given and was rejected by the stomach, after which small doses of calomel were administered. No fecal matter or gas had passed for twenty-four hours, and the bloody stools were frequent. Rectal injections of warm salt solution had been given without benefit. The condition was too extreme to urge operation, to which the parents were much opposed, and death occurred the following day.

CASE II.—May C., aged nine months, was brought by her parents to the Gray Street Infirmary in the early morning. The patient was a healthy well-nourished female child and the mother stated that she had been seized in the night with severe abdominal pain, followed soon afterward by vomiting. She had had several fecal movements, and cried almost constantly from pain. The features were pinched and the child was very ill. A distinct tumor about the size of an egg was felt on the right side slightly below the umbilical line. The temperature was normal, pulse 132. Upon making a rectal examination, blood followed the withdrawal of the finger from the rectum.

Operation nine hours after the onset of the attack. Chloroform anesthesia. Under anesthesia the tumor was well defined and the incision was made in the right semilunar line. The peritoneum contained very little fluid. The intussusception was of the ileocecal variety, the apex being well advanced in the ascending colon. The reduction was readily accomplished by expression, aided by slight traction at the last. The abdomen was closed without drainage. Duration of operation about twenty minutes.

There was one bloody stool after the operation, and vomiting occurred twice, but the pulse was reduced almost to normal in a few hours, and the pain was relieved. On the day following operation there were several rather offensive stools, but free from blood and mucus. On this day the temperature was 102° F., but fell to normal the next day and remained so throughout. The convalescence was rapid from this time and recovery complete. The child nursed from the mother throughout the whole time. The healing was by primary union.

CASE III.—Henry C., aged ten months, from Tell City, Indiana, seen with Dr. P. F. Barbour. The patient was a vigorous child, breast-fed, and had been well until three days prior to coming to Louisville. The attack had come on suddenly in the early morning with violent abdominal pain, followed by vomiting. Bloody stools were observed on the second day, and complete obstruction followed. On examination I found the abdomen distended, but a sausage-shaped tumor could be distinctly felt on the left side above the umbilical line. The child was very ill and suffered almost constant pain. The temperature was 102° F., the pulse rapid. Bloody stools were frequent.

The unpromising nature of operation under existing conditions was explained to the parents, and they refused it. Death occured on the sixth day of the attack.

CASE IV.—H. S., male, aged seven months, was brought by his parents from their home near Hanover, Indiana, to Dr. Wm. Jenkins, in Louisville, on October 11, of this year. The patient is a strong, healthy child, nursing his mother, and had never been ill. On October 8, three and a half days before, he was seized suddenly with acute abdominal pain, followed in a few hours by vomiting. He was seen at once by the family physician, who administered a dose of castor oil, presuming the trouble to be indigestion. The vomiting persisted, the features were pinched, the face pale, and on the following day blood and mucus were discharged from the bowels. The family doctor made a diagnosis of intussusception and on the third day brought the patient to Dr. Jenkins for consultation. Dr. Jenkins confirmed the diagnosis and called me for consultation.

On examination the child appeared very ill. The temperature 101° F., pulse very rapid, pallor, vomiting and frequent paroxysms of pain completed the typical array of symptoms characterizing intussusception. The abdomen was considerably distended, and no gas or fecal matter had passed from the bowels for thirty-six hours. He was placed in Norton Memorial Infirmary at once. The child's condition seemed so extreme that I did not urge operation. He refused to nurse, and when urged to do so the milk was rejected by the stomach. Twice daily warm salt solution was slowly injected into the bowel by means of a soft rubber catheter, tube and funnel, the patient being held in the mother's lap during the time almost in the inverted position. Neither fecal matter nor gas came away as the water was expelled or otherwise. The small stools of blood and mucus persisted.

On the third day after admission to the Infirmary, and the sixth day of the illness, about two hours after receiving an enema, a small fecal stool with gas passed, to be followed in two hours by a copious fecal evacuation.

Relief from pain was immediate; the child nursed with avidity, and from this time improvement was rapid. He returned home on the fifth day after admission to the Infirmary and quickly regained perfect health.

The classic symptoms of intussusception were presented by this patient, and if the diagnosis was correct the case is almost unique in the clinical history of this very fatal disease.

DISCUSSION

DR. STEPHEN H. WATTS, Charlottesville, Virginia.—Three or four years ago I presented before this Association a paper on intussusception in the adult. At that time I reported, I believe, three cases in which the intussusception was due to the presence of a tumor or tumors within the intestine, and at the same time, I discussed the etiology of intussusception in both adults and in children. I believe that the most important etiological factor in the occurrence of intussusception in children is the persistence of the fetal type of intestine, namely, a very loose ascending colon. If you will recall that most intussusceptions increase at the expense of the colon and that in certain cases the intussusceptum may even present in the rectum you will readily see that this presupposes a considerable degree of mobility in the colon which can only result from a long mesentery. Bearing this in mind it seems to me that the best way to prevent recurrence of such intussusceptions is to fasten the cecum in place which can be accomplished by suturing the outside of the cecum to the parietal peritoneum for a distance of two or three inches.

DR. HUBERT A. ROYSTER, Raleigh, North Carolina.—I desire to mention two cases of intussusception in infants in which the patients were lucky and the operator more so.

In the first case, nature shut off the perforation and, in the second place, the medical man made the diagnosis in time.

The first case was in a child, two and a half months old, whose intussusception existed for forty-eight hours. I operated under very unfavorable circumstances, but was fortunate enough to find that the perforation of the colon, which had occurred on the longitudinal line, was shut off and no damage was done. I was able to free the gut, get hold of the perforation and secure it before any leaking occurred. This case ended in recovery.

The second case presented a feature of some interest. The child was four months old, and was brought in eight hours after the initial symptoms. The physician who had the case was a recent graduate and he made the diagnosis promptly and correctly. The interesting feature was the fact that the only gangrenous portion in the whole area was the appendix. It was presenting at its tip, just in the centre of the cup of the intussuscipiens, and I first thought it was a blood clot because of its dark color; but, milking it back, I found that the appendix was gangrenous throughout its whole extent being grasped so tightly by the tissues of the bowel. Milking it out and closing the abdomen were done in about ten minutes.

DR. F. W. PARHAM, New Orleans, Louisiana.—I should like to report the case in a child, aged sixteen months, in which I was fortunate for the reason that Dr. Royster has mentioned, the diagnosis having been promptly made by an internist. I was thus fortunate in seeing the patient within the first twenty-four hours after the inception of the intussusception. The patient presented all the classical signs of intussusception and I could feel the tumor distinctly with the finger in the rectum. I could feel a long mass to the left of the rectus. I made an incision on the left side because I thought I would be better able to deal with the intussusception through that incision. Having opened the abdomen, I found a long intussusception, but could not at once make out the beginning of it. I traced it back and found it was an intussusception through the ileocecal valve. I was able without much difficulty to reduce it, and having reduced it, there was no sign of any gangrene at any point. I passed a chromic gut suture through a tenia close to the base of the appendix, and having made an incision at the right of MacBurney's point, I caught the suture with a long forceps passed through into the abdomen, pulled it through, and tied it in the iliac wound. The operation was only very slightly prolonged by this procedure. The child recovered. On account of the ease with which I was able to reduce the long intussusception, I thought it worth while to report the case.

DR. ROBERT T. MORRIS, New York City.—I would like to speak on two points:

Point 1. In addition to the anatomical difficulties which Dr. McMurtry has set forth so clearly, there may be in some cases a contributing factor in toxic influence. Some years ago, when experimenting with rabbits on the question of reverse peristalsis,

I found that if we touched a part of the bowel with carbonate of sodium it contracted in spasms. That contractive part became intussuscepted by progressive peristalsis. That led to the conclusion that in some cases toxins influencing the ganglia of the bowel wall might cause local contraction of the bowel in local spasm, and that contracted part might be swallowed by progressive peristalsis.

Point 2. In one case of desperate ileo-intussusception I made a quick anastomosis, and in addition fastened the line of intussusception with three or four sutures of Pagenstecher's thread. That stopped the intussusception, and gave relief from the symptoms immediately. The child died, however, three or four days later. It was a far-advanced case. I believe in selected cases this sort of operation might be sometimes effective.

Dr. J. Garland Sherrill, Louisville, Kentucky.—We learn more sometimes by our failures than from our successes, and if this is true, I should have learned something last year about intussusception. On May 23 I was called to see a child in the fourth day of illness with intussusception. The reason for the delay was that the family changed doctors three or four times. Finally a physician made the diagnosis and the case was referred to me. The child was in a bad condition, but I attempted operation to relieve it without success.

On June 9 I saw another case wherein a prompt diagnosis was made and the patient brought in from the country, twelve hours after the inception of the disease. Perhaps I should reprove myself, because notwithstanding the fact that early diagnosis was made I was unable to save the patient in this case.

The condition mentioned by Dr. Watts and Dr. McMurtry was present. There was an ample cecum with the gut invaginated, part of the ileum and almost entire colon being carried around to the left side. I found it was not an easy task at all to separate the invaginated portion, although there was no firm adhesion. The gut at the point of invagination was contracted, and I was impressed with the fact that I had not done the correct thing in either case when I attempted to withdraw the intussusception before making the resection. With the gut going in at this point the ileocecal valve (indicating), the invaginated part was greatly contracted, the mesentery and mesocolon were crowded into a hard mass, so that when pulled out the vessels were thrombotic. With hernia of the gut into another intestine, time may be conserved by making an incision through the outer layer of the gut or by cutting through the mesentery at this point. If we cut through the mesentery at this point (indicating) and free the gut, a long loop remains which requires resection. In most cases that have gone beyond twenty-four hours the vessels will have become thrombotic, and is it not better to make a temporary opening and later do resection? A temporary opening in children is always dangerous. Later resection is an added danger, and the question arises whether a primary resection or a later one after a temporary enterostomy, offers most for the patient.

DR. IRVIN ABELL, Louisville, Kentucky.—As illustrating the idea that intussusception may be due to a disturbance of peristalsis, I wish to mention briefly two cases that came under my observation, both of which were older than those reported by Dr. McMurtry. One was a child two and one-half years of age, and the other a child three years of age. In both of these cases the intussusception was brought on by an acute enteritis from eating green fruit. In both instances the intussusception was in the descending colon; in both the condition was recognized early, the intussusception reduced, and both recovered.

DR. LEWIS S. MCMURTRY, Louisville, Kentucky (closing).— The purpose of this paper will have been subserved if the fellows of this Association can be induced to exert their influence, as they have done on so many important practical surgical subjects, with the profession at large to popularize the knowledge that leads to the diagnosis of this disease, so that surgeons will get this class of cases earlier than they do at the present time.

There is, so far as I can recall, no surgical lesion wherein the fate of the patient so absolutely depends on early interference following an early diagnosis as does this affection.

I am familiar with Dr. Watts's cases which he presented in a paper on the etiology and I thoroughly concur in the view that there is a congenital peculiarity about the conformation of the structures at the caput coli and ileocecal junction which favors this accident.

Dr. Parham has presented a very important point, and that is, in these large intussusceptions it is very important to take some step before closing the abdomen to prevent a relapse which is so common; that the conditions preceding the occurrence of intussusception are far more frequent than the incidence of this disease. There should be some rapid method, and the one suggested by Dr. Parham is excellent, by introducing a suture and bringing the bowel back to proper position and fixing it there.

Dr. Morris brought out an unique feature regarding the effect of irritation in producing this condition. All studies seem to justify the fact that in vigorous infants the nervous system responds to an irritant by the reflex action so vital in childhood, contracting the intestine by strong peristaltic movements.

Dr. Morris and Dr. Sherrill have referred to the resection of the gut. Certainly, there needs to be an improveent in our technic in this matter. Resection of the involved intestine in an infant that has been ill for two or three days with intussusception, is almost invariably fatal, deferring the operation of resection adds very little by way of solving the problem. Resection is nearly always fatal in such cases, and we should strive to make a vigorous fight to get these patients earlier for operation.

Dr. Abell's cases are very interesting and confirm what I have already stated, that irritation is the initial factor in the causation of intussusception.

I am very grateful for the interest taken in the subject by the members.

HYDATID CYST OF THE LIVER, WITH REPORT OF TWO CASES

By George Ben Johnston, M.D.
Richmond, Virginia

WE have had two cases of hydatid cyst of the liver during the past two years, and about six months ago another case was operated on in a Richmond Hospital. This is remarkable, because of the fact that prior to 1913 only two cases of tænia echinococcus infection were reported from Virginia, and 250 from United States and Canada. The Virginia cases occurred in Alexandria and Staunton. There was, however, another case that was infected in Virginia, but was reported from Buffalo by Cary and Lyons.

During the winter of 1913–1914 several epidemics of tænia echinococcus appeared in Virginia raised hogs. In one consignment from Charles City County, slaughtered in Richmond under the supervision of the Bureau of Animal Industries, there were 46 animals, and all 46 were infected with the tænia echinococcus. In another shipment from Goochland County there were eight hogs, five of which were infected. In a number of small consigments during the winter of 1913–1914 there were one or more animals infected with this parasite. In November of this year in a shipment of sixty hogs from Charlotte County, fifteen were infected with hydatids (25 per cent.).

Dr. Hall states in Bulletin 206, U. S. Department of Agriculture, "that recent abattoir figures show an alarming prevalence of disease in domestic animals in some parts of this country, notably in certain localities in Virginia, Arkansas and Oklahoma; and the prevalence of hydatids in domestic animals is an index of the danger to which people are exposed. The bare fact that hydatids occur at all in the United States is of itself a cogent argument for the suppression of the dog nuisance as a measure necessary for the public welfare."

It may be a mere coincidence, but to me it is more than one that the sudden increase of tænia echinococcus in human beings should parallel an increase of the condition in hogs. Can there be a relation between the two? If not, are the dogs in Virginia more heavily infected than formerly? These questions are extremely interesting, but difficult of investigation.

Dr. Marshall[1] tells me that it has been his observation that hogs raised in a small pen are more frequently infected with hydatid disease than hogs raised with ample pasturage. The hogs that are particularly prone to this infection are those which are fed from the table and kitchen refuse. He explains this by the fact that the smell of food attracts the dog, in consequence of which, the farmer feeding his hogs is invariably accompanied to the pen by a dog. In this way the hogs come in close contact with dogs or with the egesta from dogs, and the dangers of infection are thereby accentuated.

If there is any relation between hydatids in men and hydatids in hogs, we would naturally look for it in rural districts, because in these districts the slaughter of animals is not supervised by the Bureau of Animal Industries, and there the hogs are more frequently infected and the offal is not as carefully dealt with as in the abattoirs where inspection is rigid.

Many may be directly infected from careless use of infected organs, but I am inclined to think that most of our echino-

[1] Bureau of Animal Industries, Richmond, Va.

coccus infections are traceable to the water supply and to raw vegetables contaminated by egesta from dogs. The disease, however, is conveyed to the dog by the eating of infected organs, and in this respect the hog is active in keeping alive this condition in certain localities in Virginia.

Our two cases came from the rural districts, and they were frequently exposed to infection both from dogs and from meat that was not properly inspected.. The case that was operated on in Richmond several months ago and alluded to above, occurred in a foreigner who had lived in this country a short while. Our cases, however, were not from the region in which the epidemics in hogs were reported. We have in mind these infected regions and are waiting to see if there will be a relative increase in infections of the tenia echinococcus among our patients living in these localities.

Geographically, tænia echinococcus is a widespread disease, and in certain countries it occurs with great frequency, especially is this true in Iceland and Australia. In the former country, according to the statistics of Galliot, one out of thirty of the entire population is infected. In Australia the returns extending over many years of the Mount Gambier Hospital show one hydatid patient for every sixty-five admitted for all complaints. In both Iceland and Australia sheep raising is done on a large scale, and a survey of the geographical distribution of the hydatid disease leads to the conclusion that sheep and especially fine-wooled sheep, such as the Merino breed, are responsible to a large extent for the infections in dogs. In Australia and Iceland 40 per cent. of the unregistered dogs were found to be infected.

I believe that the hog is playing the same role in Virginia that the sheep is playing in Australia and Iceland, and that if a search was made we would find that tænia echinococcus is more frequent in Virginia dogs than we suppose, and further that the tenia echinococcus infections are increasing

among them. According to Hall, the prevalence of hydatids
in dogs is an index of the danger to which people are exposed.
If this be true we naturally look for an increase of infections
with tenia echinococcus in man throughout Virginia.

Echinococcus in man shows two forms, the echinococcus
hydatidosus and the echinococcus alveolaris. Both of our
infections were of the hydatic type, and for this reason we
will confine ourselves more to this type of the disease.
The alveolar type is seldom seen in this country, but is
fairly common in some portions of Austria and Germany.
The alveolar type is usually a fatal infection.

The distribution of hydatids in the body, according to the
table compiled by Thomas, shows the different organs are
attacked in the following percentages: Liver 57, lungs 11.6,
kidneys 4.7, brain 4.4, spleen 2.1, heart 1.8, peritoneum 1.4.

The echinococcus cyst originates primarily from a little
tape-worm found in dogs. This tape-worm sheds off its
terminal proglottis which is filled with a large number of
eggs. This passes out of the intestinal tract with the egesta
and sooner or later the eggs are liberated from the proglottis,
and they may float about on particles of dust, or they may
be carried to a neighboring water supply. Human beings
and domestic animals drinking this water or inhaling dust
thus ladened are subjected not to a tape-worm infection but
to an infection characterized by the presence of hydatids
or bladder-like bodies located in the different organs.

The eggs which are taken into the gastro-intestinal tract
in human beings probably get into the liver through the
lymphatics, and there (liver) in the interlobular tissue they
produce these cyst-like bodies which show two separate
and distinct capsules, an inner or brood capsule which as the
name implies tends to reproduce the parasite, and an outer
or fibro-elastic tissue capsule, which is supplied by the organ
in which the cyst is located. The hydatid grows at the
expense of an organ, and strange as it may seem the organ
seems to take kindly to the growing cyst. Such cells as are

destroyed by the cyst are replaced elsewhere in the organ by a compensatory hypertrophy, and unless the cysts are quite numerous and growth quite rapid there is little loss of function of the organ. The fibrous tissue capsule surrounding these cysts is seldom thick, and is practically always vascular so as to be able to furnish the cysts with nutrition.

The symptomatology of hydatids depends almost entirely upon the pressure effects exerted upon the organ. In the liver there may be an aching about the right shoulder, a sense of weight and distention. Actual pain is rare, but if suppuration intervenes, as sometimes occurs in the liver, excruciating pains in the liver region may exist. On the other hand, not infrequently an autopsy may reveal a cyst of considerable size which gave no symptoms. The liver may enlarge and may extend below the costal arch and higher up into the thoracic cavity, especially is this true in large, deep-seated cysts. The rupture of a hydatid cyst of the liver is dangerous. The contents of the cyst may be squirted into the pleural cavity or peritoneal cavity, depending of course upon the location of cyst. With a rupture the infection may become widespread.

TREATMENT. So far as I know, surgery is the only method of treatment for this condition. Wherever possible it is always best to remove the cyst *in toto*, if this be impossible to remove, as much of the cyst as possible, and drain, and if this be impossible to aspirate the cyst. The whole question of treatment is well summed up in *Albutt's System of Medicine,* in an article by Sterling and Verco.

"1. The objections to aspiratory puncture are that it is only applicable to a small class of cases; that even in these it frequently fails in its object; that it is in itself a possible source of danger, by inducing suppurative changes, or by permitting leakage of fluid with possible consequences that we have sufficiently indicated; and that, at least, it leaves the dead organism in place. In pulmonary hydatids there is a special risk of suffocative flooding.

"2. Removal of the parasite by incision is an effectual and, with proper care, a reasonably safe proceeding; it should be the recognized and general practice.

"3· Lindemann's operation, in which, after removal of the parasite, the activity of the adventitious sac is left to drain externally, has stood the test of a large experience with favorable results, and is probably the best and safest procedure for general application. Possibly, however, Bond's operation, or some modification of it, in which, after evacuation, the emptied adventitious sac is left behind, may prove to be more satisfactory in certain cases, the proper limits of which have yet to be determined by the test of experience."

Case reports:

CASE I.—Married woman, aged forty-eight years, entered Abingdon Hospital, April 10, 1915, complaining of a mass located in upper portion of right abdomen.

Family History: Unimportant.

Past History: Unimportant.

Present illness began about two years ago with dull pain in upper right abdomen. Sometime after the pain began she noticed a small lump in the region in which the pain was located. This lump has grown steadily until it has reached its present dimension. At no time was the pain severe. She has never been jaundiced, and seldom nauseated. She has lost considerable weight during the past two years, and during the last three or four months she has been unable to attend to her household work. Examination was entirely negative, except for a mass about the size of a cocoanut lying in the right upper quadrant; this mass was tender, was movable with respiration, was smooth or symmetrical, and apparently was separate from the liver.

Urine negative. Blood examination negative.

Operation April 10, 1915. The abdomen was opened by a high right rectus incision. On entering the abdominal cavity a large cyst attached to the under surface of the liver was seen, and several smaller cysts were found to be imbedded in the liver substance. The largest cyst (about the size of an orange) was enucleated without rupture. The liver was sutured with catgut to control the bleeding, the other cysts were left. Wound closed without drainage. Patient's post-operative course was uneventful and she was discharged from the hospital on the sixteenth day. Since her operation she has been feeling quite well.

Hooklets were found in the cyst fluid.

CASE II.—Married woman, aged sixty-two years, entered Johnston-Willis Sanatorium, April 20, 1914, complaining of epigastric pain.

Family History: Unimportant.

Past History: Unimportant.

Present illness began two years ago with a pain in right shoulder and a slight epigastric discomfort. There was some nausea and occasional vomiting attacks after meals. At no time was the pain severe. She has lost some weight. She has never been jaundiced, and her bowels have moved with regularity.

Physical Examination: Entirely negative, except for a slight tenderness and a mass about the size of the fist in the epigastrium.

Urine negative. Blood examination negative.

Stomach examination: Negative.

Under ether anesthesia, April 22, 1914, the abdomen was entered through a high right rectus incision. The liver was examined and found to contain a large number of cysts, ranging in size from an orange to a walnut, and seemed to be deep down in the liver substance. The aspirated fluid was clear and colorless. No scolices were found in the aspirated fluid. None of the cysts were removed and the wound was closed and drain was put at the sight of the aspirated cyst. The patient's convalescence was satisfactory and she was discharged from the hospital May 14, 1914.

THE OPERATIVE TREATMENT OF PYLORIC OBSTRUCTION IN INFANTS—WITH A REVIEW OF SIXTY-SIX PERSONAL CASES

By William A. Downes, M.D.
New York

In April, 1914, I reported the operative results obtained in 22 cases of pyloric obstruction in infants. At that time the symptoms of the disease were given, also measures necessary to establish the diagnosis, and reasons stated which seemed sufficient to justify the opinion that surgical intervention was indicated in every case in which definite obstruction was present or seemed imminent.

Since that report was made, 44 additional cases of this disease have come under my care, making a total of 66 cases, observed in five and one-half years. This added experience has in many ways been a source of much gratification, but has not been without its disappointments. To begin with it has not enabled us to add anything new to the etiology or pathology of the disease, notwithstanding the fact, that partial or complete necropsy was obtained in every case dying in the hospital.

With one exception there was the characteristic tumor at the pylorus. All showed marked hypertrophy of the band of circular muscle fibers with the redundant and thickened mucous membrane lying in longitudinal folds. The tumor in the single exception noted above while of considerable size was less firm, and the incised muscle not more than half as thick as in the average case. These differences were noted, but were not properly interpreted. The baby continued to vomit after operation and died in 18 hours. At necropsy, Dr. Martha Wollstein, pathologist to the Babies' Hospital, discovered a small tumor, originating in the muscularis mucosa, projecting into and filling the lumen of the pylorus.

Most of the stomachs were of an average size, a few very large and 2 or 3 very small—one was so small that it would hold only 1 ounce. Edema in varying degrees, involving the pylorus and pyloric region of the stomach was present in all cases, and in a few instances it was present through the stomach wall. We believe the presence of this edema plays a very important role and is the factor which determines the definite onset of symptoms.

The theory that best explains the sequence of events in this disease is, that a true malformation is present at birth consisting of an abnormal thickening of the circular muscle of the pylorus, and that the effort necessary to force food through the narrowed and elongated pyloric lumen produces circulatory disturbance resulting in edema. As the food is increased in amount and the muscular effort becomes greater the lumen narrows down until finally at the tenth day or a little later it becomes more or less completely obstructed. In support of this theory would call attention to the fact, that after the symptoms have developed, a reduction in the amount of food with consequent relief of muscular effort, together with systematic stomach washing which removes curds and mucus, will often give temporary relief and in an exceptional case if the muscular hypertrophy is not too extensive carry the child along for a time. However, as the food is again increased all the symptoms recur.

In Case 7, typical symptoms began at 5 weeks, which under careful feeding and lavage subsided in a few days, and the child began to gain; 3 weeks later, however, after increased feedings, there was a recurrence with sudden marked depression requiring immediate operation.

As shown by Holt, definite persistent pyloric spasm without hypertrophy has yet to be proven. This author prefers to divide cases showing the symptom complex under discussion into mild and severe types, and recommends that the term "pylorospasm" be discarded. Unquestionably, there is a definite element of spasm in these cases, but it is the result of and not the cause of the hypertrophy.

SYMPTOMS. The group of symptoms which go to make the diagnosis is projectile vomiting, tumor, peristaltic waves, gastric retention and rapid loss of weight. Marked constipation is usually present, although a starvation stool or even one containing milk may occur from time to time, depending entirely upon the degree of obstruction. So much has already been said in reference to the symptoms and diagnostic signs, that I will take up but one, and that is the question of tumor.

In every case here reported the presence of a tumor, described as varying in size from the terminal phalanx of the little finger to that of the thumb was noted by at least two or more observers and so charted before operation. In a few instances where there was some doubt owing to difficulties in palpation, light anesthesia (ethyl chloride inhalation) was required. This procedure is simple and the information of such value that any slight risk is more than offset. Before administering the anesthetic a tube should be passed to the stomach. This removes the gas and makes it much easier to palpate the tumor which lies to the right and above the umbilicus. I consider the presence of this so-called tumor pathognomonic of the disease. The various house physicians at the Babies' Hospital, where most of the cases were observed have expressed the same view. The diagnosis based upon this sign alone was frequently made by them in the admitting room.

Those who state that a tumor can be found in a small percentage of cases only—have either seen too few patients with this disease for their opinion to be of value, or else have failed to make a proper examination. That vomiting, loss of weight, retention and all the symptoms of high obstruction in the alimentary canal may occur without a palpable tumor at the pylorus there is no doubt. One such case was operated upon at the Babies' Hospital, in which a heavy peritoneal band passed from a loop of the ileum across the hepatic flexure of the colon and was adherent to the duodenum in such a way as to cause complete obstruction. Without operation or necropsy this case might have been recorded as one of pyloric obstruction in which no tumor existed.

OPERATIVE TREATMENT. Obstruction at the pylorus is just as definitely an obstruction of the intestinal tract as that situated at any other part of the canal. It belongs to the obturation type which is without strangulation and is therefore without the toxemia of the more acute form. The sudden marked depression with collapse and death seen in the neglected cases is not toxic in character, but the result of starvation. With this knowledge of the disease it would seem that the rational treatment to adopt is that designed to relieve the cause of the obstruction at the earliest possible moment.

Until within recent years the operative results in pyloric obstruction were so uncertain that physicians did not feel justified in recommending surgical treatment. Now, that the disease is better understood and the operative technic greatly improved these objections no longer hold. Under the most favorable conditions and in the best hands cases treated medically are long drawn out—10 to 12 weeks or even longer, with the result always in doubt, and the knowledge ever present that without the slightest warning the baby may go into collapse and die, even though its progress had been favorable.

At the present time the opinion of most pediatricians with unbiased minds is almost a unit as to the necessty of operation in these cases once the diagnosis is established. In the cases seen and diagnosed early, some feel that a few days of careful observation with proper feeding and lavage, is justified with the hope that the symptoms may subside, others, advise immediate operation in every case. All agree that most cases surviving operation make a rapid and satisfactory recovery.

A number of operative procedures have been resorted to in the surgical treatment of pyloric obstruction, only two of which, however, posterior gastro-enterostomy and partial pyloroplasty, have given results sufficiently satisfactory to warrant adoption.

So far as I know the largest individual series of operated cases heretofore reported have been those of Richter, Scudder and myself. Posterior gastro-enterostomy was the procedure adopted by each of us and the mortality rate was 14 per cent., 24 per cent., and 32 per cent. respectively. The total number of cases in these 3 series was 61, with a mortality of 22 per cent. This was a much lower rate than any previously recorded for so large a number of cases. In my own hands, the mortality following gastroenterostomy continued above 30 per cent. This was due in part to the critical condition of the infants at the time of admission to the hospital. Operation being refused in no case, but there were a number of deaths which could not be attributed wholly to the condition of the babies. It was the effort to avoid seemingly uncontrollable fatal complications which occurred late in the convalescence of these babies that caused us to give up gastroenterostomy, at least for the time being. Therefore, in October, 1914, we decided to give the so-called partial pyloroplasty of Rammstedt a thorough trial, and our results have been more satisfactory since that date. 31 of the 66 infants included in this report had a gastro-enterostomy done, and 35 were operated according to the method of Rammstedt. The operation in 19 of those done by the latter method was modified to the extent of passing a sound through the pylorus after the muscle had been divided. The sound was introduced through a small incision made in the stomach wall

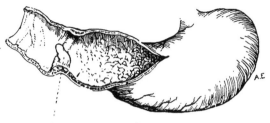

Tumor occupying pyloric opening

FIG. 1.—Tumor occupying pyloric opening. (From sketch made at time of necropsy.)

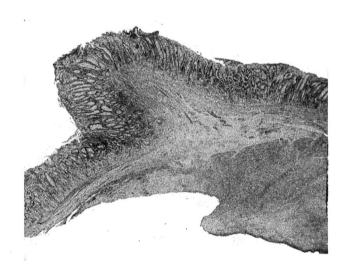

FIG. 2.—Cross-section of tumor arising from muscularis mucosæ, shown in Fig. 1.

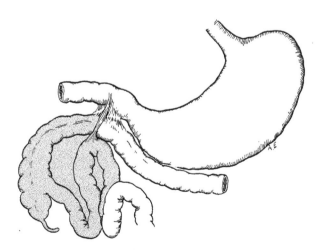

FIG. 3.—Peritoneal band passing from ileum across hepatic flexure and adherent to duodenum, causing obstruction.

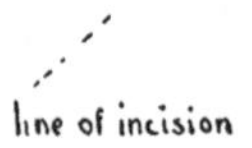

line of incision

FIG. 4.—First step of Rammstedt operation. Tumor supported.
Line of incision shown.

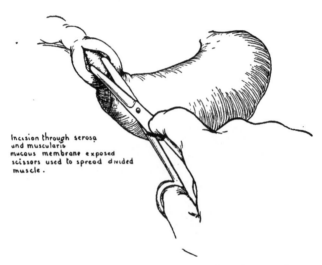

Incision through serosa
und muscularis
mucous membrane exposed
scissors used to spread divided
muscle.

FIG. 5.—Second step showing completed operation.

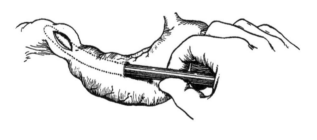

FIG. 6.—Modified Rammstedt operation. Sound passed through
pylorus after circular muscle has been divided. (This modification has
been discontinued.)

some distance from the pylorus. This procedure is similar to that recommended by Keefe, with the exception, that the sound is passed after the circular muscle is divided and not before.

The gastro-enterostomies were done according to the posterior-no loop method, with the exception of the first 2 cases where clamps were not used. Time of operation varied from 25 to 45 minutes. The partial pyloroplasty or "nicking of the circular muscle fibers" consisted in making a longitudinal incision from 2 to 3 cm. in length through the serosa and the hypertrophied circular muscle fibers of the pylorus down to the thickened mucosa. Duration of operation 10 to 20 minutes. In performing this operation the pyloric tumor should be held firmly between the thumb and index finger, and as the incision is deepened the edges of the wound gently forced apart. After the muscle is cut through, a definite line of cleavage is seen to exist between the muscle and the mucous membrane. A small pair of blunt-pointed curved scissors may be used to advantage in spreading the incision. When the muscle is sufficiently divided the liberated mucous membrane protrudes freely into the wound. There is very little hemorrhage—occasionally a small vessel may require a ligature, but as a rule the application of hot pads to the edges of the wound for a few minutes controls the bleeding. This completes the operation. The tumor is dropped back into the abdomen and the wound closed.

In spreading the incision and separating the muscle from the mucous membrane it is best to start from the stomach end of the incision as here the merging of stomach wall into pyloric tumor is a gradual one, and there is not much danger of opening the mucous membrane; whereas, the change from the thickened and edematous pylorus to normal duodenum is so sudden that extreme care is necessary, in order to avoid opening the intestine at this point. On account of this accident some operators have discarded this operation and returned to gastro-enterostomy. It occurred twice early in our series, but fortunately the openings were small and very easily closed—no bad effect followed. It is not necessary to cover the incision at the pylorus with omentum, or to attempt its closure with flaps from the muscle, nor should the effort be made to close the wound by converting the longitudinal into a transverse incision. It is very difficult to get sutures to hold in this tissue and besides there is risk of again narrowing the lumen. The fact that the mucous membrane did not give way in one of our 35 cases is sufficient proof, that any effort to reinforce the wound is unnecessary.

For fear that simple division of the hypertrophied circular muscle fibers did not quite meet all the indications in these cases, I decided to modify the operation as already stated. This was done 19 times, and in every case a No. 20 sound (French scale) passed through the pylorus without the slightest resistance. The cases in which this modification of the Rammstedt operation was done did no better than those operated by the simpler method, and it was soon discarded. Not, however, until one and possibly two fatalities resulted from its use. At times it was very difficult in the small thick-walled stomachs to properly close the incision made for the passage of the sound. In one instance a stitch gave way and the baby died of peritonitis. A second case of peritonitis occurred where this method was used, and it is very likely infection resulted from the incision into the stomach although no leakage could be discovered at necropsy.

RESULTS. The general condition of the babies subjected to the two operative procedures—gastro-enterostomy and partial pyloroplasty—averaged much the same. Several in each group were almost moribund at the time of operation. The stimulating effect of ether and the value of hypodermoclysis is well shown in these cases as most of them were in as good condition at the close of the operation as they had been at the beginning. All cases survived the immediate effect of operation—the earliest death occurring in 3 hours. The smallest baby in the entire series weighed 3 lbs. 15 oz.;

the largest 9 lbs. 9 oz.; average weight 6½ lbs. The smallest baby recovering after gastro-enterostomy weighed 5 lbs., and after the Rammstedt operation 4 lbs. The average age for the series was 6 weeks, youngest 3 weeks, oldest 20 weeks. Of the 31 cases in which gastro-enterostomy was performed, 11 died, giving a mortality of 35 per cent.; 2 died as a direct result of faulty technic; 3 died in a few hours, and 6 died in from 5 to 19 days after operation. Of the 20 cases discharged as cured 2 died within a short time from acute gastro-enteritis, and 1 died in 3 months from diphtheria. The remaining 17 cases are alive at the present time, all are will and have developed normally in every way.

So far as I can find out no late complications have followed the gastro-enterostomy. Röntgen-ray examination of several of the cases from one to three years after operation shows that the stomata are working satisfactorily and that little or no bismuth passes the pylorus, thus proving that the obstruction is permanent and that it is not influenced by this type of operation. The latter observation is also borne out by the fact that at necropsy in the case dying 3 months after operation the tumor was unchanged. It is only fair to say, that the 3 cases dying shortly after operation were in extremis and it is doubtful if the final result was influenced to any appreciable degree by the operation. It is to the group of 6 cases dying from five to nineteen days after operation, that I wish to call special attention—1 died on the 5th day of acute nephritis; 3 cases continued to vomit moderately for a few days, this gradually grew worse until death which took place on the 6th, 15th, and 19th days. The case dying on the 15th day was re-operated shortly before it died, but no cause for the continued vomiting could be found. Necropsy in the other 2 cases likewise failed to explain the persistence of the symptoms. The two remaining cases developed diarrhea, became depressed and in spite of every effort died in from ten to twelve days. In none of these cases did postmortem examination show peritonitis or in any way explain the fatal result with the exception of the one case dying of nephritis. The anastomoses were properly located, had healed, but in 3 cases failed to functionate as they should. It is on account of this unfortunate experience which is without satisfactory explanation that we decided to try other measures for the relief of pyloric obstruction.

Of the 35 partial pyloroplasties—1 was done in April, 1914, and has been previously reported. 1 was operated upon the following May, and the rest since October, 1914. 8 deaths occurred in this series, a mortality of 23 per cent.—2 died of peritonitis following the modified operation as already mentioned; 1 died 20 hours after operation with symptoms unrelieved—necropsy showed a small tumor arising from the muscularis mucosa completely blocking the pylorus. 4 cases died in from 4 to 27 hours—all were practically moribund and the result was to be expected. 1 died of inanition on the 26th day; when this baby was given more than 1 ounce of food it would vomit. The smallest and thickest walled stomach yet observed by us was found at necropsy in this case. The pylorus was patent. 27 cases were discharged as cured. Of these, 1 died in a convulsion some 10 days after leaving the hospital; up to a few hours before death its condition had been excellent—postmortem examination not obtained. 1 case returned to the hospital 3 months after operation suffering from endocarditis and pericarditis from which it died. The stomach removed at necropsy showed an elliptical cicatrix on the anterior surface of the pylorus about one-half the size of the original wound. This area was covered with serosa and appeared to be composed of serous and mucous coats only. The remaining portion of the pylorus was somewhat thicker than normal, but the tumor which had been "a typical one of moderate size" had almost entirely disappeared.

The other 25 cases have been kept under close observation and are in good condition. They have all gained rapidly and many of them are above their normal weight; in no case has there been a return of the symptoms. Roentgen examination has been made of 4 cases from 6 months to 1½ years after operation, and the stomachs have much the same appearance as those of other babies. They empty more slowly than the gastro-enterostomy cases, but at about the normal rate.

POST-OPERATIVE TREATMENT. The cases operated by the method of Rammstedt required less stimulation and reacted more quickly than those in which gastro-enterostomy was done. Vomiting was less frequent and smaller in amounts than after the latter procedure. All cases surviving partial pyloroplasty began to improve rapidly after the second or third day, some had setbacks and a few were difficult feeding cases, but as a rule they were much less trouble to feed than the gastro-enterostomies. A number of the latter developed a diarrhea, in from a week to 10 days, which was difficult to control and in 2 instances proved fatal. The pyloroplastic cases did not show this tendency and I believe the explanation lies in the fact, that the food passing out of the stomach through the natural channel at a normal rate has less tendency to cause intestinal disturbance than when it passes through the artificial opening at a rate which in many instances, as shown by x-ray is much too rapid.

Feeding is begun in the Rammstedt cases in about 2 hours, 2 to 3 drams of breast milk, alternating with water, is given every 2 hours to start with, and this is rapidly increased so they are getting from 1 to 1½ ounces every 3 hours at the end of the second day. The gastro-enterostomy cases required more care in their feeding and tolerated the rapid increase in amount less well than did the other class of cases.

CONCLUSION. I have gone somewhat into detail in comparing the results obtained in the use of gastro-enterostomy and partial pyloroplasty in the treatment of pyloric obstruction in order to bring out the advantages as well as the disadvantages of each method. From the foregoing, it seems fair to say that partial pyloroplasty has many advantages over gastro-enterostomy. The time required to do the former operation is less than half that required to perform the latter, reaction is more prompt, feeding is begun earlier and can be pushed more rapidly, post-operative vomiting is less and late complications such as diarrhea and unexplained vomiting do not occur.

The operation is simple, requires much less surgical skill than gastro-enterostomy, and most important of all the obstruction is permanently removed and the normal continuity of the alimentary tract is preserved. Specimen removed from the case dying 3 months after operation and Roentgen examination $1\frac{1}{2}$ years after operation prove the accuracy of this statement.

The method is open to the criticism that it leaves an uncovered wound, that the abdominal cavity is protected from contamination only by a thin layer of mucous membrane, and that as the scar contracts the obstruction will reform. I believe the excellent results obtained by other surgeons using this method together with those here recorded prove these criticisms to be largely theoretical. The danger of opening the mucous membrane is a real one, but with care should be avoided. To the above objections may be added the fact, that in our unique case of tumor blocking the pyloric lumen, this type of operation was inadequate. If a little more care had been exercised in examining the pylorus in this case the cause of obstruction would probably have been discovered. It is needless to say, that a gastro-enterostomy should be added if in any case there is reason to suspect that the lumen of the pylorus does not become patent after division of the circular muscle.

Continued experience and longer observation of the cases may bring out other more serious objections to partial pyloroplasty, but until that time, or until something better is proposed, operation according to the method of Rammstedt should be the one of choice in the treatment of pyloric obstruction in infants.

Finally, the success or failure of either operative procedure is determined in a large measure by the length of time lapsing between the onset of symptoms and the time of operation.

CHRONIC INTESTINAL OBSTRUCTION VERSUS INTESTINAL STASIS

By *F. W. Parham*, M.D., F.A.C.S.
New Orleans, La.

It is not my intention to discuss at length the subject of intestinal stasis, but merely to report two cases and make some comments upon them, with the purpose of emphasizing certain differentiating features.

Case I.—Miss N. K., aged forty-four years. Consulted me in 1909 and again in July, 1915.

Family History. Father died of apoplexy, otherwise negative.

Previous History. Has had most diseases incident to childhood; pneumonia twice. Was jaundiced about fifteen years ago. Menses always regular, dysmenorrhea and metrorrhagia at times. Dysentery about twenty-six years ago.

Present Illness. Beginning about twenty years ago patient says that she has been suffering from vague cramps in lower abdomen, apparently worse at menstrual period. When about eighteen years of age had a dysentery which lasted for a few weeks and then checked. Ever since then, up to present time, off and on, bowels have become loose; frequent, watery, mucus, blood-tinged stools, alternating with spells of constipation. About six years ago laparotomy was done by me, appendicectomy and drainage of gall-bladder. Nine months later she began again to suffer with colicky pains in the lower abdomen. These attacks came on periodically and were very severe, marked by distention of the lower abdomen. During the attacks the coils of intestine could be seen imprinted against the abdominal wall. The attacks lasted for variable periods, but often continued for some time, gradually subsiding with a movement of the bowel or as the result of an opiate. Numerous consultations were held with internists and a neurologist. The latter had her in exclusive charge for several weeks and gave alcohol injections of the lumbar nerve roots. All treatment, however, failed, and I determined to do an exploratory operation, suspecting the old dysenteric trouble might have left some contracting scars. A much kinked and twisted ileum just before it joined the cecum was found. Six inches were resected in one place and the lumen enlarged in another place by a Heinicke-Mickulicz plastic. She was greatly improved after this operation, in fact, seemed to have entirely recovered, remaining well until about one year ago, when attacks of colic similar to those of six years ago began to manifest themselves. Similar coils of intestines could be seen pressing against the abdominal wall and the pains were almost as intense as before, though they did not last so long. These attacks seem to be closely connected with constipation. The pain was referred always to sigmoid region. X-ray barium pictures in series by Dr. Samuels, radiologist of Touro, showed nothing noteworthy until the sigmoid was reached. Here there was a distinct halting of the stream, which only passed after a long interval. The same stop was observed when the mixture was given by rectum, and at the same point, just below the anterior superior spine of the ilium. The x-ray evidence corresponded with the point of pain reference. On July 20, 1915, I again opened the abdomen, making a left McBurney incision under novocain-adrenalin anesthesia until the sigmoid was reached. Then under ether the sigmoid was drawn out. A tumor about the size of a hickory nut was found in the mesentery of the sigmoid. It did not appear to involve the mucous lining but grew into the wall of the gut thus narrowing the lumen so that the index finger could be passed with the exercise of some force. The sigmoid with the mass was brought out onto the abdominal wall and sutured there.

On July 24, four days later, under local anesthesia, I cut off this mass after the manner of Mickulicz, level with the wall. I had intended finishing the operation acording to the Mickulicz plan, namely, by putting in enterotome, but the lower end retracted so much I thought it best not to do so but to leave it as an artificial anus. She returned in October to have the intestinal continuity restored, but I again concluded in view of the possibility of a recurrence to wait yet a few months, since she was quite comfortable and managed the artificial anus without much annoyance. All pain was completely relieved and she was regaining rapidly her health. Her only complaint was of a mucous discharge associated with rectal irritation. The opening of the low segment was closed, so that treatment for relief could be applied only through the anal end. The pathologist reported adenocarcinoma.

In this case the characteristic symptom was colicky pain occurring spasmodically, and relieved by removing the cause of an incomplete obstruction. She had been handled as a neurasthenic, but there was no stasis in the accepted sense of the term, for she was twice relieved simply by removing the obstruction.

CASE II.—Mr. R. R. P., Bay St. Louis, Miss. Aged forty-six years.

Family History. Father died at sixty-seven of inflammatory rheumatism. Mother at fifty-seven of same disease. Six brothers, three dead, one at fifty-four of paralysis, one at forty-seven of kidney trouble, one of kidney and brain trouble. Two living older than himself. One of these had had rheumatism. Both well now. Five sisters, three dead, two living. One sixty and one fifty-eight. Collateral history excellent.

No venereal history. Wassermann negative.

Previous Illness.—Typhoid fever in 1887. A long and severe attack. Had hemorrhoids following this typhoid fever. In the spring of 1906 he had a severe attack of renal colic and passed one calculus preceded by severe pain. This pain was on the right side. Six months later had another severe attack on the left side and passed another stone. Three months later had another attack and passed another stone. Spent some time at Stafford Springs and Brown's Wells and has never suffered from this trouble since that time. Fifteen years ago while driving had to get out of a buggy on account of pain in the epigastric region. In the spring of 1910 I operated on him for inguinal abscess. He stated that in September, 1909, he had stepped into a hole injuring his leg. A few days later a lump appeared in his groin. When I saw him in the spring of 1910 he had then been under treatment for about seven weeks. I had to do an extensive dissection operation on the inguinal region to eradicate the abscess and necrosed tissue. He made an uneventful recovery, his trouble extending from the beginning to the end over a period of about seventeen weeks. He remained well until about three years ago, when he had a recurrence of the epigastric pain. He was treated by an internist for some time. He was much improved, though not entirely relieved of the pain.

The pain shifted curiously from above downward until it maintained itself below the umbilicus. One year and a half ago he began to have severe attacks; bowels then became loose, and he suffered little until about a year ago, when a tendency to constipation showed itself. The pains then greatly increased. Relief usually came with action from the bowels. Distention was prominent while the pain continued. One year ago last July he had a severe attack marked by severe vomiting. (of fecal matter?) He said the vomitus was just like a passage from the bowels. These attacks lasted about twelve days. The vomiting relieved him somewhat but relief was not complete until the bowels moved freely.

He would have many actions, then constipation would begin. He went to Battle Creek in July, remaining there seven weeks. He had no severe attacks while there, but numerous light attacks. Gastro-intestinal barium fluoroscopic observations were made by Dr. Case of the whole tract. The time from pylorus to ileocecal valve was fifty hours. He left Battle Creek much improved. Arrived Bay St. Louis about August 20. He remained in the same condition, barring these slight attacks. September 15, he had an attack of fever which lasted for a day. After the fever he lost appetite and began to lose weight. Since then the attacks of abdominal pain have been more frequent.

He came to the city to consult Dr. J. B. Elliot, Jr., the first week in June and at that time called to see me, but I made no examination as I was just on the point of leaving the city. Dr. Elliot, however, had some x-ray bismuth pictures taken of the alimentary canal by Dr. Henriques. These pictures show the bismuth six hours from the pylorus to the ileocecal valve. The symptoms at this time Dr. Elliot thought pointed to the gall-bladder. It was after this that he went to Battle Creek. I extract some notes from a letter written August 5, by Dr. Eggleston, of Battle Creek Sanitarium.

"It would seem that the trouble results from partial obstruction in the intestinal tract. I say partial obstruction because some two or three days he may go on in a very normal way, but during this time he is conscious of the fact that his bowels are not moving satisfactorily, and following this he will have a severe attack of diarrhea, the bowels moving sometimes ten to twelve times within a very short period of time, sometimes within five or six hours. This, it seems, results from accumulation of intestinal contents in the terminal part of the small intestine and the beginning of the large intestine, and the cause of this it is impossible to determine accurately. We are not certain that this condition is one that can be relieved except by surgical interference."

On September 24 another letter was received by Mr. P. from Dr. Eggleston after Mr. P. had returned home. The doctor states in this letter: "In my opinion the trouble results from a temporary stasis of the intestinal contents at some point in the small intestine, probably near the ileo-cecal valve. The x-ray picture shows that the emptying time of the small intestine is something beyond fifty hours. Your clinical symptoms certainly would bear out the idea that for some reason there is a delay at some point which is followed by pain, griping sensations, and purging, with relief for a period of time when there is a repetition of this peculiar group of symptoms. Whether or not the trouble results from a spastic condition of the bowel or whether it is due to some organic change, I am unable to say definitely. From my observation of your case, it seems it must be a functional rather than an organic disturbance, inasmuch as careful attention to the bowels, which prevents a delay, seems to relieve the condition. Should a regime similar to that I recommended to you not be sufficient to relieve you, I know of nothing else than to resort to surgery, having an exploratory operation, paying particular attention to the small bowel."

When I saw him in Bay St. Louis, October 8, 1915, he was then in a quiescent condition, having only occasionally slight attacks of pain, the pain being referred to the supra-pubic region. He appeared, however, much pulled down. He had a severe attack on the night of October 13. He came over to the city and entered the Touro on Friday, October 15, and from that time was under my observation until October 30. He had during this time several light attacks, all of similar character, all marked by pain between the umbilicus and pubes, and all relieved by movements of the bowels. Enema frequently would accomplish this. X-ray pictures were taken by Dr. Samuels at Touro Infirmary on

Saturday, October 16, but the series were not very satisfactory and another set was taken beginning Monday the 18th, and finishing Tuesday morning. Description of the various series taken in June, August and October:

June, 1915, by Dr. A. Henriques in New Orleans.

There is nothing noteworthy except an apparent looping of the ileum just before it enters the cecum.

August, 1915, by Dr. J. T. Case, at Battle Creek Sanitarium.

The observations were fluoroscopically made. The notes above furnish all the information available, and indicate ileal stasis with ileocecal incompetence.

October 18, 19, 20, by Dr. Samuels, Touro Infirmary.

These seem to show a kinking in transverse colon.

October 30. Diagnosis: There seems to me little question that his attacks are connected with a partial obstruction of the bowel.

The only clues to its location and its etiology are:

1. The clinical history of typhoid, unusually severe.

2. The peculiar behavior of the colicky attacks, being preceded by constipation and relieved by a purgative or an enema.

3. The nausea which is sufficiently marked to indicate the small intestine, but not enough to point to the duodenum or jejunum.

4. The x-ray observations. These, three sets taken two months apart, are somewhat confusing. Dr. Henriques's in June seem to point to the lower ileum. Dr. Case, at Battle Creek, in August, made out a very sluggish current in small intestine, being fifty hours from pylorus to ileocecal valve.

Dr. Henriques in June, and Dr. Samuels in October, made it respectively $6\frac{1}{2}$ and 6 hours.

Dr. Henriques's pictures seem to show an obstruction by loop adhesion at terminal ileum. Dr. Samuels's seem to show obstruction by kinking in transverse colon.

The typhoid history might explain kinking or adhesions in the course of the ileum, but there is *no* item (dysentery) bearing upon ulcers which might have cicatrized in the transverse colon.

In a personal communication of October 15, 1915, Dr. Case expresses the opinion that the trouble is the result of intestinal stasis in the terminal ileum, cecum and appendix and is due, he believes, to excessive antiperistalsis with incompetency of the ileocolic valve. He does not believe there is any organic constriction.

In other words, he does not believe there is any chronic obstruction but thinks all the symptoms are to be explained by a stasis in the lower ileum.

To my mind the symptoms in the two cases now related are closely similar and ought to be explained in the same way. In the first case, the demonstration of obstruction was complete at the two operations; in the second case I had hoped to furnish the proof in this paper, but he has elected to seek other advice and since October 30 has been treated medically.[1] The signs of partial or chronic obstruction were almost pathognomonic. The colicky pain, coming on paroxysmally, and relieved by a movement of the bowel, brought on either spontaneously or by an enema, is the characteristic sign; the tympanites, the absence of stools and the vomiting are important, but may be otherwise explained. The collicky pain, however, which is severe, is not to be explained by simple sluggishness of the fecal current and its paroxysmal return is apt to continue until the cause of narrowed lumen shall have been removed. From October 30 to December 9 I had not seen the gentleman and had had no communication from him.

December 9, 1915. The above had been written when the patient sent me a long distance message saying that he was coming into town to see me again, as he was having another

---

[1] These notes have been left as written prior to his death.

severe attack. He arrive about 5 P.M., and was at once seen by me at Touro Infirmary. I found him looking very haggard, much changed from his appearance when I last saw him on October 30.

His history from October 30 was as follows: He appeared to be improving until November 25 when he had a severe attack of influenza which confined him to bed for about eleven days. He had fever December 4, 5, and 6. He improved after this attack, feeling better until the night of December 7, when nausea and vomiting began which lasted all that night. In the morning he had severe colic. Although not markedly distended he was relieved by enemata. The nausea continued all through the day and night of December 8 and 9 until I saw him about 5 P.M., December 9. He complained then of much pain all over the abdomen most marked near the umbilicus. There was a mass, soft and gaseous, on the left side just under costal arch. This could be somewhat flattened out by pressure but did not disappear. There was not much general distention.

His condition grew rapidly worse and he died the next day, December 10, fifteen hours after admission. I was fortunately able to get permission to hold an autopsy. Nothing but the abdomen was examined. The first thing observable on opening the abdomen was a movable tumor in the left hypochondrium which proved to be an intussusception, the starting point being the jejunum just one meter from the ligament of Treitz. When the intussusception was pulled out, it was found to consist of one meter of gangrenous jejunum. Further examination of the abdominal organs showed the following: (1) A very long appendix bound by adhesions which shortened the meso-appendix. There was, however, nothing remarkable. The ileocecal valve was incompetent as shown by the facility with which the fecal gas was worked back into the ileum. (2) There was a prominent pouch just at the splenic flexure due to a partial occlusion at the beginning of the descending colon. This ruptured while being taken out. The specimen was sent to the pathologist of Touro Infirmary for examination. He said the mass of tissue around the posterior aspect of the colon at this point was inflammatory tissue, and the mucous membrane showed the signs of an old ulcer which had cicatrized and had produced contraction of the lumen at this point. The gall-bladder appeared normal; the stomach was dilated but there was neither gastric nor duodenal cicatrix.

The intussusception was a late development, its incipiency dating probably from the fever beginning December 4. By December 7 the invagination had sufficiently advanced to cause obstruction high in the jejunum and give rise to the severe and persistent vomiting which continued all through the night of December 7, and through the next day and night. On the morning of December 10 he was in collapse and died about 2 P.M., The intussusception was of course, the determining cause of death. But what explanation may be given of the previous illness extending over so many years? Certainly the intussusception had nothing to do with this. The narrowed lumen of the descending colon just below the splenic flexure, in my opinion, undoubtedly explains the repeated attacks of colic and the deterioration of health consequent upon the intestinal toxemia. That it was not merely an intestinal stasis due to ileocecal valve incompetence is, I think, indicated by the record and conclusively demonstrated by the autopsy. The differentiation is often very difficult, but I believe the two cases now reported show a symptomatology so markedly in favor of true organic partial constriction of intestinal lumen that in the face of such a presentation the surgeon will disregard the best interests of his patient should he fail to offer him the benefit of an exploratory operation. If this could have been done in October not only would he have been saved from his death by acute strangulation, but perhaps we might have relieved the chronic colonic obstruction and have restored him to health. The intussusception was undoubtedly superinduced by some sudden access of peripheral colonic obstruction and, as shown at the postmortem examination, might easily have been pulled out before adhesive inflammation had fixed the invagination and produced strangulation and gangrene.

The notes on the termination of this case were concluded the day I left New Orleans for Cincinnati, where the paper was read two days later. I have left the paper exactly. as written, but desire to add a few further notes taken from a letter dated January 6, from Dr. Case, in reply to my letter giving him a statement of the postmortem findings. He also sends me three prints of x-ray negatives taken July and August, last summer. Dr. Case's interpretation of these prints is found in the extract from his letter, which is as follows:

"I find I have evidence of the following: A rather quick-emptying stomach, which is roentgenologically normal in every respect. No evidence of disease of the duodenum or gall-bladder. A very unusual dilatation of the small bowel, which led me to suspect an obstruction in the jejunum. Incompetency of the ileocecal valve with stasis in the terminal small bowel longer than fifty hours; in fact, even at the seventy-fourth hour. Poorly drained, moderately tender appendix, which was otherwise negative. After the barium meal, the head of the barium column reached the hepatic flexure by the fourth hour and the splenic flexure by the ninth hour. At the twenty-sixth hour the colon was filled from cecum to ampulla. At the fiftieth hour the colon was still filled throughout, but a plate which I happen to have made shows the filling to be much more dense from cecum to splenic region, and it also shows a little barium in the terminal ileum. I am sending you a print of this plate in case you happen to want to use it in your article. The next morning we gave the patient enemata in the effort to empty the colon, so that we might give the barium enema. The enemata was given by my assistant and a plate made during my absence from the city, but I do not see how I ever looked at this plate without recognizing the condition, for it is a very characteristic one of obstruction in the region of the splenic flexure; first, the cecum and ascending colon, and even the terminal ileum contain residue from the barium meal administered one hundred hours before, held in the colon as far as possible from the seat of obstruction by antiperistalsis, which was exaggerated in this case; second, the pelvic colon and descending colon widely distended by the enema because of difficulty encountered somewhere near the splenic flexure.

"Your conclusions as to the causation of the intussusception are very interesting. I do not know anything to disturb you in that position except that I saw what I believe was evidence of a chronic upper small bowel hindrance on two occasions, when I examined the patient on July 26 and again when I repeated the examination of the stomach on August 1."

The lesson to be drawn from these cases is especially that the diagnosis of stasis discourages resort to exploratory investigation and the possible discovery in time of the true cause of disability and its removal. The contributions of the roentgenologist are so valuable that this method of diagnosis must be constantly employed in such cases, and too great praise can scarcely be accorded the masters in this work, similarly as we acknowledge our indebtedness to the pathologists for their aid in the completion of our diagnostic data, but while recognizing fully the credit thus due these faithful workers, we must insist that sole reliance must not be placed upon laboratory interpretations. These interpretations must explain, or at least accord with the symptoms, otherwise they must be rejected. The clinical history and the examination must be given predominant place in the evidence upon which the diagnosis is to rest and all other aids must be regarded as only confirmatory.

COLON RESECTION AND ITS INDICATIONS: REPORT OF CASES WITH LANTERN SLIDES

By Frank Martin, M.D.
Baltimore, Maryland

THE colon, as we all know, is quite commonly affected with obstructive lesions due to growths, strictures, or what not; but 'the most common factor is cancer, especially of the rectum, the ascending colon, the sigmoid, and lastly, the splenic flexure and transverse colon. It so happens that I have had to deal with it in these various locations a number of times. The two factors which impress me as exceptionally important in reference to the work on colon surgery are (1) a keen insight into the vascular distribution of the colon, and (2) an accurate knowledge of its lymphatic distribution.

First, in reference to the vascular distribution, it is along the arteries that the lymph currents flow and the lymph glands chiefly lie. The large intestine is supplied by branches of the superior mesenteric artery and by the inferior mesenteric artery and their branches. The ileocolic artery, which appears to continue in the direct line of the main trunk of the superior mesenteric artery, supplies the last few inches of the ileum, the cecum, and a part of the ascending colon. It takes origin at or near the level of the third part of the duodenum, and descends, inclining to the right, to reach the ileocolic angle. The middle colic arises near the lower border of the pancreas and directs its course toward the right, in the layers of the transverse mesocolon, where it divides into branches, each of which again divides to form a series of arches, joining on the inner side of the ascending colon with the right colic, and toward the splenic end of the transverse colon in an anastomosis with the ascending branch of the left colic artery. The sigmoid arteries, one to four in number, arise directly from the inferior mesenteric artery, and radiating outward and downward in the mesosigmoid, divide each into an ascending and descending branch; these anastomosing with their neighbors, form a series of arches, from the curved side of which branches are given off, sometimes to form secondary arches, sometimes to run direct to the intestinal wall.

The so-called marginal artery (as shown so clearly in the picture of the normal colon I herewith show) is the result of anastomoses of the branches of the left colic and sigmoid arteries, extending from the splenic flexure to the lowest part of the sigmoid flexure. Here it stops for the superior hemorrhoidal artery, which in the continuation of the inferior mesenteric trunk, after the sigmoid arteries have left, does not divide into two arch-forming branches, but runs directly to the intestinal wall. It is exceptionally important to bear this in mind, for at this so-called "critical point" of Sudeck, which is at the junction betweeen the superior hemorrhoidal artery and the lowest sigmoid artery, trouble occurs if this knowledge of the blood supply is not kept in mind. Ligature of the superior hemorrhoidal artery and the lowest sigmoid artery below the "critical point" must almost inevitably result in gangrene of the portion of the rectum supplied by them. So in intestinal resections a knowledge of this cannot be overestimated (Fig. 1 clearly shows this).

It is, as said above, very important to have an accurate knowledge of the lymphatic distribution and the prominence of the lymphatic vessels. The distribution of the lymphatic gland is of great moment in all surgery for malignant conditions of the colon, because these are the agents which drain the part that is affected. Whereas a malignant disease of the colon may oftentimes remain a local one, still, through these channels, metastases occur in spite of the fact that many claim the lymphatics in this structure are few as compared to those in the small intestines. They sooner or later carry the infection, and the surgeon unfortunately meets these cases usually after this has happened, namely, late in their course, and frequently so late that they are either inoperable, due to wide-spread metastases, or offer very slim chances for permanent relief when operation is resorted to. Furthermore, they are not brought to us many times until acute intestinal obstruction demands surgical intervention.

You will all agree with me, I am sure, that under these conditions we have at best a bad surgical risk. I know of no condition more grave, nor one with slimmer chances of recovery, than a case requiring resection of the colon for cancer in the height of acute intestinal obstruction. On the other hand, when they can be operated on moderately early (and there should be no reason for delay now with the better means at our command for diagnosis, and I refer here especially to the *x*-ray, which has been of such infinite value in clearing up this trouble) surgery offers most excellent promise. It is, however, a very fortunate fact that malignant disease of the colon, barring exceptions, may remain for a long time a local process.

H. S. Clogg (*Lancet*, 1908, ii, 1007) points out, in a valuable paper, that cancer of the colon is in many cases a local disease, and that secondary visceral deposits are not the great barrier to any radical operation. Sir Berkeley Moynihan, in his recent book on abdominal operation, says. "We are, I think, entitled to believe that a carcinomatous growth of the colon by reason of its small size, its (apparently) abrupt delimitations, its long restriction to the intestinal wall, the tardy appearance of the metastatic deposits, and the paucity of the the lymph-glandular supply, should prove amenable to successful attack by the surgeon. It would appear to be true to say that if cancer is to develop in the body there are few places it could select with so happy a chance to the patient of ultimate and complete relief as the large intestine." Again, another authority, Dr. Charles H. Mayo, states in his paper, "Resection of the Rectum for Cancer of the Sphincter," which he read before this Association several years ago, "The inflammatory and cicatricial zone which surrounds such areas of ulceration acts as an effective cofferdam, preventing an early metastasis." I think these important observations above mentioned have been noted by most operators in this field, and they are observations which unquestionably add encouragement to surgery direct for the relief of cancer at this point.

During the past two years I have operated upon two cases of cancer of the colon in which the process had been of long duration, and at the time of operation there was extensive dissemination and infiltration in the surrounding tissues. In the first case an extensive extirpation of the transverse colon was done, along with the removal of the gastrocolic omentum. The infiltration even extended (apparently) into the greater curvature of the stomach, for in ligating off the attachment of the gastrocolic omentum, close to the stomach wall, there was noted infiltration of (apparent) carcinomatous tissue, and lateral anastomosis was made between the hepatic flexure and the descending colon. The patient, much to everybody's surprise, recovered *in toto*, and is still living and (apparently) doing well. This was two years ago this month.

The second case was operated on last spring, and there was such wide-spread cancer (the activity of the cellular proliferation had been infinitely more marked than is usually noted, starting from a ring-like primary stricture of the ascending colon—adenocarcinoma), infiltrating the lymphatics along the entire marginal artery of the colon, with a large nodule of carcinoma at the junction of the transverse and splenic flexure, and likewise the first few inches of the ileum from the ileocecal valve, that I did a complete resection of the colon with eight inches of the ileum. The ileum was laterally implanted into the sigmoid. Here, likewise, an uneventful recovery followed.

These cases bear out what is agreed by many, that the progress in colon cancer is slow and the cellular proliferation is not very active; in fact, it is looked upon, as I have already said, as a local disease at first. With these fortunate facts all should be stimulated to institute much earlier intervention.

As an evidence of the wisdom of this, I cite briefly the case of a man, aged forty years, upon whom I recall doing a resection of the descending colon for carcinoma which had not extended. This was done ten years ago, and the patient is still living and in good health. Whereas these observations are usually the rule, exceptions occur frequently, and I recall many cases in which the growth was rapid, a secondary metastasis of the liver occurring very early. A number of such cases in which adenocarcinomatous strictures are well removed by resection and no other invasion noted, all promised well, but liver metastasis occured with fatal results in eighteen months or two years. However, radical procedure should be undertaken always and at the earliest possible moment, as it offers the only promise. We all know the pathetic picture of those cases which rely on the use of the *x*-ray and radium as a means of help. They are distinctly of no value, and there is nothing we can offer save the knife.

CHOICE OF METHODS FOR OPERATING. These vary in the clinics of the different operators; some prefer the end-to-end method, some the lateral anastomosis. Of course, the thing of moment is to get well around the growth and do a wide-spread extirpation. After that is thoroughly done the procedure of restoring the lumen is a minor one, provided the anastomosis is well done. The ideal method is end-to-end anastomosis, which can be done perfectly well, even though we have to anastomose the lumen of the small intestine into the large bowel.

The first case I recall doing in my series was an adenocarcinoma in the descending colon; a wide-spread excision was done and an end-to-end anastomosis made by use of the Murphy button. This was used, I might say, because it was reported to me, falsely, that the patient was badly shocked and a time-saving device required. At the completion of the operation I found this not true, however, and an uninterrupted recovery followed. This was many years ago, and I know the patient to have been alive five years afterward; but I am unable to report further, as I have lost touch with the case. This was the first and only colon resection in which I have used the Murphy button. I have used it a number of times in rapid resection of the small intestine when speed was demanded.

Since then I have always employed a lateral anastomosis by suture, except in four cases of resection of the entire cecum, part of the ascending colon, and a small portion of the ileum. In these cases, lateral implantation of the ileum into the ascending colon was resorted to. The chief objection to an end-to-end anastomosis (which after all is the most ideal method) is that the blood supply may be encroached upon sufficiently to possibly produce small points of necrosis at the suture line, and the chief cause of defeat in all intestinal work, namely, leakage, occurs. Whereas, in lateral anastomosis, if the work is neatly and carefully done, such an occurrence is not liable to follow, and obviates the difficulty which occasionally arises in dealing with the mesenteric attachment.

In this series of fifty-odd cases there have been but five complete resections of the colon, and I have embodied at the end of this report complete histories of these five cases. Colon resection in its broad sense, for the relief of cancer, which we seem to have always with us, is an undisputed surgical problem; but the wide diversity of opinion in the surgical world comes with the radical operation for colon resection as practised by Sir William Arbuthnot Lane, for the cure of that vast array of conditions assumed to be caused by "intestinal stasis." All say that Lane's operation is radical work, and it is radical work; but to emphasize how striking the diversity of opinion is, you will hear the remarks, "Lane is too radical; he is ahead of his time; his colectomy is unwarranted." But usually, when a man of authority is applied to for an opinion, I find there is not one who condemns the man or his method *in toto*, and no unfavorable opinion is noted. The time has not yet arrived, in my opinion, when we can either condemn the operation or accept it without hesitation, as Lane would have us do.

Lane, unquestionably, is a genius and a wonderfully able and skilful surgeon, and all of his work has been distinctly worth while and along markedly advanced lines. The few words of comment made by Dr. Charles H. Mayo in his discussion of the article written by Dr. John G. Clarke on the "Removal of the Colon for Obstructive Fecal Stasis, with a Report of Eight Cases," read at the Atlanta meeting of the Association two years ago, clearly shows how much Lane's opinions in the past have been thought of. He said on this occasion: "Lane at this time occupies a more enviable position than any other living surgeon in regard to his work. He was the first man to open the jugular vein and wash out clots in sinus thrombosis, following mastoid abscess. He has done more to put bone surgery on the map than any other living surgeon. His work on cleft palate has led to much discussion for relief to the condition." Lane's work and methods have been widely discussed and their influences broadly distributed. Adverse criticism has become less of late, particularly in England. This goes to show that his name and work are held in high regard in this country.

Never before in the history of surgery has the subject of intestinal surgery claimed more wide-spread attention. The colon with its fecal stasis is truly the bane of modern civilization. Whether the abnormalities of the colon produced by malpositions, kinking, and adhesions are of congenital origin, or whether produced by "bad workmanship on the part of nature," as our English friend would have us believe, it is a tremendous portal of entry for disease in consequence of the lack of free drainage and the bacterial activity produced and generated here and carried far afield; therefore, it is justly held responsible as the primary source of infection. Lane emphatically states that it is the cause of all diseases except cancer, and that the only medicine to relieve this condition is Russian oil. If that does not succeed, there is but one operation, namely, colon resection. His belief is that unless free drainage can be secured absorption is going to continue. If the obstruction is such that it will not drain by the use of Russian oil, then the colon should be removed. Now in just what percentage of cases does the profession at large look to the colon as the responsible factor in auto-intoxication, or as the portal of entry, as the cause of the vast army of disorders, is the great question at issue.

Authorities by no means agree as to how intestinal stasis causes alimentary toxemia, and not a few even deny that it is responsible for the toxic manifestations which are attributed to it, and are looking only at the teeth, tonsils, sinuses, or what not as the chief portals of entry in every case. But be that as it may, there is one fact that can be affirmed without fear of contradiction, and despite the difference of opinion, the condition is so frequent and prevalent as to warrant the belief that there is an intimate relationship between intestinal stasis and alimentary toxemia.

Alimentary toxemia is defined in the following words by Dr. F. W. Andrews: "The absorption from the alimentary canal by chemical poisons of known or unknown composition in sufficient amounts to cause clinical symptoms, the blood having served as the channel of distribution to the tissues which are poisoned." And many there are who believe that fecal stasis is directly responsible for many maladies both of mind and body. The clinical picture in these cases is so well depicted by Lane, as well as by other noteworthy contributors, such as Smith, Goldthwait, Reynolds, Clarke and many others in this country, that there is no need to touch on this.

J. E. Goldthwait, of Boston, is as ardent an enthusiast as Lane, of England, although he believes by his specific methods of treatment that he can relieve this condition without colectomy. In a series of brilliant papers, Goldthwait shows how faulty posture of growing children and of women and young girls tends to weaken the skeletal supports and to place at a disadvantage the ligaments and muscles of the abdomen and back. J. G. Mumford, gives credit to Glenard for the angulation theory of stasis and auto-intoxication. In consequence, he cites the fact that "a great number of persons are the subject of congenital ptosis, and the anatomist long ago pointed out that one person in every five is born with a mesentery upon the entire colon, and that the stomach also is more loosely attached. When such attachments fail to retract, the victim carries through life a gastrocolonic ptosis." This is entirely in accord with the theories advanced by Lane as to the mechanics and the alterations which are undergone by the gastro-intestinal tract.

Lane stands foremost as the most ardent enthusiast in attributing auto-intoxication to stasis. In his article on "Chronic Intestinal Stasis," he states that unless the capacity of the several tissues of the body to resist entry of certain organisms is inhibited by the auto-intoxication resulting from intestinal stasis, it is impossible for these diseases to develop. Therefore, to meet these diseases, he adopts means to improve the drainage scheme, whether simply mechanical or operative, with the most excellent results. This is nowhere better exemplified than in the extraordinarily rapid disappearance of large tubercular glandular masses in the abdomen; after disconnection with the large bowel the disease disappears and the health and weight of the patient improves accordingly. On eliminating the supply of poison the color of the skin changes with remarkable rapidity, the deep brown or coppery tint disappears in these cases (if they have simulated Addison's disease) and is replaced by the warm red color indicative of health.

The great difficulty in the treatment of chronic intestinal stasis and its results, so Lane says, is to recognize when it is too late to interfere; in other words, when the end result has assumed such proportions that the removal of the primary cause does little or no good. Again, as regards the influence of these toxins or poisons on the nervous system, Lane has seen a patient, who has been confined to bed for many months, having neither capacity nor desire to stand or walk, and whose mental condition was such that she was regarded by many as an imbecile, become a happy, active, and intelligent woman within a few weeks after removal of the large bowel.

I might add that during the Clinical Congress of Surgeons of North America, held recently in London, the most sought after man there was Lane, and he, of course, attributes everything to the colon. He gave us every facility for not only seeing him operate and remove colons by the score, but we were able to see his patients before operation and afterward. I saw him do in one morning three colectomies, and I must admit they were most skilfully and masterfully done, maintaining in his clinic that the cause of such things as stomach ulcer, gall stones, tuberculosis, goitres, chronic arthritis, and, in fact, the vast and entire army of maladies result therefrom. He actually closed cases with a gall-bladder full of stones upon whom he had done a colectomy, and mentioned to the audience the gall-stones would be taken care of now that the colon was out. He showed a boy with a supposed tubercular arthritis of the wrist-joint sent in to Guy's Hospital for amputation of the forearm. The x-ray pictures clearly showed a disorganized joint.

He left the splint on and removed his colon. This boy was shown at his clinic some few months following the operation, with a cured wrist. A case of large goitre was shown to be rapidly reducing in size following a colectomy. A young woman with wide-spread universal arthritis, with every joint in her body locked, was shown a month following a colectomy, and the remark he made was that she was progressing toward recovery and could already use her fingers and hands to some extent; and so I could mention many other cases. I fail to remember the number of colectomies he has already done, but it is a vast number, and he is apparently doing them now without mortality.

His short-circuiting operation, or the ileosigmoidostomy, he has abandoned, and said that in his latter cases he would not have performed that operation could he have gotten the consent of the patient to remove the colon. As a matter of fact, I saw him do three colectomies on cases upon whom he had formerly done the short-circuiting operation (or ileosigmoidostomy).

Dr. Nassau (*Annals of Surgery*, 1913) calls attention to a picture that is worthy of mention because it is so commonly noted by all of us, and so closely allied to this particular subject, namely, that when doing our common operation, appendectomy, how often do we see cases where the appendix is little at fault, but we have presented in many of these cases enormously distended ceca which are religiously left undisturbed, the bearers of which had complained constantly of annoyance from vague pains in the right iliac fossa, and other cases of ventral fixation, nephrorrhaphies, gastro-enterostomies, in which ptosed and dilated colons were observed at operation, and in whom there had been but little abatement of symptoms, or no improvement in the general health.

I am not going to take up your time further with any of the serious scientific problems which may speak for or against this operation as a justifiable procedure. Nor am

I going into the long list of symptoms as given in the advertising pamphlets sent out by the different houses, setting forth albolene, Russian oil, liquid paraffin, and so on, for although I am not an ardent enthusiast of so radical an operation as colon resection, I am convinced that there are cases manifestly calling for just such radical procedures.

This paper is based generally upon my own personal observations and impressions gained from seeing the work of others. I have not attempted to make an exhaustive review of the numerous contributions to the literature on the subject, and I believe my chief reason for reporting on this matter was the encouragement offered by the splendid result obtained in the first case in which I found it necessary to perform such a wide-spread resection. Briefly, the case of this patient is as follows:

A young woman, aged forty years, was brought from the country to me with so-called appendicitis. I operated on her at the Union Protestant Infirmary and did the ordinary appendectomy. It was noted at the time that she had an enormous cecum very much ballooned, and the whole colon seemed to be redundant and big. I remarked at the time that I thought that was probably the cause of her discomfort, and the appendix probably played no part in it. I was just leaving for my vacation and did not see her afterward. During my absence from town, she was brought back to the Union Protestant Infirmary, and operated upon again on account of abdominal pain, by another surgeon. An ovary was removed, a ventral fixation of the uterus was done, and an exploration of the entire abdominal cavity was made, and the abdomen closed. No relief followed and her discomfort continued. She entered the Union Protestant Infirmary again later on and was treated for stomach ulcer without relief. All during this time she continued to have symptoms and the supposition was that it was stomach ulcer that was causing them. The following winter she was brought to me; she had become very ill, vomiting, inability to have bowel movements, tender over the left abdomen and over the ileum, kidney secretion had decreased until she almost had suppression; she was emaciated and markedly weak from lack of nourishment. The x-ray findings in her case were (as will be shown on the screen) as follows: Following large doses of bismuth, showed kinking at the pylorus, also a lot of bismuth in the cecum and ascending colon. It showed a large cecum and a redundant loop of the ascending colon folded back on the cecum and in this loop the bismuth seemed to be retained and stayed there. Pictures were taken again at the end of twelve hours, showing it still there, as though the kinking or this folding of the colon back upon the cecum had obstructed the cecum so that there was not any through passage of the bismuth on through the large bowel. This was so convincing that I resorted to a resection to overcome the intestinal stasis from which she was suffering. A good recovery followed, and later on she was brought back to me still without free drainage from the colon. X-ray pictures again showed interference at the point of anastomosis. I went in the second time and freed that, and from that time on she has had complete relief, gaining back her health slowly after the source of her absorption was removed.

This case was done three years ago, and only recently have I seen the patient who tells me she is perfectly well, and in her presence I asked her husband what he thought of the result, in order to get his opinion, which had all along been most depressed, and he assured me with a great deal of gratitude that he considered his wife a well woman. This case excited my interest because the patient's condition was of such gravity that we feared an operative death, and undertook it with the greatest anxiety. This was long before I had seen any of Lane's work, and I was guided purely by the x-ray findings and clinical condition of the patient. If there ever was a case indicating fatal issue from absorption this was one, and distinctly warranted the operation.

FIG. 1   FIG. 2

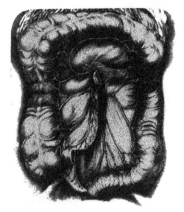 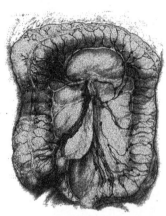

Description of two normal colons, I–II, and description of the X-ray findings before and after operation, and specimens removed from patients.

FIG. 1.—Shows a normal colon, with its blood supply and its marginal artery, also the junction between the superior hemorrhoidal artery and the lowest sigmoid artery, which has been called by Sudeck the "critical point." The importance of the marginal artery, in so far as the procedure of intestinal resection is concerned, cannot be overestimated.

FIG. 2.—Shows an accurate arrangement of the lymphatic glands of the colon, a knowledge of which is so essential to all sound surgery of carcinoma of this portion of the intestine.

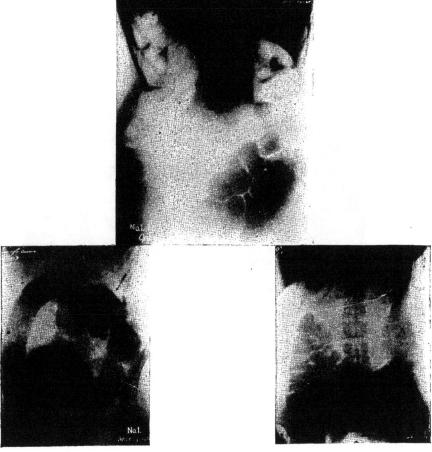

FIG. 3

FIG. 4   FIG. 5

FIG. 3 (before operation).—Picture taken twenty-four hours after bismuth was give
showing complete obstruction to the onward passage of the bismuth enema at a redunda
loop of colon in the right iliac fossa below and behind, the cecum constricted at its upp
portion. This loop consists of part of ascending and part of transverse colon bound t
gether by adhesions and kinked off, obstructing the lumen so the bismuth meal
retained.

FIG. 4 (before operation).—After colon enema, showing rectum, angulation at sigmoi
high angulation of splenic flexure, dilated transverse and ascending colon, and cecu
Incompetency of ileocecal valve, with quantity of bismuth enema in terminal ileum.

Fig. 5 (after operation).—Shows a distended, redundant sigmoid, descending and le
half of the transverse colon. On the right the cecum and ascending colon are smal
and the point of anastomosis following resection is marked by an arrow. The termin
ileum as it approaches the ileocecal valve is shown in the picture, filled with bismuth.

FIG. 6

FIG. 7

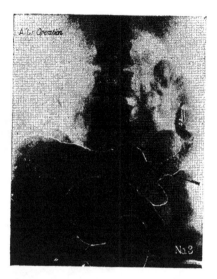

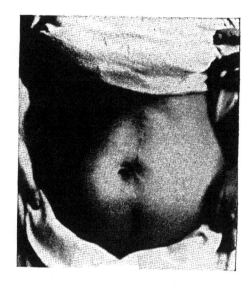

FIG. 8

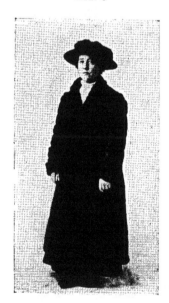

FIG. 9

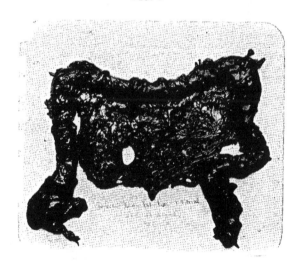

FIG. 6 (after operation).—Shows the anastomosis between the terminal ileum and the sigmoid, the enema having passed through the anastomosis freely, distending the terminal ileum.

FIG. 7.—Shows scar.

FIG. 8.—Shows patient in much improved condition.

FIG. 9.—Shows picture of specimen after its removal.

FIG. 10

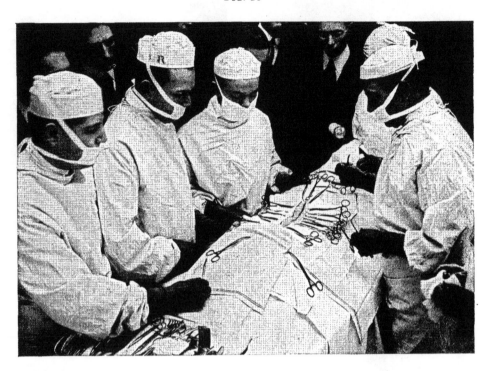

FIG. 10.—Shows superficial skin incision, which is to the left of the midline running through the left rectus, well above the umbilicus, down near the symphysis, and likewise shows the gauze clamped to wound margin, thus completely covering the skin surface, the operator standing on the left side.

FIG. 11   FIG. 12

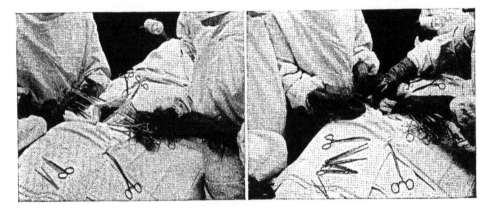

FIG. 11.—Abdomen opened and clamps on the skin margin used as retractors.
FIG. 12.—Ligating vessels near ileocecal valve preliminary to section of ileum.

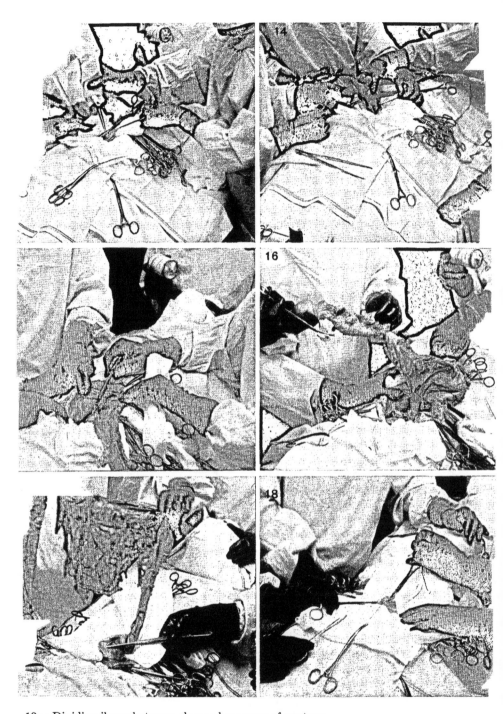

. 13.—Dividing ileum between clamps by means of cautery.

. 14.—Ileum divided, cecum delivered, thus marking the beginning of resection.

. 15.—Shows cecum and ascending colon turned out on abdomen, the hepatic flexure freed
hments, and the duodenum uncovered at the point where the scissors are pointing. I call atte
lly to this: If in ligating off the mesentery the peritoneum covering this section of the duoden
ged by ligating the mesenteric attachments of the hepatic flexure too close to it, it is liable
ed by duodenal obstruction, from which the patient is not likely to recover; or, furthermore, i
neal covering is torn off this section of the duodenum, or unduly traumatized, as might
count of the close proximity of the duodenum in this vicinity, obstruction will likewise occ

. 16.—Shows the resection of the colon well under way.   The cecum, ascending colon, and he
e have already been freed from their attachments, as shown in the picture, in the hands c
ant.   The illustration also shows the method used in isolation and quickly ligating large v

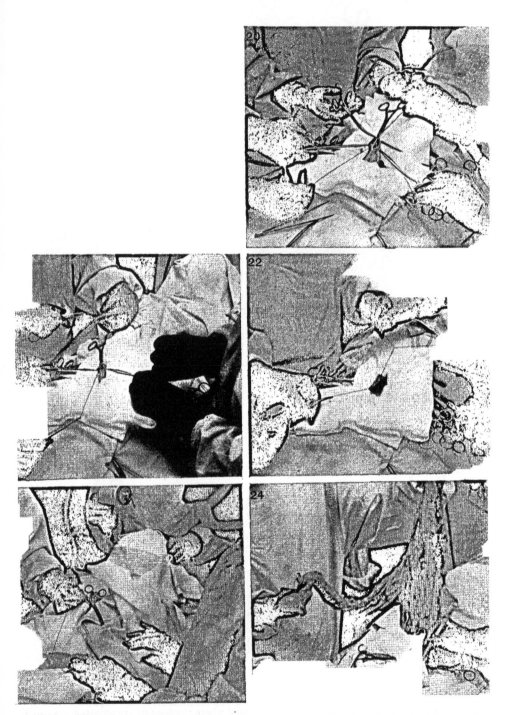

19.—Shows the continuous posterior Lembert suture completed and the incision made :
  oid corresponding in size to the opening in cut surface of the ileum before further sutu
eum into that opening is begun.
20.—Complete suturing of one side and beginning of the Connell stitch.
21.—Connell stitch near completion.
22.—Anastomosis completed and posterior and anterior continuous stitches about to be
  ompletion.
23.—Shows the lateral implantation completed, and the sigmoid slightly ballooned in co

INDICATIONS. I thoroughly agree with the opinion of Clarke that we should not be too optimistic concerning Lane's theories and practices, for there is unquestionably a considerable element of danger, and a good legitimate working basis would be to attempt relief by this procedure only after other agents had failed, provided obstructive symptoms are evident. He applies the same rule to intestinal stasis as to cases of movable or floating kidney; "no obstructive symptoms, no operation." Whereas this will not apply absolutely, it is a good working basis. I believe that when the x-ray examinations show very definite angulation at the splenic and hepatic flexures, with large redundant colons filling the pelvis, associated with evidence of toxemia, in which relief does not follow other known means, then colectomy should be resorted to, and resorted to before the cases become so toxic that they cannot undergo or withstand the operation with safety.

MORTALITY. In Lane's work, published in 1909, on "The Operative Treatment of Chronic Constipation," he states: "Except in patients who are supremely toxic and feeble, the removal of the large bowel is not accompanied with any special danger to life. If the patient is very toxic, and the resisting power to organisms is correspondingly lowered, there is a considerable risk of infection of the incision in the abdominal wall. I have lost more than one patient in this way. I believe that infection takes place from the bowel which is being excised to the wound if it is allowed to rest upon it. I attempt to avoid this by fixing sterile impermeable cloths, not to the skin edge as I usually do to render infection from it impossible, but to the peritoneum, shutting off the divided soft parts from any possible contact with the bowel whose circulation has been impaired during the process of excision. The peritoneal cavity seems quite able to escape this infection. If, however, the obstruction be acute and the intestines and abdomen be distended, the risks are those of the condition calling for interference rather than of the operation itself." These are Lane's opinions as to the dangers of the operation. The probabilities are, however, in the light of wider experience and fuller knowledge, that if better judgment is used in deciding which colon had better be removed and which had better be left, and if greater care is exercised in the carrying out of the various steps in the technique of the operation and postoperative treatment, there will arise a course in between, as it were, the ultraconservative and the ultraradical, which will at all times be open to the well-balanced, thoughtful surgeon and which will lead to a decreased mortality rate and a lowering of the percentage of unsatisfactory results in operating. It is purely a question of respecting your blood supply and making careful and neat approximation to assure against leakage.

COLON RESECTION FOR CONSTIPATION ALONE. I cannot accept the opinion that an operation of such gravity should be resorted to for control and relief of this condition *per se.* From my limited experience, I should unreservedly say that not only is the removal of the colon too hazardous an operation, but one that is totally unjustifiable in these cases for the probable outcome of relief. Do I believe in any operation for the relief of this condition? Yes, most certainly I do, and have done many with excellent results, namely, partial or limited resections and have achieved excellent results in those cases of long, angulated, redundant sigmoids by resection of this portion of the colon at fault. Some of the results have been really brilliant. I am not overoptimistic or overenthusiastic and distinctly believe in adopting the "mid-path," or the conservative side of this problem, and I might say that my attitude is strengthened by the fact that out of some fifty-odd cases of colon resections, I have seen fit to do but five radical colectomies.

ILEOSIGMOIDOSTOMY. In regard to this procedure, I might say that in none of my cases have I seen a condition that I considered warranted the so-called short-circuiting operation of Lane's (ileosigmoidostomy) and therefore have never performed an ileosigmoidostomy operation. It has never appealed to me in any way, and my only experience has been with one case in which I attempted to save the life of a patient practically dying from obstruction following several months after this operation had been done at another hospital.

BRIEFLY SUMMARIZED. 1. So far as cancer of the colon is concerned, this is an undisputed surgical problem, and it should be dealt with by operative intervention, and widespread resections done; the sooner the better.

2. It seems to me that in analyzing the results of colon resection for other than malignant causes the most critical and careful judgment should be excersied and no case reported favorably unless the case has been kept under the strictest surveillance for a considerable period; for its merits are not to be judged by its immediate, but by its ultimate results.

3. The operation is distinctly of the major type and should be undertaken only in obstinate and exaggerated cases; but they should not be waited upon so long as to bring about a toxemia that will, of itself, defeat the good effects of the operation.

4. It is distinctly too hazardous, as I have said before, to be undertaken purely for the relief of constipation alone. I feel that it is best in these cases to deal with the localized obstruction, or the actual sharp angulation, which is presented in so many of these obstinate cases, rather than do a complete and total resection.

5. There are dangers attending it and they should not be lost sight of. They are in the majority of cases remote postoperative ileus as well as immediate obstruction. These are the most common causes of the fatalities, as well as most of the ill effects that may follow.

6. Theoretically, the colon is, fortunately, a part of the human anatomy which can be dispensed with without

inflicting serious damage to the physiology that is the better part of it. It is needless to call attention to the fact that in most cases a considerable portion of the colon is always left, the sigmoid, and in a good many cases a part of the descending colon, if necesssary, which is sufficient to compensate for and take on the function of the portion that has been removed, and with this amount maintained, and free drainage established, intestinal toxemia ceases.

7. I have not observed that thirst in any of my cases was complained of, in spite of the physiologists pointing this out as one of the theoretic dangers. This is purely fallacious and incorrect, as is likewise their statement in maintaining that diarrhea is a concomitant. This I have not observed to be a fact, nor have I seen any serious physiological derangements in those cases that are done while there is still chance of recovery. They have gained in strength and in weight, and in cases Nos. 1 and 3 they have been made useful citizens, whereas before they were bed-ridden.

8. The chief dangers that we have to keep before us are in the operation *per se*, and in the possible immediate and postoperative obstructions that are liable to follow.

CASE No. 1.—Mrs. G. W., aged forty years, married, was admitted to my service at St. Joseph's Hospital, February 6, 1912, complaining of severe attacks of pain in the upper abdomen, vomiting, and retention of food, with marked weakness and loss of weight.

Past History. Patient was brought to me July 14, 1911, giving history of pain and discomfort, for the last ten days, over her appendix region. She entered the Union Protestant Infirmary and I removed her appendix, following which she made an uninterrupted recovery. At the time of operation it was noted that the cecum was enormously distended and the whole colon redundant, and I expressed the opinion that she was probably suffering more from retention in colon than from the appendix. During the summer of 1911, while I was away, she was again brought to Baltimore and operated upon at the Union Protestant Infirmary. The right ovary was removed and a ventral fixation was done. Examination of gall-bladder, kidneys etc., revealed nothing of importance, and her abdominal wound was closed. She returned home unimproved, and a few weeks later came back to Baltimore under the care of a stomach specialist, complaining of severe pain in her upper abdomen. Her stomach was repeatedly washed and anodynes given for her pain during her stay of ten weeks at the hospital. She again returned home without improvement.

Present Illness. Her present illness dates back to the summer of 1911. The clinical picture is one of a patient exhausted from vomiting and suffering from severe abdominal pains. These pains are periodical in character and located chiefly in her upper right abdomen. She was brought in with a probable diagnosis of gall-stones. The gastric contents were analyzed and found to be normal. *X*-rays were taken following large doses of bismuth with the following results; stomach emptied itself very slowly, a distinct kinking was noted at the pylorus, the cecum and ascending colon were found to be markedly dilated and a redundant loop of the ascending colon folded back on the cecum, and produced a pouch in which the bismuth accumulated and was retained, showing the cecum had been obstructed below this point, due evidently to the kinking of the bowel. Heart and lungs present no abnormality of significance. The kidney output, very low. Patient pale and anemic, and has lost considerable weight due chiefly to her starvation.

Operation. On February 8, under ether, abdomen was opened by a right median line incision. The pyloric end of the stomach came into view, and it showed a distinct kink due to traction from below. The pylorus was found to be somewhat constricted and much thickened. Further examination revealed many adhesions tying fundus of the gall-bladder to the pylorus. These adhesions also extended to the free border of the liver and the hepatic flexure of the colon, tying all these structures in a mass. The adhesions were all removed, thus freeing the hepatic flexure at the colon, and relieving to a great extent the kink at the pylorus. The omentum and a loop of small intestines were adherent to the parietal peritoneum in the cicatrix, resulting from previous lower abdominal incision. These adhesions were finally relieved with much difficulty, especially where the small intestine was caught. When the omentum was freed, the ascending colon itself was found to be tied to the scar a distance of three or four inches and almost completely obstructing the bowel at this point. This was also freed and further investigation showed that the ascending colon was very long and redundant. It took about two hours to free the abdominal adhesions, which were largely the result of former operations, and I had a shocked patient to continue with, but concluded it was best to go on and do a partial resection of the colon, because of the marked redundancy of this organ. About twenty-four inches of the bowel extending between the cecum below and over to the left arm of the transverse colon near the splenic flexure above, was removed. The mesenteric vessels were tied, a purse string was put around the colon, it was clamped, cut across with a thermocautery near the splenic flexure, the end invaginated, and the purse-string suture tied. This was reinforced by a few mattress Lembert sutures, and the same method of resection was done just above the cecum. A lateral anastomosis was then made between the cecum and descending colon just below the splenic flexure. The abdomen was then closed with drainage.

CASE No. 2.—Miss F. O., aged thirty-seven years, American, was transferred to my service at St. Joseph's Hospital November 24, 1914, with a general vague history of illness dating back more than four years, which principally consisted of obstinate constipation, indigestion and pains in abdomen. The obstinate constipation dates back even further and has been the predominating symptom in her case. The pain was not definitely localized in any particular part of the abdomen, save that it was more pronounced in the left lower abdomen, in the ileocecal valve, and complained of very much less when the bowels were freely moved; but they are never moved without the use of strong purgatives. As this symptom has grown gradually worse, it has now become very obstinate. She is a small woman, anemic and very nervous. I offered the operation on account of this obstructive form of constipation and on account of the x-ray findings which showed a marked angulation at sigmoid, high angulation of splenic flexure, dilated transverse and ascending colon and cecum. Incompetency of the ileocecal valve with quantity of bismuth enema in terminal ileum also noted.

Operation. Anesthetized with ether, abdomen opened by long rectus incision; ileocecal area was then sought and brought up into the wound and the blood supply to the last two inches of the ileum ligated and severed between ligatures. The ileum was then clamped and severed by means of electric cautery several inches from the ileocecal valve. The ascending colon which was markedly dilated was then delivered into the wound and bloodvessels in mesocolon, beginning from below upwards, were doubly ligated close up to the bowel margin. The same procedure was carried on until the colon was freed around to the sigmoid flexure, and anastomosis was made between the end of ileum and through upper portion of sigmoid flexure as is indicated and shown in the figures. The bowel was then severed by cautery and the opening beneath the anastomosis closed by interrupted silk sutures. A rubber tube was then passed into the rectum and through the anastomosis, three inches above it (as in all these cases) six ounces of Russian oil were then injected and kept in. I might say that in this case, as in all the cases, I employed subcutaneous salt solution through the entire operation and a 1000 c.c. was taken up. Daily afterwards six ounces of the Russian oil were given through the tube and the tube left in for eight days. After this, the tube was removed and patient given night and morning two ounces of oil by mouth for ten days. The wound healed under one dressing, and patient made an uninterrupted recovery. The lantern slides show the specimen which was removed, and x-ray plates before and after operation.

CASE No. 3.—Mrs. R. E. C., aged thirty-nine years, married, entered hospital in my service November 17, 1914, with symptoms of pronounced abdominal pain and long-standing chronic and obstinate constipation. This history dates back to a number of years. She is rather a slender, frail, little woman, and has recently grown so weak and feeble that for a number of months she has been a bed-ridden sufferer. She has rather a pathetic history, in that during her illness of five or six years she has gone through with a great many surgical procedures. The first operation was supposed to have been a gastro-enterostomy for gastroptosis. No relief was gotten and in June 1913, a second operation was done and no evidence of the gastro-enterostomy was found. The appendix was removed and abdominal adhesions severed. The rest in bed following this opera-seemed to help her to some extent, but in a short while her symptoms again recurred, and in April, 1914, she was again operated upon for abdominal adhesions, this time by myself, and I found adhesions running from the incisions and fixing the stomach pretty definitely to the abdominal wall, and also the colon to the abdominal wall. It was noted, however, at this operation that she had an enormously redundant and large looping transverse colon down into her pelvis. Nothing was done in the way of its relief however, and she was kept in hospital at rest for quite a little while, hoping that it would improve her general condition. The constipation was not improved, however, and no apparent help was gotten. She continued to complain of her nervousness and general weakened condition associated with headaches, loss of appetite and dizziness. When I was applied to again to go in and see what I could do, I told them, judging from what I had seen at the former operation, that the only thing I thought would be of help to her would be removal of the colon, to get rid of her obstructive constipation; so on November 19, 1914, I operated and took away her colon, using the technique that I have herewith described, and closed her without drainage. She made an uninterrupted recovery. The lantern slides show pictures before and after operation. I might say the x-ray findings in her case before operation show a long circuitous aberrant sigmoid, distended transverse colon, and incompletely filled cecum and ascending colon, probably due to impaction. Also a high angulated splenic flexure and tremendously tortuous upper rectum and sigmoid. Recent report from her physician is that she had some diarrhea five weeks after returning home from hospital. Previous to operation she had nervous attacks bordering on hysteria, but never becoming unconscious from same. Since operation has been quite free from these attacks, although at times still nervous. She looks improved and expression of face is infinitely more healthy. She has lost that haggard expression and her general appearance and conduct nearer normal. She has gained in weight and is sufficiently strong to get about and do many of her household duties.

CASE No. 4.—Miss L., aged thirty years, Irish, admitted to my service at St. Joseph's Hospital, November 16, 1914, suffering with general arthritis. Every joint in her body locked. She had had rheumatism for many years, tonsils were removed three years ago without any benefit. Present illness dates back seven years, to an attack of rheumatism from which she has never recovered. The second bad attack began three years ago. She entered the Women's Hospital and stayed sixteen months. Plaster casts were applied, limbs were baked, she was put to sleep and the muscles forcibly stretched by passive motion, without improvement.

I mention this to show that she has been through all methods of treatment and was in the most pitiable state, in fact, in such a condition that I hesitated, for I thought her toxic condition would make her a bad surgical risk. At this time she could not move any joint and was completely helpless, in fact she had not a joint that was not invaded. This condition has been present for the last four years, but it grew worse and worse as time went on. X-ray picture before operation showed a large rectum, circuitous aberrant sigmoid, causing angulation of descending colon as it passes the crest of the ileum. The splenic flexure was high and transverse colon narrow, and on its hepatic end had an angulation as it approached the flexure. The ascending colon and cecum were dilated. The aberrancy was so great that the cecum and sigmoid were touching, one overlying the other. On account of the x-ray findings and on acccount of the apparent helplessness of the case, unless something radical was done, I offered them operation. She went through it very comfortably without shock.

Operation November 24, 1914. This went well, done by the same method as the others, but I noted at the time I was tying off the hepatic flexure that the peritoneum over the duodenum was interfered with, but it did not occur to me that it would interfere with the duodenum. She was anastomosed as the others were and closed without drainage. For several days all went well, then vomiting began and persisted in growing worse and worse. There was no ballooning of the abdomen, no evidence of trouble about the wound which healed primarily, and there was no apparent infection, so with the absence of distended abdomen and wound closing as it did, I inferred this was a duodenal obstruction where the peritoneum had been stripped off, and I felt I could not remedy it. On the eighth day she died from exhaustion from vomiting. I had no means of getting a convincing autopsy, but feel death was due to duodenal obstruction where the peritoneum had been interfered with at the time of getting away the hepatic flexure.

CASE No. 5.—Mrs. J. W. A., aged sixty-seven years was admitted to my service at St. Joseph's Hospital, May 11, 1915, suffering from pain in her abdomen, occasional vomiting, and slight distension of abdomen. Four months ago she began to experience pain and discomfort in the right side over region of the appendix, which however has gradually grown more pronounced. Three weeks ago she stated that she could see and feel a large mass in her right side which would grow very large and finally disappear, thus relieving her pain markedly. She consulted her physician who also thought by abdominal examination he could palpate a lump in the abdomen. X-rays were taken and the doctor's diagnosis verified before she came to the hospital, as follows: An obstruction in the ascending colon as it joins the cecum. Absence of the shadow of the cecum due to an annular carcinoma at this point. Upon entrance into hospital it was noted that her general condition was poor, rather thin, has lost considerable weight in last three months. Her chief complaint is a dull pain in abdomen and inability to keep food on her stomach, with marked constipation. The slightest amount of food seems to increase the pain and bring about marked fulness and distension of the abdomen. Bowels have been irregular for the last three months, and during last ten days has had great difficulty in getting movement of bowels. Bladder active, urine shows slight trace of albumen, otherwise normal. Heart and lungs in good condition.

Operation May 13, 1915. Anesthetized with ether, abdomen opened by a vertical incision near the midline, extending through upper and lower abdomen, and about ten or eleven inches in length. Abdomen was explored and a large annular carcinoma of ascending colon, three inches above ileocecal valve was noted. Also a large hard carcinoma was noted in the mesenteric attachment near the splenic flexure. Smaller nodules of metastasis were seen through the mesentery of entire colon, extending into the mesentery of the ileum a distance of six or eight inches. Resection was begun eight inches from the ileocecal valve, including the ileum and the metastatic invasion of the mesentery. Bloodvessels were ligated independently and separated between ligatures. The ascending, transverse and descending colon were likewise removed in similar manner around to the sigmoid flexure. The end of ileum was then anastomosed by lateral implantation into side of sigmoid, a purse string put around the bowel two and a half inches above and the intestine crushed and tied off with a catgut ligature. The resected portion was incised just distal to the ligature and removed. The stump was then invaginated, purse string tied and stump reinforced with a few interrupted mattress stitches of fine silk. The opening in mesentery behind the anastomosis was then closed with four interrupted silk sutures. A tube was then passed through the anastomotic opening into the small intestines and six ounces of Russian oil (paraffin) was injected and the tube clamped to prevent oil from escaping. Abdomen closed without drainage. She made an uninterrupted recovery. The wound healed per primam and discharged from hospital three weeks following operation. No reaction whatever followed the operation, temperature never going above normal during entire convalescence. Bowels moved daily. Russian oil (6 ounces) was injected into bowel through tube in rectum daily, tube remained in anastomosis six days. Specimen showed an annular carcinoma (adenocarcinoma) of ascending colon. The lumen of the colon was so strictured that it was almost completely obstructed. The opening was so small that it would only admit the point of a lead pencil. A nodule of carcinoma was also noted in the wall of the colon near splenic flexure, and carcinomatous glands were observed all along the lymphatics in the mesentery and along the wall of the ileum.

REFERENCES

J. E. Goldthwait. The Relation of Posture to Human Efficiency and the Influence of Poise Upon the Support and Function of the Viscera. Boston Med. and Surg. Jour., December 9, 1909, *et seq.*

J. E. Goldthwait. The Cause of Gastroptosis and Enteroptosis, with Their Possible Importance as a Causative Factor in the Rheumatoid Diseases. *Ibid.*, May 26, 1910.

J. E. Goldthwait. The Recognition of Congenital Visceral Ptosis in the Treatment of the Badly Poised and Poorly Nourished Child. Amer. Jour. Orth. Surg., November, 1911.

J. G. Mumford. Surgical Aspects of Digestive Disorders, 1907.

Sir W. Arbuthnot Lane. Operative Treatment of Chronic Constipation, 1909. Chronic Intestinal Stasis, London *Lancet*, December 21, 1912, 11 No. 4660, pp. 1701–1770.

Dr. Nassau. Annals of Surgery, 1913.

H. S. Clogg. London *Lancet*, 1908, ii, 1007.

Sir Berkeley Moynihan. Abdominal Operations, 1914.

DISCUSSION ON THE PAPERS OF DRS. DOWNES, PARHAM AND MARTIN

DR. JAMES F. MITCHELL, Washington, D. C.—I should like to say a few words about this really remarkable paper of Dr. Downes which carries with it a lesson that must be brought home to all of us, namely, that these cases are occurring everywhere. There are a few of us who are seeing only a scattered case now and then which comes to the notice of someone, but Dr. Downes's paper shows that where medical men especially are on the lookout for them more and more, these cases will be turned over earlier to the surgeon for operation.

I believe that most of our marasmic babies that go on and die with a diagnosis of marasmus are cases of pyloric stenosis. This paper should be brought to the attention of medical men, and might have been read before them rather than before surgeons, because it is through these men that these cases are neglected and do not get into the hands of surgeons as early as they should.

Personally, I have seen four of these cases, all coming through private practice, and the last one is especially interesting as bearing upon what Dr. Downes has just said. The first three cases I reported two years ago at the Atlanta meeting. They are now six, seven, and three years of age respectively. They are all healthy babies. A posterior gastro-enterostomy was done in all three of them. This operation is not particularly difficult, although there are some drawbacks, and if we can establish a natural current we feel we are doing better work.

The last case I had was some two months ago, and emphasizes very strongly the etiology of tumor formation, as brought out by Dr. Downes, that is, the first thing is the obstruction and the size of the tumor, which may depend upon or be due to the straining on account of the obstruction. This baby I operated on when it was two weeks old. It is the youngest case, so far as I know, that has been subjected to operation, Dr. Downes's youngest case being three weeks of age. It is by far the most interesting case I have seen because there was no visible tumor, although there was said to have been a palpable tumor, which really was not palpated, so far as I could make out, because it did not exist at the time of operation. This baby weighed eight pounds at birth, a large, healthy boy, and when it was about four days old began vomiting. Vomiting became more and more pronounced until at the age of two weeks he had lost two pounds, and was vomiting practically all his food. The little patient was seen by Professor Howland, who thought he could make out a definite tumor. Peristalsis was quite evident and characteristic. The so-called bony ball rolled across the upper abdomen. I could not feel a tumor although I examined the patient very carefully. The symptoms were so definite that we decided upon operation. At the operation we found a definitely thickened pylorus, but not the olive-shaped translucent, edematous tumor which was found in the later cases. This is a very early stage, the stage of obstruction, which is exaggerated into the edematous tumor, as Dr. Downes has described. I did not fell justified in doing a gastroenterostomy, and after talking with Dr. Downes about his other cases in which the Rammstedt operation was done, we decided to do that. We found it exceedingly easy. A slit was made longitudinally, and instead of scissors, we used an artery clamp which was introduced down to the mucosa and spread apart, opening up completely the constricted pylorus. No covering was used, no attempt was made to suture it. This child went on to a splendid recovery. He was troublesome for a few days in the way of feeding, which was started immediately after operation, but he is gaining rapidly in weight and is improving in every way.

This splendid modification in treatment is going to revolutionize operative intervention in these cases, and it seems to me we are going to get better results.

The one important lesson to be drawn from this paper is that these cases exist everywhere, and we are overloooking them and they do not get into the hands of the surgeons as early as they should.

DR. DEAN LEWIS, Chicago, Illinois.—Dr. Downes has had a rather unique experience in the operative treatment of congenital pyloric stenosis and it is difficult to select any points for discussion which he has not already touched upon. I have operated upon nine cases. The first five recovered and developed normally. One of these died nine months after operation, and in reporting with Dr. Grulee the pathological condition of the pylorus, I made the statement that babies stood posterior gastro-enterostomy well and that the mortality associated with this operation should be low. Three cases which followed died. The sixth baby died of peritonitis which followed opening of the abdominal wall on the fifth day. The seventh baby died as a result of perforation of the line of suture of the gastro-enter-ostomy on the seventh day. The eighth baby died 48 hours after operation. The autopsy did not reveal any definite cause of death. There was no peritonitis and the line of suture of the gastro-enterostomy orifice was good. The ninth baby, which has made a good recovery, was an exceedingly poor operative risk. This baby had a bad rhinitis with a fairly high temperature, but had been losing so rapidly that we were afraid to postpone the operation. Chloroform was used—as a rule ether has been given and is the anesthetic of choice.

I have had more trouble with the abdominal wall than with the gastro-enterostomy and great care must be employed in closing the incision. An incision carried to the right of the median line is probably more easily and effectively closed than one through the broad part of the linea alba.

A congenital pyloric stenosis once established is permanent. This is indicated by the observation made by Grulee and me upon a pylorus of a baby which died nine months after successful gastro-enterostomy in which the pylorus had been at rest. This would seem to indicate that any medical treatment instituted with the idea of relieving the stenosis is futile and that if persisted in for any length of time reduces to a minimum the chances for surgical relief.

The diagnosis has been based upon projectile vomiting and peristalsis. If a baby presents these symptoms beginning three or four weeks after birth, the indications for surgical intervention are definite. We have not been able in all cases to palpate a tumor.

Posterior gastro-enterostomy is not a difficult operation in babies. It has, I believe, one advantage over the Rammstedt operation. If the mucous membrane beneath the hard hypertrophied pyloric tissue should be injured repair would be exceedingly difficult and a gastro-enterostomy would probably have to be resorted to. There is more chance to repair errors in technic in the gastro-enterostomy and unless the mortality is markedly reduced by the Rammstedt operation, I believe that I shall still employ the posterior gastro-enterostomy.

DR. JOHN YOUNG BROWN, St. Louis, Missouri.—Just a few words in regard to the paper of Dr. Downes. Surgeons are practically agreed as to the time and method of treating cases of congenital pyloric obstruction.

I quite agree with Dr. Mitchell that this paper should be presented before a society of practitioners. I can no better illustrate the importance of this than to refer to a paper recently read by Dr. Scudder of Boston before the American Association of Pediatricians. Although he demonstrated the pathology of this condition and outlined the correct method of treatment, and presented arguments which would have readily been accepted by the State Association of Plumbers, the discussion that followed showed that his views were not accepted, and a majority of those present still urged the medical care of these cases.

My experience with this condition has been limited to four cases in all of which I did a posterior gastro-enterostomy, and encountered no technical difficulties in the operation. The mortality in these cases was 50 per cent. Two of the patients came late for operation and I feel that I possibly might have saved them, if I had done a two-stage operation, doing a jejunostomy quickly, and later doing a posterior gastro-enterostomy.

DR. ALEXIUS MCGLANNAN, Baltimore, Maryland.—After several years of hoping and searching, I had my first case of congenital pyloric stenosis last week in a white child. I did a posterior gastro-enterostomy. The baby lived forty-eight hours. It vomited continuously. At the postmortem examination we got the entire gastro-intestinal tract and found the anastomosis was perfect. The cause of death I do not know. There was no reason for death so far as we could make out from the postmortem examination. The tumor was extremely hard and edematous and very white.

With reference to the frequency of this disease. In Baltimore I have access to an asylum for colored children where there are admitted probably eighteen to twenty children a month. For several years the most important cause of death in that institution was marasmus. We made postmortem examinations for several months on all children who died there in the hope of finding congenital pyloric stenosis, feeling we had missed it in the diagnosis of marasmus. We kept on making these postmortem examinations for many months without running across such cases, and none has occurred in this large children's clinic.

DR. A. J. OCHSNER, Chicago, Illinois.—Just a word in connection with Dr. Parham's paper. We have studied a lot of these cases, and we have come to this rule: we make the diagnosis from the history and clinical examination and write it down. Then we make an x-ray diagnosis, and if it is positive we accept it. If it is negative, we pay no attention to it. I am sure that is what Dr. Parham's patient should have had, because if you depend primarily upon a diagnosis with the x-ray, you are bound to fall into trouble all the time. You should do it the other way, write down the diagnosis, then accept the x-ray diagnosis if it is reasonable and confirms your diagnosis based on clinical examination.

DR. WILLIAM A. DOWNES, New York City (closing).—I thank the gentlemen for their consideration of my paper. It is up to us to educate medical men along lines with which we are treating pyloric obstruction by operation. Unfortunately we had eight or ten cases in which I had observed in the hospital ward which were kept in the medical service hoping they might make medical recoveries.

NOTES ON FOCAL INFECTIONS

By Robert T. Morris, M.D.
New York

BETWEEN the accurate laboratory work of Rosenow and the accurate application of principles made by Billings, to the subject of focal infections, we have on the other side the charming flights of poetic fancy of Lane, and between these two sides the profession, at the present time, has not obtained its equilibrium in this very important subject. I know this particularly well, because in a concrete way cases of ulcer of the stomach are being sent to me for operation again after operation has already been done, and yet the question of focal infection has never been brought up by the family physician or by the surgeon who operated.

Two months ago in a case that came on from Vancouver the surgeon had done gastro-enterostomy for ulcer of the stomach. The ulcer recurred and the patient came to New York. I did a second operation for that patient. The patient returned home benefited, but came back with recurrent ulcer. In this case, after careful investigation, there were found four tooth roots with various cultures of the Streptoccocus viridans, and these were found for the first time only two weeks ago. That patient was suffering from neglect on part of two surgeons, and I was one of those surgeons. I was the one who did the second operation, and did not at that time give enough attention to the question if any focal infection occurred at the tooth roots. Rosenow's work shows us that a selective affinity of certain groups of cells for certain toxins will lead to such cell destruction at these points that we must be ever on the alert for every possible focal infection which may furnish toxins for excretion by the duodenum and stomach. We shall find an explanation for many of our cases of ulcer of the stomach and duodenum, the excreted toxins having a selective affinity for cells at that point. Commonly a proliferative endarteritis develops leading to secondary changes. This matter of proliferative endarteritis at a point where toxins are engaged in a selective process, I brought out some years ago. In that part of the enteron where we have a terminal arterial system, proliferation of the inner coat of an artery occurs as the result of excessive excretion of toxins at this point. When this arterial proliferation occurs in a single terminal artery we have a roundish ulcerating area in consequence. There are few cases of ulcer of the stomach or duodenum coming into your practice today in which you may not get positive or negative testimony bearing upon the question of these toxins emanating from affected tooth roots, and the patient knowing nothing about it. A patient may have colonic infection, such as Mr. Lane has described, without knowing anything about it. That brings me to another point, and a very important one, namely, that Lane has concentrated too much attention upon the abdomen, like some of the ascetics of India, and with about as satisfactory a result. Therefore, I would make this point, that we are not to concentrate our attention upon the colon in searching for focal infections. We must look over the periphery of a large circle of causes in order to find a possible focus which is sending out toxins that are being excreted at a certain point where there is selective cell affinity for these toxins. I mention this point particularly because so many of these cases are being overlooked. On making inquiry I often find that the question of focal infection has never been taken up in a large way in connection with such cases. It is more apt to be taken up by some one who has fanciful ideas about the importance of some one area of focal infection, but the entire subject has not been gone over. This is true of our cases of dyspepsia in general, using the term "dyspepsia" as a blanket diagnostic term. If you can have a blanket diagnostic entity, dyspepsia is that. In all of these cases we must look for various focal infections, and very often at such a distance as a single tooth root, with the Streptococcus viridans confined in such a way that it cannot make its escape by way of some nearby opening. Its toxins must find exit through the circulation, and thus the toxins are excreted by mucosa of the pylorus or duodenum.

Another point in this connection is the question of cancer. It has not been brought up prominently in relation to focal infection. According to very recent work with œnethera among plants, physiologists have shown that in the primrose under toxic overstimulation certain fertilizers cause a bizarre chromatin arrangement in plant cells. We may have haploid or triploid arangement of the chromosomes in the nuclei as a result of toxic influence.

It seems to me that one new line for observation in studying cancer is this: we may have the loss of one of the chromosomes out of the cell nucleus, and something like haploid development as a result of the toxin influence upon the cells in cases of cancer. That is a postulate. The idea is based upon this observation, that during the past year I have made note of a group of patients with cancer who also had foci of infection which might be domonstrated and during this time I found that practically all of the cases of cancer of any form whatsoever were patients in whom focal infection could be demonstrated. We know cancer must begin from one cell which has gone wrong, and we know that this one cell has something wrong with its nucleus. We know from our study of plant physiology of the cell nucleus that any number of chromosomes may go wrong as the result of toxic influence. I bring this point up as a suggestion because it is one that is acutely before us today. We find that irritation plus toxic enzyme constitutes the "dual unit" in cancer causation.

We are not to look for a defect in the colon in explanation for as large a proportion of these cases as does Mr. Lane. We must look for all distinct focal infections. In a patient allergic to the influence of toxins, we may have intestinal stasis as one symptom of the presence of those toxins which cause vagatonia. We have intestinal stasis in vagatonic patients because the vagus is overstimulated, and being overstimulated holds in check the enteric drivers. The vagus may be constantly overstimulated because of toxins which may be traced to the Streptococcus viridans from a tooth root in one given case. The colon itself then becomes a second focus for more toxins. On the other hand, you may have a number of focal infections at a distance furnishing toxins which overstimulate the autonomic system and its plexuses, and these toxins may proceed from the colon or from some distant source, as an infected endometrium or seminal vesicle. The point I wish to make is that in our study of focal infections today, no matter whether we are dealing with arthritis or with intestinal stasis due to vago-tonic impulse or autonomic stimulation as symptoms, or whether we are dealing with ulcer of the stomach due to selective cell affinity for toxins at this point, we must keep ever in mind very clearly two concepts: (1) the fanciful poetry of Lane, which has enlarged our range of vision enormously, and (2) we must keep also in mind the careful, accurate scientific work of Rosenow with the practical applied science deduced from his facts by such men as Billings.

A FURTHER STUDY IN THE USE OF IODIN
IN COMBATING THE PERITONITIDES

By J. A. Crisler, M.D.
Memphis, Tennessee

At first blush the proposition of pouring an alcoholic solution of iodin into the peritoneal cavity, for any cause whatever, strikes the trained surgeon with amazement and horror, while men who would advocate such a measure are set upon as cheap notoriety seekers, if not indeed criminally insane. I had a part of this same feeling concerning my associate Dr. Eugene Johnson, some ten years ago, when he first worked out the idea and I studied the matter long and carefully before adopting it.

Bichloride of mercury, ether, formaldehyde, and other poisonous and irritating drugs have been vainly tried for the same purpose and justly abandoned. The iodin treatment of peritonitis, however, as hereinafter set forth, has come to stay with us as far as we are individually concerned.

You will be welcome to expend upon us your most fitting words of condemnation, for such is our abiding faith. However, rash and misplaced criticisms upon the iodin method does not raise the standard of surgery, nor lend a helping hand to those who suffer.

Wrapping one's self in a cloak of self-sufficiency and proclaiming discredit upon the heads of those who are conscientiously trying to reduce and are reducing the mortality from peritonitis is unworthy of men in high station. Surgeons of lesser note have automatically inherited the more virulent cases of peritoneal infections, since the great teachers of surgery and the better clinics, especially of the North and East, have of necessity rightly divorced themselves from every pus case possible.

Geographical situations, poor transportation facilities, malaria, illiteracy, hookworm, and other factors help make many of our cases hopeless to the ordinarily accepted regime of treatment. Surgeons in our section of the South, who claim to be saving over 75 per cent. of their cases of real peritonitis, without the aid of the iodin method, are fooling themselves, or else have but few exceptional cases.

We have read papers on this method before the Southern Medical Association at Hattiesburg, Miss., Jacksonville, Fla., and Lexington, Ky., and before the St. Louis Medical Society, the Kentucky State Railway Surgeon's Association at Louisville and the Tri-state Medical Association at Memphis, besides numerous smaller medical gatherings; therefore most of you are familiar with every detail of the method.

TECHNIC. We use a 2.5 per cent. solution of iodin (crystals) in 95 per cent. alcohol, and as soon as the incision is made and the cavity reached (if pus is discovered in the peritoneal cavity) this solution is poured in immediately so as to thoroughly flood the infected area before any attempt is made to liberate the pathological tissue. By this means we have learned not to fear a spread of the infection through mechanical means. The principal feature in this method up to now is to make ourselves feel perfectly sure that the iodin reaches well beyond the areas infected and also that we are operating in an immersed field, from which no further contamination can reach the healthy portions without first coming in contact with the solution. The amount of the solution that we use is dependent upon the extent of peritoneal infection; that is to say, if the infection is partially or completely localized, two or more ounces may be sufficient to flood the field and render the necessary service. If, however, there is a widespread of infection as in diffuse, septic peritonitis, we retract and elevate the abdominal incision and literally pour the entire abdomen and pelvis full of this solution, taking great care to make sure that the drug reaches all of the fossæ and recesses within the abdominal and pelvic cavities. This may require from 8 to 32 ounces or more of the solution. After the focus of infection is dealt with, we take large towel sponges and insert these into the most dependent fossæ and gently mop out the excess solution and débris, avoiding scrubbing and trauma. Of course, in every case we employ abundant drainage, Fowler position and Murphy drip. If there is profound toxemia we also use saline hypodermoclysis in order to more rapidly eliminate the toxins.

OBJECT TO BE ATTAINED. We are all familiar with nature's defensive elements that are primarily active in an infected area within the peritoneum. This defensive process is manifested by the abundant outpouring of leukocytes around the focus of infection. These phagocytes are victorious in so long as they are able to encompass and combat a given number of the invading bacteria. In progressive cases, however, these are soon overcome and are no longer defensive, but become offensive in that they have been mastered by the virulent infecting organisms. A case may end by localization of the infective processes, provided the spread of infection is not too rapid and the resisting forces of the economy are in good fighting order. If this does not obtain, or if the localized abscess ruptures into the general cavity, we have a more extensive infection, which may go on to diffuse or even general suppurative peritonitis.

Our large experience in the use of this drug and the clinical manifestations after its use in these cases lead us to firmly and conscientiously believe that the infected fluids that are free in the cavity are at once sterilized and that the absorption of toxins, which after all, is the *sine qua non*, mortuary factor of peritonitis, is immediately terminated for at least twenty-four hours; also an outpouring of serum and new phagocytes is immediately encouraged. We are strengthened in this belief by the fact that a high temperature in these cases almost invariably falls in a few hours down to normal or nearly normal. Then too there is an abundant serous drainage following, which is in excess of the usual drainage common in other methods. This tends to disgorge and in a measure wash out the subserous, cellular tissues, which may receive some beneficent, antiseptic effect through a process of osmosis directly from the iodin that has come in contact with the inflamed serosa.

Byron Robinson correctly describes the peritoneum as a veritable lymph sac. If it were not for stasis and clotting in these lymph capillaries, every case of intraperitoneal infection, however mild, would be rapidly fatal. By the iodin method of treatment these lymph capillaries are immediately coagulated, we think for a period of at least twenty-four hours, during which time there is no absorption of toxins from the peritoneal surface lymphatics.

In our investigations of the elimination of the iodin element it has never appeared in the urine earlier than the eighteenth hour after its use in the abdomen, and then only in very small quantities. The height of elimination (which is almost entirely through the kidneys) is attained about the seventy-second hour. We conjecture from this study that the absorption of toxins is held in abeyance for a like period. All the facts brought out by these studies, including clinical, physiological, and chemical, combine to show the truth of this assertion. During this period there is developed in the patient an autoresistance and toleration quite sufficient to overcome the disease.

Since it would be impossible to incorporate all these studies in so short a paper, we take the liberty of submitting the urinary reports of one which accentuates the points above mentioned. This is from the case of a boy, aged twelve years, who had an extensive streptococcic peritonitis and differs from the others in no material respect as far as urinary findings are concerned, except a slightly larger output of the iodin through the urine (of course in the form of iodides). Thirty-two ounces of the iodin solution was pured into the abdomen.

Specimen A.   April 11, 1913, 3 P.M. contains no iodin.

Specimen B.   April 11, 1913, 6.30 P.M. contains no iodin.

Specimen C.   April 12, 1913, 12.30 A.M., contains no iodin.

Specimen D.   April 12, 1913, 6 A.M., contains trace of iodin.

Specimen E.   April 12, 1913, 12 M., contains in 90 c.c. 0.0766 gram iodin.

Specimen F.   April 12, 1913, 5 P.M., contains in 110 c.c. 0.1269 gram iodin.

Specimen G.   April 13, 1913, 7 A.M., contains in 110 c.c. 2.5384 grams iodin.

Specimen H.   April 14, 1913, 5 P.M., contains in 120 c.c. 0.3807 gram iodin.

Specimen I.   April 15, 1913, 8 A.M., contains in 100 c.c. 0.0634 gram iodin.

Specimen J.   April 17, 1913, 6 A.M., contains in 190 c.c. 0.2855 gram iodin.

Specimen K.   April 19, 1913, 8 A.M., contains in 90 c.c. 0.0317 gram iodin.

Specimen L.   April 22, 1913, 8 A.M., contains no iodin.

It will be seen from this that the elimination is at its height between the third and the seventh days. Its combination with the salts of the blood is very interesting from a physiological and therapeutic standpoint. In some cases as high as 40 grains of iodides to three and a half ounces of urine have been found.

From December 1, 1914, to December 1, 1915, we operated upon 678 abdominal cases with 23 deaths. In this number of operations we had 104 pus cases. In other words, slightly over 15 per cent. of all of our abdominal cases were due to pus in the abdomen, either localized and walled off or free with no effort at walling off. In these 104 pus cases we had 31 cases in which there was free pus in the abdomen, with no localization of walling off whatsoever. In this latter series we had one death, this case reaching us in a moribund condition and utterly hopeless.

The remaining 30 in this series we classified as follows: Gangrenous appendicitis that had ruptured (peritonitis still local though no walling off), 9; cases of peritonitis involving the pelvis and abdomen below the umbilicus, 5; cases of general peritonitis, 16.

It is in such cases as the last 30 mentioned in this series that the iodin method is so definitely indicated and has given us the most satisfaction. Some of these cases may have recovered by simply removing the source of infection and giving the abdomen abundant drainage, because the outpouring of white cells and serum may still have been defensive. On the other hand, these fluids may have become virulently infected, in which case the outcome for recovery, without the iodin method, is only speculative. After its use we have less temperature, less distention from gas, and we think less pain and nausea.

There are three arguments against the use of iodin in the abdomen, all of which deserve mention.

CONCLUSIONS. 1. Nearly all cases of peritonitis will get well without its use. (?) If this argument is true, as has been rashly advocated, then the subject needs no further discussion. In our hands we know beyond the question of a doubt that we have lost cases of peritonitis before using this method under the most careful and worthy surgical efforts of which we were capable. We know that since using this method we have not lost cases that were seemingly parallel to the others in every respect. We really feel so sure of our position that we no longer fear the outcome of these desperate cases so long as the patient reaches us with even a fighting chance for life.

2. As to the question of toxicity from the drug when used in the abdomen, we have this to say most emphatically, that we have never seen the slightest toxic effect, at any stage, nor have we seen the slightest evidences of iodinism in any case, even though we have washed out the abdomen with as much as a quart of the solution and have made but little effort in removing the excess remaining in the various fossæ. This includes many hundreds of cases.

3. How is it possible to use an irritating chemical of sufficient antiseptic strength to destroy bacteria in the abdominal fluids, pouring it over and soaking it into the delicate endothelial linings, without producing an excoriation, from which, if the patient survived, there would be innumerable adhesions, producing a condition that would be probably worse than the one for which the remedy was intended to cure? This is the most difficult argument of all to answer, and deserves the most credit and consideration at our hands. To begin with, we have all seen the resulting effects in way of adhesions which followed a cured case of peritonitis without the use of our method, and have been astonished at the multitude of adhesions, and have wondered how the intestinal tube could possibly functionate in the midst of these. Following the use of the iodin method, we are able to report 42 secondary operations (done mostly for ventral hernia) wherein we were enabled to view the results as to adhesions. In none of these cases have we found, at any time, any serious adhesions whatsoever beyond the ordinary omental adhesions in the hernial sac and around the hernia opening. So gratified have we been with these findings, and also with the general condition of our cases, upon whom the secondary operation has not been done, that we have been led to hope and even believe that the iodin method in treating peritonitis actually prevents adhesions. Whether or not the prolonged weeping of the peritoneum accounts for this we are unable at present to say; nor, indeed, do we know that the 42 cases mentioned would

be a sufficent index upon which to base a conclusion, even though these represented some of our worst cases in which the solution was used most liberally.

In order to make clear the strength of the iodin solution used the following explanation is given:

A 5 per cent. solution of pure iodin crystals in 95 per cent. alcohol is made. This is the stock solution. The nurse in the operating room dilutes this with equal parts of 95 per cent. alcohol, giving a 2.5 per cent. solution; this is the strength used in all operations.

In order to make it perfectly clear I will compare it with the official tincture both in strength and composition.

Official tincture of iodin:

7 per cent. pure iodin crystals.

5 per cent. potassium iodide dissolved in 95 per cent. alcohol.

The object of the potassium iodide in the official tincture is to increase the stability of the solution as well as the solubility.

From this it is seen that the strength of the iodin solution used in all operations, insofar as iodin content is concerned, is 29 per cent. of that of the official tincture, or a little less than one-third; in addition it contains no potassium iodide.

DISCUSSION

Dr. Robert T. Morris, New York City.—This paper must not go without discussion, because it is revolutionary. Dr. Crisler is either right or wrong. When he presents such definite data as he has presented, it places us upon the defensive and it is a very serious defensive point which we must meet. We cannot overlook a paper of this sort. *A priori*, we know this: iodin upon the peritoneum causes adhesions. The reason why we know it is because in our work with rabbits if we did not get all of the iodin carefully removed from the skin before operating, upon the second opening of the abdomen there was found adhesion of peritoneum where a little iodin got upon the peritoneum. One of the best and most expert operators in New York gave up the use of iodin in preparing the skin of the abdomen because where it got through the incision it caused vicious peritoneal adhesions along the line of incision. This however was in cases in which we did not have an extensive infection already present, such as has been described by Dr. Crisler.

Some years ago, when I brought forward the point of leaving pus in the free peritoneal cavity, and giving little attention to it, my idea brought about the same sort of criticism that I would now feel like applying to Dr. Crisler.

As to the thyroid group of patients, there are patients who are sensitive to iodin, particularly patients with exophthalmic goitre, whose adrenals are driving the thyroid gland ahead too fast. In these patients a very little extra iodin will upset the entire chromaffin system.

Dr. J. Garland Sherrill, Louisville, Kentucky.—Dr. Morris says that this paper of Dr. Crisler and the method he employs are revolutionary. We have had a good many debates in this Association upon the subject of peritonitis. At the Birmingham meeting of this Association, held about ten years ago, I presented a paper on the subject of "Perforative Peritonitis Due to Rupture of the Appendix." At that time the professional mind was somewhat chaotic. Dr. Blake and others were urging drainage of the abdomen; Dr. Morris was getting in and getting out quickly, and Dr. Murphy just at that time began a similar method, incorporating in his treatment the Fowler position and the introduction of saline solution in the rectum, and so forth.

If I had the opportunity to read my paper now, I would make a few changes in it, but dating from that time the professional opinion has become more or less crystallized upon this subject. We realize that the contention of Dr. Morris is true, that you can leave an enormous quantity of fluid, which becomes discolored, in the abdomen, in cases of acute perforative peritonitis from the appendix, and the patients do well. The tissues are good to us in their ability to withstand traumatism and infection. In this condition, if we use a substance like iodin, we must realize that iodin on the unbroken skin will often produce a blister in the dilute solution in which it is employed. If it will produce a blister upon the unbroken skin, it can do cellular damage to the wall of the intestine. As Dr.

Morris says, if the iodin is active in the peritoneal cavity, it must not be absorbed, otherwise we will get evidences of iodin absorption and the effects of iodism. If it is not absorbed it must act locally, and it acts not under the peritoneal surface but on top of it, and if Dr. Morris's contention is true, infection lies in the tissues, and not on top of the tissues of the peritoneum, then the iodin cannot reach the focus of infection. It will tan the peritoneum, and it may stop absorption, but whether it will stop absorption of toxins is a problem that cannot be well decided at this time. However, those of us who are not using iodin can report a series of cases with even better results than Dr. Crisler has given, namely, 42 cases of secondary operations for ventral hernia and other adhesions. I claim, furthermore, that if you open the abdomen, close the entrance of bacteria into the abdominal cavity, put in a drain, close up, put the patient in the Fowler position, and give a sufficient quantity of salt solution, that patient will be in a comfortable condition and in a few days will be out of bed. If you can improve on that, we can take the risk of putting poisonous substances in the abdomen. The surgical profession should adopt the simplest method that will reach the desired end, and I believe the simplest method is that universally adopted throughout the country.

My personal experience with appendicitis in the last 200 cases has been most satisfactory, including all forms of the disease, in which we have operated upon the patient when received regardless of the time or character of the peritonitis, and have lost only one case in this series. I would like, however, to get rid of that one death, but do not believe it can be done by using iodin. I have seen sloughs in the abdomen by using iodin upon the abdominal wound. In iodin we have an irritating substance which may do damage, and we have a much better method to be applied. I remember twenty-five years ago or more we used bichlorid of mercury solution in the treatment of tuberculous peritonitis. We have abandoned it now because we get just as good results without any substance being put into the abdomen in such cases.

DR. WILLIAM R. JACKSON, Mobile, Alabama.—Iodin is a necrotic agent. In one per cent. solution it necrotizes. We think when it is used we diminish the pyogenic process. Normal salt solution or any other isotonic solution would be much better. At first iodin was applied to the abdomen by Grossich for the purpose of preparing the field of operation with the view of destroying all bacteria. We have something much better now in *oil of creosote*, which will destroy the Staphylococcus albus in a short time; and so far as infections of the skin are concerned we get very little of them into the interior anyway. Therefore, iodin or any coagulant, or necrotizing chemical agent, put in the peritoneal cavity naturally produces chemical trauma and adhesions, therefore it is a dangerous agent. Like Dr. Morris I believe when pus is pent up for a long time, it is a benign agent. Our pathologists and biochemists have taught us recently that this fluid when pent up for a long time is bacteriolytic and will destroy bacteria and toxins, so the relief of tension, phagocytosis, and chemotaxis will do the rest.

DR. CHARLES M. ROSSER, Dallas, Texas.—I would like to ask Dr. Crisler, in the first place, if in a case of gangrenous appendicitis he has followed the usual rule of simply draining and allowing the appendix to remain to be removed subsequently or whether in connection with this particular treatment he has been able to complete the operation at that sitting. In the second place, I would like to ask him whether he has used iodin in tuberculous peritonitis with success. In the third place, whether he has experimented with alcohol alone without iodin, and if so, has he reached the same result?

Those are questions that naturally come to our minds, first, in view of this discussion as to what is general peritonitis. The doctor himself does not answer that; therefore, do we know whether he is handling general peritonitis cases, or whether he is handling the sort of cases we are losing or cases we have been successful with. If the same line of cases, is he able to do a more complete operation than we have been able to do without the use of iodin? The third question is only one of scientific interest, and he no doubt has made the experiment.

DR. BRANSFORD LEWIS, St. Louis, Missouri.—I know little or nothing about the use of iodin in the abdominal cavity, but I want to relate a personal observation of a case I saw in Dr. Crisler's hands. In former years, when I was younger in medical work, I had five years' experience in the City Hospital service of St. Louis. I had unpleasant experiences and a bad memory of the cases operated on at that time. Apparently, it made no difference whether we opened them up and drained them, or whether we drained them and gave them the benefit of posture; they nearly all died. I do not remember a single patient that lived, if he was in the extreme condition of the one I wish to mention.

I saw Dr. Crisler operate on a young man, about twenty-five years of age, about a year ago when I was in Memphis. The patient was a robust young farmer who had had a perforating appendicitis. After refusing for five days to be operated on, the young man was brought to the hospital at Memphis with a pulse of 140, which was merely a thread. He was gasping, his belly was greatly distended, and when Dr. Crisler opened him up, I should estimate that a quart of viscous, foul-smelling pus was removed, which to my mind indicated the man's doom. I remarked to Dr. Crisler that there was hardly any hope for the case. Dr. Crisler said, "Well Doctor, I think he is going to get well." Personally, I would not have given ten cents for his chances to get well. However, the patient went through the operation and I was astonished at the result three days later when I returned from a trip to Arkansas. The patient was thriving and was asking for his meals regularly, and he got well. I never saw any patient in such an extreme condition get well before, and I want to do Dr. Crisler the justice of relating the facts.

Dr. Louis Frank, Louisville, Kentucky.—I have been familiar with Dr. Crisler's work for some years, and, astounded by his statements, was led to carry on some experiments with the use of iodin within the peritoneal cavity. Our subjects were dogs, the peritoneum normal. Whether or not the results would tally with those in an inflamed cavity, is, of course, conjectural. However, tincture of iodin, injected in quantities of from five to ten c.c. into the normal peritoneum of dogs, almost invariably produced death within a very short time. Upon autopsy, such areas, with which the iodin had come in contact had the appearance of being charred or burned; in other words, the tissues were completely dehydrated, the endothelia being destroyed.

Aqueous solutions of iodin, as well as grain alcohol, produced death with similar local changes. Application of tincture of iodin to localized areas, such areas being marked to enable them to be recognized later, always produced endothelial destruction. In animals that had lived sufficiently long, adhesions were always found between such areas and other viscera or the parietes. Whether the same results obtain in pathological areas, we cannot say but it has seemed to us impossible to confine the action of tincture of iodin to abnormal structures when it is used in the way described by the essayist.

After having heard a paper, similar to the present one by the same essayist several years ago, though having in mind the results of my experimental work, I nevertheless used tincture of iodin in several cases, applying it locally and confining the application directly to the infected areas. I did not pour it into the abdomen, and I was very careful not to have it come in contact with the normal peritoneum. In these cases the only difference I noticed with regard to convalescence was that these cases required longer time to heal and the suppurative process was more prolonged than by our usual manner of treatment in similar cases.

I feel sure in my own mind that the use of iodin is not a means *per se* of lowering mortality, and I feel sure that the explanation of Dr. Crisler's lowered mortality is due, not to his iodin but comes in spite of it, as a result of the perfection in his technic due to a more extended experience in such cases and to better methods of drainage. The essayist is modest in giving the credit entirely to iodin.

Those of us who have been doing work for any number of years have no trouble in recalling a mortality of twenty, fifteen and ten per cent. in appendicitis cases. With improved technic and methods, with improved methods of securing bacterial and toxin elimination we have lowered the mortality to two and three per cent., and should our mortality today rise above this, we would make most careful search of our methods, realizing that something is wrong. I am sure that in the cases reported, the improvement comes not from any peculiar value of the iodin in those cases where there may be a colon, a streptococcic, or a staphylococcic suppuration, which may have existed for any length of time, but comes from the fact that Nature has had an opportunity, of which she has taken advantage, to put up a proper defence by increased leukocytosis and an increased immunity.

To be of greatest value the test of the method which the essayist has given us, or of any other agent used in peritonitis, must come from its use in acute infections due to trauma, such as gunshot wounds, in which the infective material has been suddenly introduced, and in which Nature has had no time or opportunity to put up a defence, and these cases should be permitted to reach the most dangerous stage before the value of iodin can be definitely determined, for we know that interference early in such cases is followed by good results, while in later interference the outcome in a large per cent. of cases has been fatal. Should this latter class of cases recover by the treatment indicated by the essayist, then we will believe in the value of his thesis.

DR. J. A. CRISLER, Memphis, Tennessee (closing).—I wish to thank the gentlemen very much for their generous discussions, some of which I greatly appreciate. Every time we read a paper on this subject we immediately stir up a hornets' nest in the camp of those blessed few who never lose patients from peritonitis. As stated in the paper, we have no appeal that can reach this class of men, for if they do not lose patients from peritonitis, they have nothing to gain by adopting the iodin method of treatment. In our section of the country we have a large population who are not educated to the importance of early operations and are inclined to delay these necessary procedures until they are desperately ill. Poor railroad facilities, malaria, and hook-worm help to further these unfavorable conditions in many cases. So it seems to us that we have proportionately more desperate intra-abdominal conditions to deal with than are encountered elsewhere. Surely the more northerly sections of our country do not have to face similar conditions. Louisville, however, is not so remote from our section and I am gratified to know that Dr. Sherrill has made such a wonderful record as he has just stated, wherein he lost only one case out of two hundred operations for all forms of appendicitis. He probably will not be able to repeat this record, nor can any of the remainder of us ever hope to do as well. It is a pity that he could not have used the iodin method on this one that died and made a clean score.

Dr. Frank thinks that the two cases upon which he used the iodin method (both of which recovered) were a few days longer in their convalescence than cases wherein he did not use it. We have found there is only a few minutes difference.

We do not think that our technic has improved in any measure insofar as the operative procedures are concerned and feel sure that we are saving these desperate cases that we hitherto lost, by the use of the iodin method as set forth in the paper.

As to Dr. Jackson's discussion, I will not refer to it further than to say that he is dealing with imaginary nightmares instead of with cold facts.

I fully agree with Dr. Morris and Dr. Frank that iodin poured into a healthy peritoneal cavity might produce all sorts of adhesions. It might produce death. I do not know. From what Dr. Frank says, I think it probably would. I have no desire to pour it into a healthy peritoneal cavity and try it. The same should obtain with regard to rabbits, cats, dogs or any other animals who have no infection in the peritoneal cavity.

In answer to Dr. Rosser, I will say yes, we invariably remove the pathological tissue in cases of gangrenous appendicitis. We always remove every appendix we go after unless perchance it helps to make up the wall and we feel that it had disintegrated sufficiently to take care of itself. In all "unwalled-off" cases we remove the pathological tissue.

While our experience in tuberculous peritonitis with the use of iodin is not large, still we have used it liberally in such cases with great satisfaction. Dieulafoy used it in 1848.

As for gunshot wounds and traumatic injuries we have had very little experience, comparatively speaking. We have had a few cases of gunshot wounds of the abdomen and have reported on them, with satisfactory results, and in every case we used the iodin solution liberally with supreme satisfaction.

TYPHOID PERFORATION PERITONITIS: REPORT OF AN UNUSUALLY INTERESTING CASE

By *F. D. Smythe*, M.D., F.A.C.S.

Memphis, Tennessee

"Typhoid fever is disgracefully prevalent in the United States."

Five hundred thousand persons are annually infected, and of that number forty thousand die.

One-third of all the deaths from typhoid are due to perforation peritonitis.

Hospital statistics show a mortality of 2.5 per cent. plus from perforation.

We have no way of determining the percentage of deaths from perforation, from typhoid, in private practice. Perhaps, however, it is not quite so high as in cases treated at the hospitals.

Time of Occurence of Perforation. More than half of the perforations occur during the third week of the disease. Perforation may occur, however, as early as the last of the first week or as late as the second month.

Period of greatest danger, third week.

Location of Perforation. Perforation is found in the majority of cases in the last twelve inches of the ileum. (Hart and Ashhurst.) Quoting from their record:

"Out of 362 cases it was found in 73 per cent. within twelve inches of the cecum; in 4 cases, 2.10 per cent., only was it situated more than three feet from the cecum. In

7 cases the colon was perforated. In 5 cases perforation of the ascending colon, 1 of the transverse colon, and 1 of the sigmoid. There were 3 cases of perforation in Meckel's diverticulum and 8 perforations of the appendix."

In the majority of my cases the perforations have been multiple, and with two exceptions the cases have been late ones; more than twelve hours after the initial symptom pain occurred. Generally speaking, the perforation is single; in a few cases, however, they have been found very numerous.

DIAGNOSIS. Complete record of the clinical course of the case should be kept so that the attendant's attention will at once be fixed upon any variation, however slight.

Diagnosis of perforation in known cases of typhoid is easily made in the majority of cases, though operation should never be performed without a careful examination of the chest. Most of the errors committed in diagnosis have resulted from neglect on the part of the surgeon to examine the chest.

In the absence of history of previous illness, as in the ambulatory cases, the cause of the peritonitis is not so readily determined. Though failure to attach proper value to symptoms, the presence of an existing peritonitis should not escape the attention of the physician and surgeon. The objective findings are sufficient within themselves and but little time should be devoted toward an effort to determine the particular viscus at fault prior to operation.

The earlier operation is performed after perforation occurs, regardless of the cause of the perforation, the better, the less the risk, the less morbidity follows, and the less mortality there will be.

SYMPTOMS SUSPICIOUS OF PERITONITIS. Symptoms suspicious of perforation appearing, a surgical consultant should be summoned at once. Delay in so doing until the next regular visit, or for the appearance of pathognomonic evidence is inviting disaster.

SYMPTOMS SUGGESTIVE OF PERFORATION. Severe pain in the abdomen after the tenth day.

Thorough physical examination should be made at the earliest possible moment.

In the event of abdominal rigidity, operate at once.

In the absence of abdominal rigidity, keep constant vigil; total white and differential count at hour intervals for six to eight hours if suspicious symptoms only exist.

PATHOGNOMONIC SYMPTOMS OF PERFORATION. Symptoms, subjective and objective, pathognomonic of perforation and peritonitis are:

Subjective: (a) Pain in the abdomen, usually in the hypogastrium or right lower quadrant.

(b) Pain most severe in the hypogastric region, in the majority of cases of typhoid perforation, though it may be, and often is, located elsewhere.

(c) Pain is persistent, increasing in severity, often shooting and paroxysmal.

(d) Nausea with or without vomiting.

(e) Urgent desire to go to stool, efforts often ineffectual neither flatus nor feces passing; copius dejecta rare.

(f) Vesical tenesmus, very common, though not so pronounced as intestinal torma.

Objective: (a) Patient restless; facies denote physical distress; forehead moist, large drops of cold sweat often present.

(b) Position in bed indicative of effort on the part of patient to relieve tension.

(c) Palpation reveals rigidity pronounced, if not general, rapidly increasing and soon becoming so.

(d) Tenderness upon pressure everywhere, most pronounced at or near site of perforation.

(e) Temperature and pulse altered but little, if any, immediately after perforation occurs. Generally slight acceleration of the one and lowering of the other. Both variable, and too much importance should not be attached to pulse or temperature.

(*f*) Blood count of no value immediately after perforation, unless the patient's blood has been repeatedly examined for some hours prior to suspected perforation.

POSITIVE INDICATIONS FOR OPERATION. Positive indications for operation are:

1. Typhoid after first week, usually the third, with sudden pain in abdomen, severe, persistent, growing progressively worse; muscle spasm.

2. Pain at first local, rapidly extending, with or without nausea and vomiting.

3. Tenderness upon pressure, local and general.

If the above finding exists, preparations for operation should be begun without delay regardless of the pulse rate, temperature, or blood findings. The sooner the operation is performed the better for the patient, as in gunshot-wound perforations.

Operation should be performed in hospital cases within from half an hour to two hours after perforation occurs. Operations performed within that period may be classed as early operation. Operation four to eight hours after occurrence of perforation in hospital cases is late operation and is evidence of inexcusable delay.

Early operation would result in reversal of the recovery and death rate, that is, it would read 80 to 20 and not 20 to 80, our present statistics.

REPORT OF A CASE OF TYPHOID PERFORATION WITH UNUSUAL AND INTERESTING HISTORY. CASE 1.—Male, aged forty-two years. Residence, Memphis. Occupation, merchant.

Previous Illness. None, except chicken-pox and measles in childhood. Five years ago he developed a hernia, right inguinal, incomplete. Never strangulated or irreducible.

While engaged in a friendly wrestling match he experienced sudden and severe pain in hypogastrium, extending upward and outward toward right quadrant. Pain excruciating, followed almost immediately by vomiting, copious.

Vomitus consisted of a large dinner he had just eaten. Urgent desire to go to stool. No gas passed, no feces. Collapsed while at stool. Was carried to his home, near by. Continued to suffer pain in abdomen, most marked near symphysis pubis.

When seen by his physician, two hours later, temperature was 99.8°; pulse, 74. Suffering severe pain, restless, nauseated, though not vomiting. Right lower half of abdomen rigid and painful upon pressure. Pain continued independent of pressure.

Diagnosis. Acute peritonitis. He was referred to hospital for operation.

Seven hours after onset of trouble he entered the hospital. Temperature, 100°; pulse, 84. Very restless and complaining of severe abdominal pain. Nauseated, but did not vomit.

Physical Examination. Patient well developed, well nourished. Facies indicative of considerable suffering. Heart and lungs normal. Abdomen slightly distended, lower half. Spleen not palpable. Muscular resistance general. Increased tenderness upon pressure over hypogastrium and involving right lower quadrant.

Blood count made while preparation for operation was going on. Polymorphonuclears, 74; total white count not submitted.

Clinical Diagnosis. Peritonitis, secondary to perforation of hollow viscera, probably due to rupture of an incarcerated segment of intestine at site of old hernia. Perforative appendicitis or typhoid ulcer perforation.

Under ether anesthesia right rectus incision.

Upon entering the cavity a dark, offensive fluid escaped. Intestines distended and very red. Numerous flakes of fibrin present. Appendix examined at once, no trouble of consequence found, though engorged. Examination of ileum discovered perforation near the jejuno-ileal junction. Perforation about the size of a pinhead. It was single.

It was sutured at once upon discovery—through-and-through marginal seroserous reënforcement. The cavity wiped out carefully; provision for drainage made with four large tubes, one directed upward, toward either flank, emerging through stab wounds, the other two directed downward to bottom of pelvis, emerging through lower end of incision.

Progress of case satisfactory. Patient discharged cured, fifteen days.

CASE II.—This patient, operated upon by Dr. Battle Malone and reported by him to the Mississippi State Medical Association in 1903, presents so many points in common with my case that I am by courtesy of Dr. Malone including it.

M., male, aged thirty years. Suddenly seized with violent pain over the lower portion of abdomen at 6 o'clock in the morning. He had eaten a hearty meal the evening before, and had felt unusually well for several weeks. His pulse was 78; temperature, 100° to 100$\frac{2}{5}$° F. when the doctor saw him, a short while after the perforation occurred. Some tympany present, but little rigidity over hypogastrium— more marked over right lower quadrant, greatest tenderness around McBurney's point. Neither pain nor rigidity in the epigastrium. He had never had a similar attack.

Diagnosis: Acute appendicitis of the fulminating type.

Patient was ordered sent to the hospital and preparations made for immediate operation. The operation was performed at 9 o'clock, three hours after onset of attack.

A three-inch semilunar incision made. Upon entering the cavity a quantity of mucus filled with flocculi escaped; fecal odor was absent. The appendix was at once examined and it was evident that it was not at fault. The ileum was very much congested, also the colon. One perforation the size of an ordinary pinhead was found six inches from the ileocecal valve. Perforation closed by transverse Lembert sutures. Drainage provided for by insertion of two gauze wicks.

Widal reaction, taken on March 18, two days after perforation, negative; twelve days later specimen gave a typical Widal reaction.

Provision for drainage discontinued on the fifth day and patient made an uneventful recovery, leaving the hospital on the twenty-first day after operation.

Dr. Malone's case was a very interesting one and his patient's life was saved by the prompt diagnosis of perforation, though the cause of the perforation was not suspected until after operation, and like mine, Widal was not obtained until after the third week of the disease.

Points of special interest concerning the subject of typhoid perforation peritonitis are that perforation peritonitis is responsible for one-third of all the deaths from typhoid, and that 2.5 per cent. of typhoid patients have perforation, and that 100 per cent. of perforation peritonitis cases die in the absence of prompt surgical intervention; and that operation should be performed as early as possible after diagnosis.

In my own case I want to call attention to these important facts:

1. Diagnosis of peritonitis.

2. The man felt sufficiently well to engage in a wrestling match as a matter of choice when the perforation occurred.

3. He had not lost a day from his work nor missed a meal.

4. The only evidence of trouble prior to perforation was an estimated loss of about ten pounds in weight and a feeling of malaise for two weeks preceding the perforation.

5. That immediate operation was urged by his family physician, Dr. Joe Clifton, of Memphis.

6. The diagnosis of peritonitis was made from the pain in the abdomen, its severity and persistence, plus rigidity.

7. Tenderness upon pressure.

8. Collapse.

9. Vomiting early with intermittent nausea.

10. Widal made daily for seven days and proved negative. On third day after operation blood culture was made with negative result, and on the eighth day a positive Widal was obtained.

11. But few, if any, conditions exist where gentleness, accuracy and speed count for so much as in typhoid perforation peritonitis.

DISCUSSION

DR. WILLIAM R. JACKSON, Mobile, Alabama.—Perforation of typhoid ulcer is a serious thing to the surgeon. It will test his bravery, his skill and vim as a surgeon. A patient soon dies on the table. When a patient has a pulse of 140, a temperature of 103° F., and all at once severe abdominal pain, and the abdomen becomes rigid, with tympany rapidly increasing, you know by these symptoms you have perforation. If the patient's vitality is too low to give a general anesthetic, local anesthesia comes into play.

I have had four cases of perforation from typhoid ulcer. The first two were operated under general anesthesia. In these two cases I found so much thickening of the intestinal wall and so much infiltration and induration that sutures could not be placed. In many cases due to perforation, where there is a hard infiltrated condition and perforation in the centre the size of a lead pencil or not so large, you cannot suture. Drainage is all you can do. If you have a desperate case, you can make a small incision under cocain, put in drainage, and the patient will get well more often than if you had cut him wide open and looked for the perforations.

DR. FRANK D. SMYTHE, Memphis, Tennessee (closing).—I have nothing to add that was not brought out in the paper, though I beg to differ with Dr. Jackson, and think one of the essential features of the operation is closure of the perforation. Where the perforation is not closed the case would in all probability terminate fatally.

The object sought by the surgeon is to accomplish closure of the perforation or perforations and provide for thorough drainage. Unless those objects be accomplished our efforts in behalf of the patient would prove in vain.

SALPINGITIS SECONDARY TO APPENDICITIS

By JAMES E. MOORE, M.D.
Minneapolis, Minn.

THE writer's experience goes back to the time when we had perityphlitis, pelvic hematocele, and pelvic cellulitis. We first learned that perityphlitis was due to an infection in the appendix. We next learned that what was termed pelvic cellulitis was due to an infection, and some time later that the infection began in the Fallopian tubes and that whatever of pelvic cellulitis there was, was secondary to the tubal infection; and still later we learned that in the majority of instances pelvic hematocele is due to an ectopic pregnancy. It is now well established that infection of the Fallopian tubes is the most common condition in the pelvis requiring surgical treatment. The entrance into the tubes from the uterine side is very small, and it would seem as if it were one of Nature's wise provisions to prevent the entrance of bacteria into the peritoneal cavity through the natural channels. On the contrary, the fimbriated extremity of the Fallopian tube is wide open, and if any bacteria are present in the peritoneal cavity it would be very easy for them to gain entrance to the tube. The tubes normally are sterile, although occasionally they are found to contain bacteria without symptoms of infection. Under normal conditions the uterine end of the tubes are further protected by a sterile uterus, and they do not become infected until after an infection of the uterus. In other words, the tubes are not liable to infection from the uterine side except under abnormal conditions. Is it, therefore, not rational to conclude that when abnormal conditions obtain within the peritoneum that the tubes may be infected from the peritoneal end? When abscesses were first found within the tubes the contents were reported as sterile, but better technic has enabled us to demonstrate various forms of bacteria in these abscesses.

In 1886 Westermark first discovered the gonococcus in these abscesses. Following this discovery the profession went to the extreme, as it too often does, and many articles were written supporting the belief that all cases of salpingitis were due to the gonococcus infection. At the present time it is well established that while the majority of cases of salpingitis are due to a gonococcus infection, there are many due to infection from other bacteria. The bacillus coli has often been found in salpingitis and has been considered due to intestinal adhesions. Kelly says that bacteria may escape from the appendix and infect the tube, and quotes a case of Robb's in which one tube in a double pyosalpinx gave a negative culture and on the other side the tube was closely adherent to an inflamed appendix and contained streptococci. Salpingitis is often complicated by appendicitis. May not one be the cause of the other?

In a recent paper by Goldstein[1] 328 cases of salpingitis are reported, of which 197 gave positive evidence of gonococci; 43 were of puerperal origin, and 86 from other sources. In 12 cases the appendix was firmly attached to the right tube and ovary, and in 5 of these the right tube only was involved, which would seem to be positive evidence that the tube was infected from the appendix.

Some years ago the writer's attention was first called to the possibility of appendicitis being the cause of salpingitis by the following case: A single woman, aged thirty years, was brought from one of the smaller cities of Minnesota

---

[1] Surgery, Gynecology and Obstetrics, August, 1915.

to Minneapolis for operation with a diagnosis of salpingitis. She was taken to a gynecologist who firmly believed that the only cause of salpingitis was infection from the gonococcus, and in the absence of any evidence of infection in the vagina and the presence of an imperforate hymen concluded that it was impossible for the patient to have salpingitis, and discredited the attending physician's diagnosis. The patient was then brought to the writer, who found that the patient gave a history of repeated attacks of inflammation in the lower abdomen and pelvis, and by rectal examination a solid mass could be made out in the pelvis. The vagina was healthy and the hymen intact. There was no history of disease or unnatural discharges from the vagina at any time. The diagnosis of salpingitis was confirmed, although the possible cause was not understood. Operation was performed by the writer, who found evidences of repeated attacks of appendicitis, found the appendix closely adherent to the right ovary and tube, and both tubes distended with pus. The appendix and tubes were removed, and the patient fully restored to health. It is evident that the infection had not extended to the uterus, because it was left and has never caused symptoms. This led the writer to conclude that this was a case of salpingitis secondary to appendicitis. This occurred many years ago at a time when facilities for careful bacteriologic examinations were not at hand, so that we had no means of knowing what bacteria were present. Since that time the writer has observed a number of cases that have confirmed his conviction that some cases of salpingitis are due to an infection from the peritoneal side caused by an appendicitis, but only two more cases will be cited to emphasize the point we are trying to make.

CASE II.—A woman, aged thirty-nine years, married a number of years and had never conceived. She spoke a foreign tongue little used in this country and it was difficult to get an accurate history, but we learned that she had had repeated attacks of abdominal inflammation which resulted in chronic invalidism. Upon entrance to the University Hospital a physical examination showed marked tenderness over the lower half of the abdomen, particularly over the pelvis, and in the left pelvis a mass could be made out which was evidently an inflamed tube. A median incision was made and a large hydrosalpinx of the left tube removed. On the right side the ovary and two-thirds of the tube were absent. There were extensive adhesions and the appendix, which had undergone many changes from inflammation and was tightly bound down, was removed. This woman had had no previous operations, but owing to our inability to talk with her we were unable to get a satisfactory history of an abscess having discharged through the bowel. Yet it seems to me that the only way that the absence of this right ovary and tube can be accounted for is that there has been an inflammation beginning in the appendix and extending to the right tube and ovary, which ended in extensive abscess and sloughing, and was all discharged through the bowel. The uterus did not seem to be enlarged or infected, but was retroverted. It was fastened forward by the use of the round ligaments.

CASE III.—A trained nurse, aged twenty-three years, was admitted to the University Hospital July 10, 1915, complaining of pain in the pelvis and right lower abdomen. She had a temperature of 102.5°, leukocytes 22,900, polymorphonuclears 84 per cent. Upon physical examination there was marked tenderness over the lower abdomen and pelvis, but no muscular rigidity. Deep pressure over the right iliac region together with pressure in the loin elicited severe pain. This was the location of her severest pain. Upon vaginal examination the uterus was found freely movable and not sensitive. The right tube was distended but floating freely, and was not particularly sensitive. It was decided that the pelvic condition did not account for the temperature and blood picture, and from the pain elicited by pressure over the right loin and right lower quadrant of the abdomen a diagnosis was made of acute retrocecal appendicitis. This diagnosis was based upon the location of the pain and tenderness and the absence of muscular rigidity. An incision was made and the appendix found behind the cecum and extraperitoneal with the exception of a very small portion of its tip. It was dissected out and removed, and upon section proved to be full of pus. The patient gave a history of having had like attacks before and there were many adhesions, showing there had been a previous appendicitis. The right tube could be felt quite markedly distended but freely movable. The left tube was normal. The distended tube was not removed, and the abdomen was closed. By midnight her temperature had dropped to 100°, and the next morning was 99°. Leukocytes and polymorphonuclears dropped promptly and were gradually reduced to normal. After this time the temperature ranged from normal to 101°, most of the time being about 99°, which could be accounted for from her salpingitis. On the fourteenth day after the operation she was allowed to sit up and her temperature immediately rose to 102°, with return of pain in the pelvis. This again disappeared when she was put to bed. On August 21 she had been sitting up some days with comfort and was allowed to go home with a temperature of 99°. In other words, her convalescence gave a picture of a convalescing subacute salpingitis. There was no history of vaginal infection, and smears were negative. It seems to the writer that the only rational conclusion to be arrived at in this case is that this woman had appendicitis which infected the right tube. The left tube, it will be remembered, was normal.

We believe that these cases demonstrate that infection of the Fallopian tube may occur from the peritoneal end. and that when it does it is usually due to appendicitis. We believe that it should be accepted as an established fact that a certain small percentage of cases of salpingitis are due to appendicitis, so that when looking for possible causes of a pelvic inflammation we may take this fact into consideration.

DISCUSSION

Dr. O. H. Elbrecht, St. Louis, Missouri.—I wish to report two similar observations in children, one a girl about twelve years of age, who had an attack of appendicitis, and came to operation about a month later. In her case the right tube was about as thick as my thumb and filled with pus.

The other case was a girl, seven or eight years of age, in whom the right tube was infected as we see it in an acute case of salpingitis, but before the tube was closed and filled up. In both of these cases the hymen was intact and there was no history of vaginal infection of any kind.

In children we get positive evidence of this complication which may escape our observation in suppurative appendicitis, as in the last case Dr. Moore reported, where they do not make as rapid a convalescence as we would like to have them do. If there is general infection in that region of the peritoneal cavity, it seems plausible that an infection can start from the fimbriated extremity, and result in a well-defined salpingitis or pyosalpinx. Some years ago I reported a case which to my mind is comparable to this conditon, in a twin pregnancy at full term. The woman was delivered of twins, and died on the sixth or seventh day from peritonitis with two well-formed pus tubes, one of them the size of a lemon, the other about the size of your finger, both fimbriated extremities being closed. The peritonitis was the result of contraction of the uterus after delivery to which the omentum was firmly fixed, also the tube; and in its contraction possibly by the expulsion of the placenta by Credé's method, tore the omentum from this tube, thus rupturing it and causing peritonitis. Here was a twin pregnancy with double pus tubes. The explanation of the impregnation in that case was this: One side was undoubtedly a salpingitis when impregnation took place, and the infection on the other side occurred later probably by way of the fimbriated extremity thus making a double pus tube of it. If it occurred through the uterine end, then why should pregnancy have proceeded without abortion?

Dr. J. Wesley Bovée, Washington, D. C.—While it is recognized that tuberculous peritonitis will usually spread into the Fallopian tubes by passage through the fimbriated extremities, it is also well known that the colon bacillus *may* pass in to them in the same direction and from the vermiform appendix as well as some other portions of the intestinal tract. We have, on the other side, overwhelming evidence of infection of the tubes coming in through the uterus and through the blood and lymph channels. The vermiform appendix that is attached to an inflamed and closed Fallopian tube simply by coming in contact, I consider as having been in bad company, that is all. I think in these cases of closed fimbriated ends of tubes, the infection has come from the lower direction. In the cases Dr. Elbrecht mentioned, I believe that one of these tubes was closed, perhaps both of them, before pregnancy occurred. We do know pregnancy may occur through a closed tube, provided the tube has a glued fimbriated extremity. It seems to me, that we are also going to get far away by emphasizing the fact of the hymen in a child acting as a marked defense against gonorrheal invasion of the vagina. What can we say about the many cases of gonorrheal vulvovaginitis we find in infants? I wish we would take all these points into consideration before we lay much stress on this matter, although I grant, at the same time, the possibility of infection of the Fallopian tubes from the appendix is possible.

DR. THOMAS S. CULLEN, Baltimore, Maryland.—I agree thoroughly with Dr. Moore that in many cases the salpingitis is secondary to disease of the appendix, and that in the majority of such cases the adhesions are on the right side while the left tube and ovary, unless there has been a bad appendix, may be normal. In quite a percentage of these cases we find the right ovary adherent while the tube is normal. When the tube is involved secondary to the appendix the fimbriated end may still be open indicating that the inflammation came from the outer surface of the tube instead of from the tube lumen.

DR. ROBERT T. MORRIS, New York City.—After what has been said, I would like to make this point: I believe that in studying typhoid fever cases we will find we often have para-enteral anërobes to deal with. That brings up the question that these para-enteral anërobes in the cases described by Dr. Moore may be found to be present and exerting a malign influence.

PLASTIC OPERATIONS FOR ACQUIRED
DEFORMITIES OF THE FACE

By J. Shelton Horsley, M.D.

Richmond, Virginia

Plastic operations on the face are usually not life-saving procedures, but the curing of a facial deformity not only relieves the physical discomfort of the patient and assuages his mental anguish, but gives relief to the inhabitants of the community in which the patient lives. The necessity for seeing daily someone with a hole in the frontal sinus, a retracted lip, or a deformed nose, is by no means an agreeable prospect. So if a philanthropist be one who makes two blades of grass grow where one formerly grew, plastic surgery of the face may be considered a philanthropic field. Surely it is of more importance to the community than the placing of monuments or the beautifying of streets.

Surgery of the neck and plastic surgery of the face probably demand more skill than any other kind of surgery. It is essential for one who operates upon the neck to be a good operator and to know anatomy well. Plastic work on the face demands some knowledge of anatomy and physiology, but particularly requires a kind of ingenuity to meet unusual conditions and to make things fit, which is not essential in most major surgical operations.

General considerations, such as the age and health of the patient, must be given due weight. The age of the patient is of great importance, as flaps can be successfully transplanted with a smaller amount of nourishment in the young than in the old. In the matter of dressing, dusting the wound with boric acid powder and leaving it open is all that is necessary. If there is much oozing, a compress of dry gauze may be kept on for a few hours. When any of the cavities of the face are involved in the wound, hexamethylenamin is administered before and after operation, as it tends to sterilize the secretions of the mouth and nose.

While general principles can guide in plastic work on the face, each case is truly a law unto itself. Though the same principles may be followed in a certain group of cases, no two of them will be done exactly alike. For this reason a report on plastic surgery of the face, and particularly for acquired deformities, should deal largely with reports and illustrations of individual cases.

Dividing the face into regions and taking them from above downward, we first have the deformities of the forehead. I have had three cases which illustrate a very striking deformity following the loss of a portion of the anterior bony wall of the frontal sinus, all of them resulting from trauma. In such instances it is necessary to find if the infundibulum, or communication between the frontal sinus and nose, is well open. If so, the skin can be readily turned in with the epithelial side down and the small amount of discharge together with the exfoliated epithelium can go through this communication to the nose. If it is not sufficiently large, a curved probe is passed through the frontal sinus, the infundibulum, and out of the nose and by means of a string tied on the end of the probe, a gauze strip is drawn through the infundibulum. The gauze, when sawed back and forth, will increase the size of the opening to the desired caliber. As the bone in this region is quite fragile, this procedure is better than any attempt to use metal instruments. If the defect in the wall of the frontal sinus is large, two small skin flaps are outlined around the depressed margin with the base of the flaps at the margin of the opening. The flap is then cut through to the pericranium. The skin external to the incision is undermined and the pericranium cut down to the bone at some distance from the incision into the skin. The flaps are then elevated and turned into the opening with the epithelial surface inside, the pericranium being over-lapped like a double-breasted coat. This will fill even a large defect. The skin to cover the raw surface is brought from the adjacent portions of the forehead, depending upon the manner in which the scar tissue runs and upon the tension. A vertical flap with the base over one eye-brow may be used, making the lines of incision when the flap is in position about parallel with the normal creases in the forehead. In one instance where the defect was not very large, I made a long transverse incision, mobilizing the skin of the forehead, and covered the flaps that had been inverted by sliding the whole forehead down. If the defect is large, however, or particularly if it extends more vertically than transversely, this cannot be done.

Deformities about the eyelid often fall into the hands of the eye specialist. A rather interesting case, however, came under my care in which the patient was severely injured by an explosion in a mine. The bones of the nose and upper part of the face were comminuted, and after healing had taken place it was found that there was a sagging down of the left eyelid, so that it was impossible for the patient to see with the left eye. An examination showed that the muscles of the eyeball were normal, but the inner canthus was considerably lower than the corresponding inner canthus of the right eye. The problem, then, was to raise the inner canthus of the left eye, and if this did not relieve entirely, to shorten the upper lid. An incision was made along the bridge of the nose and through the left eyebrow. A piece of bone including the ascending portion of the superior maxilla, to which the inner canthus is attached, and a small portion of the lacrimal bone was found separated and displaced downward. It was loosened from its new position and replaced at its normal level. A hole was drilled in the nasal

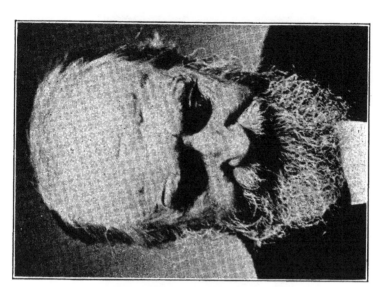

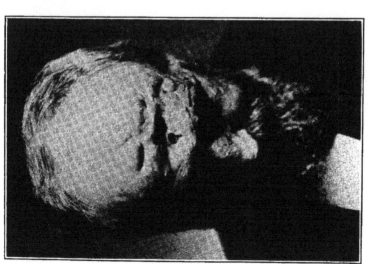

Fig. 1.—Deformity due to accidental discharge of shotgun which blew away a portion of the anterior wall of the frontal sinus. Note the opening into the frontal sinus. Photograph taken about a year after the injury.

Fig. 2.—Photograph of the patient shown in Fig. 1 about two months after operation.

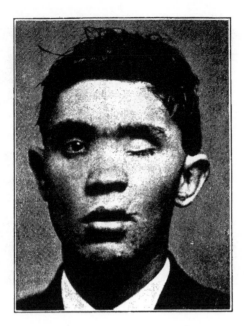

Fig. 3.—Closure of left eye due partly to displacement of fractured bone to which inner canthus of the left eye is attached, and partly to injury to the levator palpebræ.

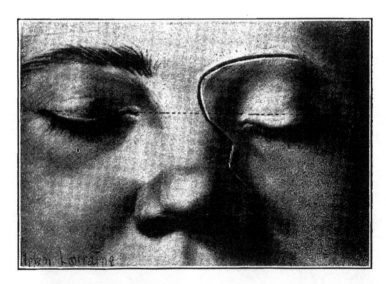

Fig. 4.—Drawing of patient shown in Fig. 3. Note that the left inner canthus is lower than the right. The skin incision is shown.

bone and in the fragment, and the fractured bone was fastened in position with kangaroo tendon. Healing was good, except there was some discharge of pus opposite the kangaroo tendon. The scar was very satisfactory. This improved the condition, but still the lid could not be elevated enough; so under novocaine, a transverse section of the upper lid, including skin and tarsal cartilage, was removed. The wound healed nicely and the patient now has use of the eye.

There are occasional instances in which injury is so extensive and so many portions of the face are involved that the case cannot be classified regionally. In one such case the skin for the eyelids was made by freeing the tarsal cartilage, suturing the lids together, and then transplanting a flap from the forearm, leaving it with a pedicle attached for about ten days. After this time, the pedicle was severed and in a few days the flap was split, making both an upper and a lower lid. If necessary, the method of transplanting a flap from the abdomen to the hand and then from the hand to the face can be used. In this case a number of operations were performed, the lips being made by a large flap from the upper arm which was split so as to form part of the upper lip as well as all of the external portion of the lower lip.

Defects of the cheek are sometimes difficult to close. When it is impossible to slide flaps from the margins of the opening without too much tension, a flap can be taken from the forehead by dissecting the attached anterior temporal artery and transplanting it beneath the skin. A lower eyelid was made by Monks, of Boston (*Boston Medical and Surgical Journal*, October 20, 1898), by undermining the skin between the region of the eyelid and the origin of the anterior temporal artery, dissecting a flap from the forehead with the anterior temporal artery attached, and carrying the flap and its artery under the undermined skin to its new position. For large defects, the method of transplanting the anterior temporal artery with a frontal flap seems peculiarly desirable. The artery should be dissected with considerable tissue around it and transplanted to its new bed by means of an incision that merely goes through the skin and not deep enough to sever the branches of the facial nerve. The skin, of course, should be undermined on each side so as to cover the artery without tension. The flap should be stabbed in several places to facilitate the oozing of blood. The chief objection to this operation is that there is too much nutrition, and until a venous supply forms which will carry off the excess of arterial blood, there is danger of the artery pumping the flap so tight that thrombosis and gangrene will occur. If the defect involves the mucous membrane of the mouth, the inner raw surface can be lined with mucous membrane from the tongue, as suggested by Willard Bartlett, or a flap may be turned up from the neck with the epithelial surface inside.

Deformities of the nose are conspicuous and sometimes difficult to deal with on account of the inability to give the shape that cartilage would. In one instance in which the nose completely collapsed because of traumatic destruction of the septum, I transplanted a piece of rib. The rib was split and the half covered with periosteum was moulded and inserted between the mucous membrane and the skin of the nose like a rafter, each end of which rested on a superior maxillary bone. In a patient with a defect of the nose following a paste applied by some advertising cancer doctor, the ala was thoroughly freed and a flap taken from the septum including mucous membrane and some cartilage. In order to lower the point of the nose, a section of cartilage was removed from the septum. The flap was left attached to the septum near the tip of the nose, and was then brought up into the defect. Thiersch skin grafts were applied to the raw surface. They did not take except in one small place, but the healing was satisfactory. After about two weeks

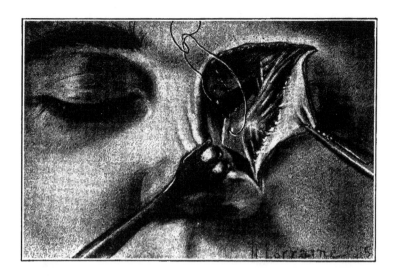

Fig. 5.—The misplaced bone has been loosened, holes have been drilled, and kangaroo tendon to hold fragment in position is about to be tied.

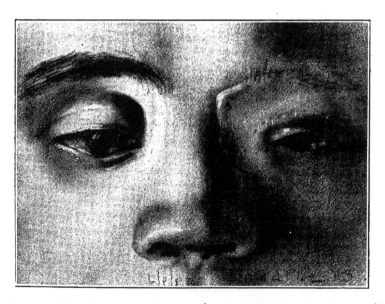

Fig. 6.—Result after both operations. Note the scar in the lid, where part of the lid was resected to take up the slack in the attachment of the levator palpebræ.

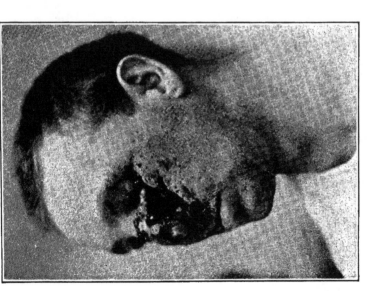

Fig. 8.—Appearance of patient shown in Fig. 7, about two weeks after operation, in which a frontal flap was transplanted with anterior temporal artery. Note the scars where the anterior temporal was dissected and transplanted.

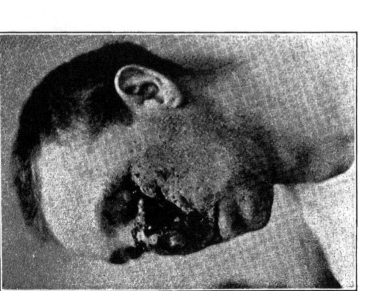

Fig. 7.—Defect in cheek resulting from wound with shotgun. The opening is into the nasal cavity.

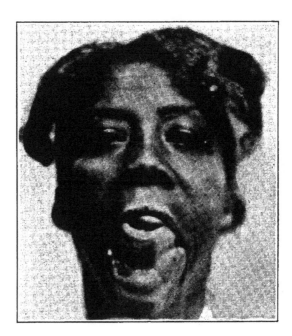

Fɪɢ 9.—Deformity from burn in an old negro woman. Relaxation of the tissues due to age permits the pulling down of the soft tissues of the lip while the lower jaw remains in the normal position. In a younger patient the same burn would produce the deformity shown in Fig. 13. This patient refused operation.

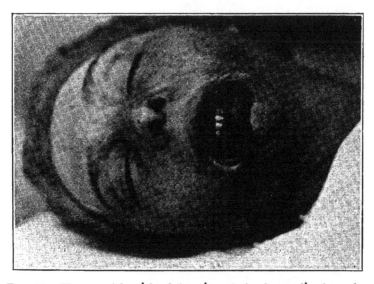

Fɪɢ. 10.—Young girl with deformity of the lower lip from burn. Note the eversion of mucous membrane. Photograph was taken just before operation while the patient was under ether with rubber cap on her hair.

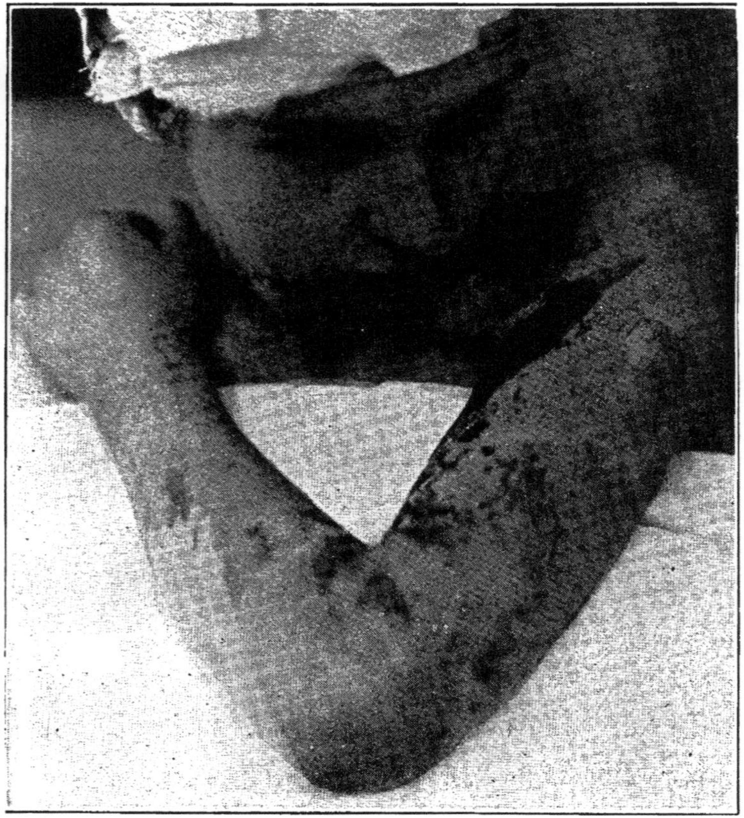

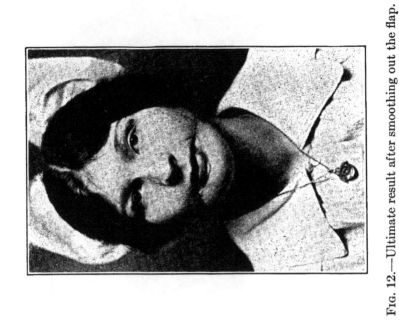

Fig. 12.—Ultimate result after smoothing out the flap.

Fig. 11.—Same patient as shown in Fig. 10, just before cutting the pedicle of the flap used to reconstruct the lower lip.

the base of the flap was cut and pushed up on a level with the rest of the nose. The nutrition of the flap was poor at its base (after being cut) and there was probably too much pressure from the gauze which was inserted within the nose to hold up the base of the flap. There is still a small opening at this point, which I think can be closed. The septum is necessarily crooked, but the general appearance of the nose when viewed either from the full face or from the side is fairly satisfactory.

I have had one patient, a Greek, with a very peculiar deformity of the lower jaw. It was probably congenital in origin, though it increased greatly with his growth. It was remedied by removal of the redundant bone down to the inferior dental canal, through an incision about an inch below the jaw.

Deformities of the lip resulting from operations for cancer may be corrected in a number of ways, following the rules laid down in the textbooks. I have found, however, that a long V-shaped excision with the apex rather narrow, and loosening of the tissue on each side, is a simple and effective measure. If too much constriction occurs, the corners of the mouth can be split and the mucous membrane sutured to the skin. Fortunately, cancer of the lip occurs in middle-aged or elderly persons, in whom the skin is greatly relaxed and the lower lip usually sags down; consequently, the appearance of the lip is often improved by such an operation. In younger persons, in whom burns often produce deformity, the skin can be slid up from the neck, if the burn is not too extensive, or can be transplanted from the arm, leaving a pedicle for about two weeks. All of these cases will require slight operations later on to smooth down the region where the pedicle was cut. Thiersch grafts will promote healing but do not prevent the contraction following burns; therefore the whole skin should be used.

Owing to the relaxed condition of the tissues in the old, a burn will often produce a different type of deformity here from that which is found in the young, in whom the tissues are firmer and more closely connected and tend to move as a whole.

In a case of a young girl it was necessary to make practically the whole lip except the mucosa, and a very satisfactory result was obtained by reconstructing the lip from a flap transferred from the arm. If only the lower part of the lip is involved, flaps can be slid up from the chest, or from the neck, sometimes cutting them twice in order to get them into position, "waltzing" them, as it is termed by Halstead.

A complete defect such as is left by noma, involving skin, muscle, and mucous membrane, can usually be corrected by a quadrangular flap which is turned down from the cheek, the mucous membrane being included. In a case of this kind, the base of the flap was external to the outer angle of the mouth and the lateral incisions ran up parallel to to the nasolabial fold. The flap was turned into the defect, which consisted of a complete destruction of almost half of the lower lip and part of the cheek, and the vermilion border of the lip was constructed at subsequent operations.

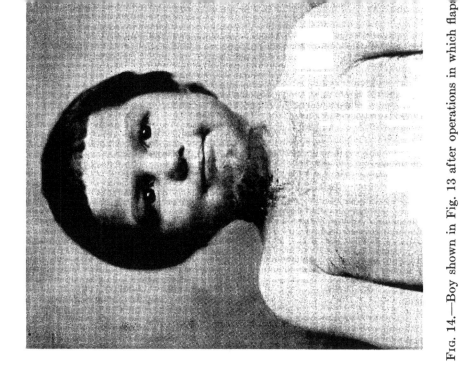

Fig. 14.—Boy shown in Fig. 13 after operations in which flaps

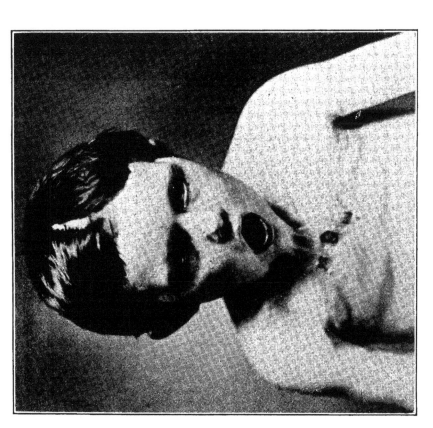

Fig. 13.—Boy with deformity resulting from burn on the lower

IN CASES OF SYMPTOMS WITHOUT GALL-STONES, WHAT DISPOSITION SHALL BE MADE OF THE GALL-BLADDER?

By Le Grand Guerry, M.D.
Columbia, S. C.

Borderland cases, we believe, constitute the most neglected field of surgery. By this we mean literally cases in which it is extremely difficult to know both before the operation and after the abdomen is open, exactly what course to pursue. Cases that are included in this larger group of symptoms without gall-stones, constitute a large proportion of what, for the want of a better name, we are disposed to class as borderland.

When our Association held its meeting at Hot Springs, Va., I read a paper on the subject of interstitial pancreatitis, in which the question was discussed from the standpoint of treatment. We wish very briefly today to view the same general topic, from rather a different viewpoint. My experience with these cases is surely not unusual and I am convinced from extensive observations that my difficulties in this class of work constitute the common lot of the general surgeon. A broad statement it is to make, but nevertheless it is true, in every clinic that I have visited in this country during the last five years there have been cases of symptoms without gall-stones operated on, and on inquiry, the same statement is elicited, namely, that the work is unsatisfactory and a large percentage have recurrence of symptoms. October, 1915, I saw one of the truly great surgeons of America operate on three of these cases at one morning's clinic, and then the day after do two more of them, and his testimony is, that in at least 25 per cent. he fails to give permanent, symptomatic relief.

There seems to be confusion in the minds of some of us as to exactly what constitutes chronic pancreatitis, or really whether such a disease has any existence as a matter of actual fact. In what is to follow we simply assume the existence of this disease as a definite pathological entity and point to the fact that it is described by Adami, Moynihan, Mayo Robson, Opie, Deaver, Mayo and many others. In the 1915 copyrighted revision of Stengel and Fox's *Text-book of Pathology* we find the following: "Chronic indurative pancreatitis, or cirrhosis of the pancreas, may be hematogenous in origin, resulting from syphilis and alcoholism, or it may be caused by prolonged irritation exercised through the pancreatic ducts, calculi, either biliary or pancreatic, in consequence of frequent entrance of intestinal contents or partial stenosis of the ducts. In the latter case it may be secondary to duodenal catarrhs or obstruction of the pancreatic duct." (Page 688.)

We grant that the disease is extremely difficult to diagnose and at times perhaps impossible but this constitutes no sufficient reason for ignoring it or not trying to learn more about it. Its existence being proven, it is fairly up to the medical men to learn more of it. We submit the following:

1. In an article in the *Boston Medical and Surgical Journal* by Whitemore, in which he reviews all of the gall-bladder cases operated on at the Massachusetts General Hospital during a period of ten years, we find the following statement: "59 cases had a cholecystotomy for cholecystitis, 29 of them have remained perfectly well and 16 have had recurrence, one patient who is now well had several

recurrences, and 13 are dead, showing 27 per cent. of recurrence in cases traced."

2. The results in all cases at the Johns Hopkins Hospital, in which the gall-bladders were drained and no stones found, show that in about 25 per cent. of the total number of this group they fail to give permanent symptomatic relief. These figures are not absolutely accurate, but approach very nearly the truth.

3. Dr. J. M. T. Finney, in a personal communication, permits me to say that in his own private work, and this statement is meant to apply to all cases he has operated on in his career as a general surgeon, that where he drains the gall-bladder and does not find stones present, that 25 per cent. would be a conservative estimate of the number of cases that, sooner or later, in one way or another, have a more or less marked recurrence of symptoms.

4. Stanton, in an article in the *Journal of the American Medical Association,* August 5, 1911, pages 441 to 444, and quoted by W. J. Mayo in the *American Journal of the Medical Sciences,* April, 1914, reviews a series of 350 patients that have been operated on for gall-stones and cholecystitis; where stones were present, over 90 per cent. have gotten a satisfactory result, while in the cases in which the gall-bladder was drained and no stones found only 50 per cent. remained cured.

5. My own personal results in about 100 cases show that in about 30 per cent. of the cases of symptoms without gall-stones operated on we fail to get permanent symptomatic relief. Surely any method of treatment in which, by frank confession, we are failing to cure from 25 to 30 per cent. of cases must be fundamentally wrong somewhere. It almost raises the question as to whether the method is justifiable at all or not. We wish now to call attention to a very interesting series of experiments conducted by Dr. Archibald, of Montreal, Canada. These experiments have for their

object the demonstration of certain new factors in the causation of pancreatitis. Of course, what we need fundamentally to know is more about the etiology of this disease. It may be possible, as Dr. Finney suggests, in addition to the more common etiological factors, there may be some disturbance in the normal functions and correlation between the activities of the structure of this region and the gall-bladder, duodenum, stomach, pancreas, etc. We are, of course, all familiar with the classical work of Opie in which he proved the injection of bile through the duct of Wirsung into the pancreas would cause pancreatitis. This injection, of bile being due to the presence of gall-stone in the ampulla of Vater, which prevented the bile from going into the duodenum and under force of pressure from behind, injected into the pancreatic duct.

Archibald's contention is that many of these cases of pancreatitis are not due primarily to bacterial infection but to the injection of bile through the pancreatic duct into the pancreas, due to spasm of the sphincter muscle which surrounds the ampulla of Vater. "The key to the situation," says Archibald, "seems to my mind to lie in the presence of this sphincter muscle. That there existed such a sphincter it was easy to prove. With a cannula in the common duct of the dog, and a manometer attached, it was immediately found that this sphincter would resist a pressure of 600 mm. of water before becoming paralyzed— roughly about six times that under which the bile is secreted. Later, I observed that Oddi had described this sphincter from the anatomical and also the physiological side as long ago as 1885, but his work, in an Italian journal, has received but scant attention." Archibald calls attention to two important facts: Fact 1 is the great natural strength of this sphincter muscle, and Fact 2 the possibility of bringing about a condition of spasm of this sphincter. This we conceive to be a very plausible explanation of certain of these cases, because assuming the condition of the sphincter muscle and the possibility of creating a condition of spasm of the muscle which in turn would close the ampulla, it is easy to conceive that in varying degrees and in varying limits and in varying amounts the closed muscle would be as likely to produce injection of bile into the pancreas as would a gall-stone that blocked the opening of the common ducts into the intestinal tract. This work is so interesting that we will quote verbatim the following experiments:

"Experiment 51, Cat 12. Papilla closed by pressure of handle of dissecting forceps on the flat. Then, fearing to close off the pancreatic duct also, the duodenum above and below the papilla was converted into a pocket by ligature and suture, and the fluid allowed to distend this pocket for one and a half hours at a pressure of 800 mm. The pancreatic ducts later showed the iron present even in their finest ramifications.

"Experiment 53, Cat 13. In this animal the sphincter was unusually strong. It did not allow the passage of any fluid under 320 mm., and did not become paralyzed under 700 mm. There were four applications of HCl, each causing a temporary spasm. (There was no mechanical interference at any time.) There were several rises of pressure to 700 mm.; the injection of the pancreas shows well.

"Experiment 58, Cat 16. Here no HCl or other stimulant was used, but there were sudden rises of pressure up to 800 mm. in half an hour. The solution is found in the pancreas, but only slightly.

"Experiment 59, Cat 4 (Weed's solution). The pressure was raised suddenly eight or nine times in the course of an hour to 700 mm. No stimulation by acid or pinching. The sphincter showed a tendency to become paralyzed after six or seven rises, finally letting fluid through continually at 230 mm., the minimum pressure at the beginning. The iron is found only to a slight degree in the pancreas.

"Experiment 65, Cat 18. This experiment only lasted five minutes, being interrupted by the death of the animal, probably from the anesthetic. The minimum pressure at which fluid was let through was 220 mm., it was raised suddenly once only to 700 mm., with the result of an immediate profuse spurt through the papilla. The cat then died. At postmortem the injection solution was found in the main ducts and even between the cells in fine lines in a large part of the organ." Dr. Archibald considers this last experiment the most important, "since it demonstrates that the sphincter is able under the stress of a single sudden pressure, even without the stimulation of acid—in other words, by its own unaided strength—to force the solution into the pancreas before it yields." The above experiments are extremely interesting, are well worth study, and we are constrained to feel they throw additional light on the cause of this vexing problem.

When we remember that the normal pressure under which bile is expelled by the liver is about 100 mm., Freese having shown that the normal contractile strength of the gall-bladder being represented by 100 mm., an additional force is lent to the contention of Archibald. We greatly wish that more time could be spent on this aspect of the paper, but as our time is limited, we must approach the real task that we have set before us. What shall we do with the gall-bladder when we are operating on this class of cases?

In the first place, it is evident that 75 per cent. of these cases are cured by simple drainage of the gall-bladder, since the figures we have obtained show that from 25 to 30 per cent. represents the cases that are not relieved. Manifestly, then, it would be unwise and unnecessary to subject the 75 per cent. that can be cured by a simple method to the greater risk of a more serious operation. As we see it, out of every 100 cases, 75 remain well after cholecystotomy and 25 per cent. are not relieved permanently. The trouble comes, however, in the great difficulty of deciding at the time of the operation whether or not the individual case will be one of the 75 or one of the 25 per cent. Could we determine this accurately in every case the whole subject would be much simplified. Clinically, we feel that when any given case presents definite symptoms without gall-stones, with slight fever, occasional attacks of jaundice, varying in intensity, the abdomen being opened in such a case, we find a pretty definite indurated head of the pancreas, a dilated and distended gall-bladder and choledochus, no stones, black, tarry bile, or even infected bile, we are very much disposed to place such a case among the 25 per cent. that are not cured by simple drainage of the gall-bladder.

Secondly. In what cases shall the gall-bladder be removed? We do not feel that the advocates of cholecystectomy in these cases have completely made out their case. I am willing to grant that a certain percentage of these cases will be relieved by removal of the gall-bladder, the so-called strawberry gall-bladder, the cases in which there is an infection of the gall-bladder itself; but as we have already seen, probably a good many of these cases can be caused by conditions other than infection of the gall-bladder wall. This is fairly proved by the experiments above related and by the investigations of pathologists which show that the infection may come from the blood stream. It may be luetic, alcoholic, or from other sources. Of course, what we stand in greatest need of is some reliable guide which will enable us at the time of operation to classify the case and suit the operation to the patient and not the patient to operation. Another reason why the gall-bladder should be removed only on definite and positive indications; in my own personal work I have had five cases with marked recurrence of symptoms after the gall-bladder had been removed. Morris Richardson is reported to have said once, while on a visit to New Orleans, that among other reasons why he was glad to be in New Orleans was, that some of his gall-bladder cases in which he has removed the gall-bladder were coming back to him with recurrence of symptoms, and he did not know what to do with them.

Of the five cases I have operated on after the gall-bladder has been removed the results have been as follows:

In two cases the patients died on the third and fourth day after an effort on my part to establish communication between the common duct and the duodenum or stomach. I do not know how the rest of you feel about this matter, but to me an anastomosis of this sort, especially in a case that has been operated on two or possibly three times, comes very near to being an impossible undertaking. Certainly this is true in my unskilful hands at least. The third case was alive two months after, with a permanent biliary fistula. The other two cases are well, one two and the other three years after an anastomosis between the common duct and the duodenum. Here at least are three, possibly five, other good reasons why the indiscriminate removal of the gall-bladder is unwise. Gall-bladders that are in themselves badly diseased, gall-bladders incapable of function, gall-bladders the seat of an infection, especially if it is thought the infection is a contributing cause of pancreatitis, should be removed. It is unwise to remove the gall-bladder if the patient can be relieved without it, and particularly is it unwise to do so unless the patency of the common duct is established beyond question. We believe that the last-mentioned point is fundamental.

In the third place, accepting the work of Archibald, it would seem reasonable that division of the sphincter of the ampulla has a certain definite field of usefulness. As a matter of fact, Archibald has so treated cases, experimentally, with good results.

In the fourth place we believe that certain of these cases are best treated by the establishment of a permanent communication between the gall-bladder and duodenum.

Of course the opening between the gall-bladder and intestine will probably not remain open if the common duct is normally patent. In fact, there is no indication of this type of operation unless the common duct is either the seat of stricture or unless the enlargement of the head of the pancreas is so definite as to amount to practically the same thing. When we recall that in about one-third of all cases the common duct really tunnels the head of the pancreas we can see the reasonableness for this method of treatment. Apart from my personal cases mentioned above we have done the operation of uniting the gall-bladder and duodenum in an effort to side-track the bile around the head of the pancreas in at least fifteen cases. In these fifteen cases there has been one operative death. Two cases in which the gall-bladder has been subsequently removed, one of these removals being due to the closure of the cholecystenterostomy opening. One case unbenefited and the rest permanently cured.

In conclusion, then, our feeling is that this disease is like most other diseases: there are no hard-and-fast lines to be drawn, and that the best results will be obtained by a judicious selection of the operation to suit the individual case.

CHOLECYSTOSTOMY VERSUS CHOLECYS-TECTOMY

By Charles H. Mayo, M.D.
Rochester, Minnesota

AFTER the many years in which operations have been done on the gall-bladder and ducts it would seem that our knowledge of the pathological conditions, the indications for medical treatment or for surgery would be quite settled. Medical treatment, though apparently fairly successful in cholecystitis which has a periodic recurrence of symptoms, yet has often led to delay and later operations for secondary complications. Instead of general progress in surgery, secondary operations for diseases of the gall-bladder and ducts have become so frequent as to be a subject of comment, and many who suffer from such diseases delay operation knowing that while the percentages of cures are high there are failures, and other operations may be necessary.

An investigation of the 370 cases of diseases of the gall-bladder and ducts coming to operation in our clinic during four months, from July to November inclusive (1915), showed that 48 (13 per cent.) patients had already been operated on for these various conditions. It was also noted that the majority being women, naturally there had been many previous operations, such as removal of the appendix, of the right ovary and fixation of the right kidney.

Nevertheless, considered all in all, gall-bladder surgery has made great progress during the past twenty-five years. Culled, as most of the cases were in the early period, from diseases of the stomach it is found that the condition is a common cause of reflex irritation, vying with the appendix in creating gastric symptoms.

Early in this period the operations cholecystotomy, cholecystostomy, cholecystectomy and drainage of the duct were developed. Too often only advanced cases were diagnosed, and secondary complications of infective disease of the ducts and pancreas led to a high mortality. Thus the surgery of this region suffered for a time from a vicious circle; late operation and complications gave a high mortality, while the high mortality led to delay. Through improved technic and a study by sight of the progress of the disease in the living, the operation, usually cholecystostomy, became a safe procedure and resulted in a large percentage of cured patients, with many others improved.

After a safe technic had been developed the number of cholecystectomies as compared to cholecystostomies increased for a time, amounting to one-third of the operations performed. Later a great effort was made to save the gallbladder and nearly 80 per cent. were preserved. With growing knowledge of the subject and influenced by a recurrence of symptoms which showed many failures to cure, cholecystectomy became the rule and now nearly 90 per cent. of diseases of the gall-bladder are so treated, only some special circumstance of infection, perforation, great age or general condition leading to the choice of cholecystostomy. Should further symptoms develop, cholecystectomy is advised as a later procedure.

It is hardly fair to base our judgment as to the present state of surgery on reports including the relative value of results in cholecystectomy or cholecystostomy which were made during the imperfect and developing period of the early surgery of these diseases, say twenty to ten years ago, or including a proportionately large series of unproved medical cases so diagnosed. Knowledge of the subject has progressed so far that the diagnostician prides himself in stating that the disease is cholecystitis with gall-stones or cholecystitis without stones, common duct stone, cholecystitis with secondary pancreatitis, cystic gall-bladder or empyema of the gall-bladder, perforating gall-bladder or cholecystitis with gastric syndrome. Previously the gall-stone was the entity, now it and the other conditions are all secondary to cholecystitis which may be acute, chronic or quiescent. When formerly a vague idea of infection was conceded this was generally believed to be of a so-called catarrhal type, whatever that may have meant to the mind of the user of the term.

As to the origin of the supposed surface infection of the mucosæ there has been much discussion as to whether it arose from an ascending infection through the ducts from the duodenum or by way of the lymph channels or that bacteria from the intestine passed by the portal of circulation through the liver to be distributed by the bile. These possible facts or fancies have given way to the theory of a rear attack by vascular borne bacteria to the capillary base of the mucous cells of the gall-bladder, a theory which has been proved by Rosenow in numerous instances. He has shown that the bacteria of local diseases have as selective an affinity for similar environment as have the bacteria of the general and well-known infectious diseases. Of bacteria cultivated from the tissue, not the contents, of diseased gall-bladders taken from man and injected into the veins of animals with an even chance at all of the body tissues, the effect was to produce cholecystitis in 68 per cent. of 41 animals so treated.

When the etiology of the disease is considered gall-stones must be relegated to the second place in diseases of the gall-bladder and ducts, and a focus of infection should be searched for.

The diagnosis must be based on the known conditions which make it possible to recognize cholecystitis as an entity, yet the infective beginning of the disease may be so mild as to be unrecognized until stones develop and mechanical obstruction ensues, or the disease may occur with far graver conditions of infection than occur with stone. The roentgenological evidence in the diagnosis of such conditions, while often of value, cannot become a factor of great reliability since it recognizes the secondaries of but one group of cases.

Briefly reviewing the anatomy of the gall-bladder, we find that it is an elastic, muscular sac, attached to the liver, and connected to the common duct at an acute angle by the cystic duct. It is bound to or connected with the hepatic duct in such a manner that when it contracts upon its contents the fluid pressure is the same in the gall-bladder, cystic and common ducts. The gall-bladder does not completely empty itself like the urinary bladder. It is capable of enlarging its capacity to several times the one to one and a half ounces which is normally found in it.

Although man has a gall-bladder, there are several animals, including the deer and horse, that have none. It is stated that such animals have somewhat larger ducts, a condition proved clinically to occur in man and in animal after removal of the gall-bladder (Mann).[1] There are about 30 instances of failure of development of the glands reported in man, also it is often found that certain persons have had cystic, shriveled or functionless gall-bladders for a long period preceding operations. As to the usefulness of the gallbladder, some claim it is an unnecessary or obsolete organ and others that it is a disappearing one. Others claim that the mucus added to the bile from the gall-bladder is of functional importance and renders the bile less irritating to the ducts of the pancreas should it enter them.

The bile is formed at a rate approximately of an ounce an hour and delivered through the common duct. This duct does not empty directly into the duodenum but enters the muscular wall and passes for a short distance between the

---

[1] In manuscript.

outer wall and the mucous lining. Any pressure within the bowel thus flattens the duct and prevents regurgitation. Coffey, from much experimental study, states the mechanical development of this method of entrance is so perfect that the duodenum may burst before any fluid or gas can enter the common duct.

Man is a diverse feeder, eating many things which tend to form gas. This, however, is not serious, as the gall-bladder is capable of symptomless distention to several ounces and by contraction acts on the delivery of bile as the elastic ureter does on the flow of urine into a full bladder. However, if there is infection of the gall-bladder he will suffer from so-called gas with stasis in the duodenum often associated with pyloric spasm and epigastric fulness or pressure. The gall-bladder, being thick-walled in chronic disease or inflamed with bacteria and infiltration of its wall, can no longer expand and contract without its owner being conscious of the fact. Most patients develop a special or possibly unconsciously selected diet, learning to avoid greases, fried foods, raw apples, etc. They also often have idiosyncrasies to special foods of slow digestion or gas production; the so-called qualitative food dyspepsia in contradistinction to quantitative food dyspepsia which occurs following heavy or large meals and gives symptoms one to two hours after eating. These symptoms are induced by interference with peristalsis or the peristalsis of inflamed areas, and occur with chronic appendicitis with concretions, with Lane's kink, with incarcerated, incomplete hernias and with adhesions. Some patients complain but little even when gall-stones are present, the original infection having subsided. They suffer less from dyspepsia, as the gall-bladder can expand and contract almost normally. The symptoms then are mechanical, due to obstruction by the stone or to its passage. In some cases, especially cholecystitis, a gastric syndrome with attacks much like those due to gastric or duodenal ulcer occurs. The conditions can usually be differentiated, although we have been unable in some cases to differentiate diseases of the gall-bladder, of the appendix or duodenal ulcer, since all three of these may exist in the same patient. In duodenal ulcer especially the Roentgen rays are often of great aid. We must occasionally be content with the diagnosis of a lesion with possible reflex symptoms to be proved at exploration if the symptoms warrant the procedure.

It is undoubtedly true that with reference to gastric symptoms the crux of the situation is concerned wholly with the question of infection. Gall-stones in gall-bladders free from infection (though it was present when the gall-stones were formed) may give symptoms from obstruction or the movement or passage of the stone, but they do not produce gastric symptoms or at least such symptoms are not a major complaint. When gastric symptoms are a prominent feature in these cases, infection is the rule whether stones are present or not, and spells recur followed by free intervals just as they do in gastric and duodenal ulcer and in appendicitis when they are the result of infection. A large percentage of the patients who are free from infection may be cured by drainage of the gall-bladder. Because of adhesions and fixation of the gall-bladder and consequent impairment of function due to the operation for drainage a few of these patients may later be liable to cholecystitis. When infection is lacking, even if there are stones present, the glands along the cystic, common and hepatic ducts should be found but little enlarged on palpation. Patients in the second or infective group should have the gall-bladder removed at the operation whether or not stones are present, since the infection is the essential element. In these the glands of the cystic, common, and hepatic ducts should be found enlarged.

For many years we overlooked cases of cholecystitis without stones. Some of these patients had colic and frequent mucous obstructive attacks or local tenderness, yet did not have stones. Often there was a better external appearance of the gall-bladder than in those we were saving after removal of the stones and the gall-bladder was not even opened upon exploration. Two such patients later developed large stones, as was found several years afterward. Wider experience of the subject led to opening and draining the gall-bladder and in some cases if grossly diseased it was removed, especially the strawberry gall-bladder. Many such patients were relieved while the drainage continued, but symptoms recurred when drainage ceased.

Temporary drainage of the gall-bladder in cholecystitis did not give a satisfactory percentage of cures, and as our diagnostic ability improved a gradually increasing number of cholecystectomies were done in cases of infection. The persistence of reflex gastric symptoms after cholecystostomy, if no other cause is manifest, is evidence that the gall-bladder should have been removed.

If cholecystitis is an infection of the wall of the gall-bladder from which bacteria can usually be cultured, then the lymphatic glands draining such an area should show the evidence of such infection. The glands along the common, hepatic, and cystic ducts should be enlarged in such cases, and if not enlarged some other cause for the symptoms should be searched for. These glands also drain the duodenum and the head of the pancreas as well as the gall-bladder, therefore these structures should be examined for ulcer and pancreatic involvement. The latter, however, is often secondary to an infected gall-bladder and may present a lympho-edema such as is seen in the arm from blocked lymphatic return after removal of the axillary glands following operation for cancer of the breast. The general surgical problem of the present period is the search for the local focus of chronic local infectious processes and already great progress has been made.

In 2940 cholecystectomies prior to November 1, 1915, we discovered 130 cases of papillary gall-bladder. Papillary growths of other mucous surfaces have a tendency to cancer; just what their relationship may be in cancer of the gall-bladder is not known. Approximately 85 per cent. of cancers of the liver are metastatic. Of the 15 per cent. of primary cancer the great majority are associated with gall-stones and have their origin in the gall-bladder or ducts. Cancer of the gall-bladder in some cases, for example impacted stone and possibly in papillary cholecystitis, is undoubtedly avoided by cholecystectomy.

TABLE SHOWING THE RELATIVE MORTALITY OF CHOLECYSTECTOMY AND CHOLECYSTOSTOMY

	CHOLECYSTECTOMIES.			CHOLECYSTOSTOMIES.			
	Total operations.	Cancers.	Deaths.	Percentage deaths.	Total operations.	Cancers.	Deaths.	Percentage deaths.
1907–1909 . .	304	..	4	1.3	1085	.	15	1.4
1910 . .	111	2	..	...	426	2	7	1.7
1911 . .	100	2	3	3.0	481	2	4	0.8
1912 . .	211	7	4	1.9	427	1	3	0.7
1913 . .	261 ⎫	2	5	1.9 ⎫	204 ⎫	3	10	4.9 ⎫
1914 . .	817 ⎬1767	..	5	0.6 ⎬1.2%	157 ⎬435	...	4	2.5 ⎬3.4%
1915 . .	689 ⎭	..	11	1.6 ⎭	74 ⎭ .	...	1	1.4 ⎭
st 10 mos.)								
Totals. .	2493	13	32	1.3	2854	8	44	1.5

It will be seen from the above table that the mortality following cholecystectomy is less at present than that following cholecystostomy (1.2 per cent. as against 3.4 per cent.) for the last three years, or including all cholecystectomies, 1.5 per cent.

In a series of form letter inquiries sent to patients on whom cholecystostomy had been done during the past several years, none more recent than one year, 242 replies were received which showed that 53 per cent. of these patients were cured, 38 per cent. improved, and 9 per cent. not improved. Of the patients who were cured (129) 49 per cent. had stones, 11 per cent. had stones and empyema, 18 per cent. had stones and cholecystitis, and 22 per cent. had cholecystitis.

In a series of form letter inquiries sent to patients on whom cholecystectomy had been done during the past several years, none more recent than one year, 219 replies were received which showed that 71 per cent. of the patients were cured, 22 per cent. improved, and 7 per cent. not improved. Of the patients who were improved (48) 57 per cent. had stones and cholecystitis and 43 per cent. had cholecystitis alone.

CONCLUSIONS. Cholecystitis is an infective disease of the gall-bladder. The bacteria are in the tissues of the gall-bladder.

Infection may be mild, acute, chronic, or recurring.

Gall-stones may occur in mild infections.

Gall-stones may cause mechanical obstruction.

Colecystostomy (with removal of stones if present) gives a high percentage of cures only if the infection has subsided.

Colecystectomy with or without stones in diseased gall-bladders or existing cholecystitis gives a high percentage of cures.

Reflex gastric symptoms are caused by the infection.

The infection may through local peritonitis cause adhesions to the bowels, stomach or liver to abdominal wall.

Symptoms of mild gastric trouble may be nearly constant, may increase with exacerbation of infection and subsidence of attack, much like those of ulcer.

The etiological factor may be a small local focus primary in the mouth, secondary in the appendix.

Typhoid bacteremia may also be the etiological factor.

DISCUSSION ON THE PAPERS OF DRS. GUERRY AND MAYO

DR. WILLIAM R. JACKSON, Mobile, Alabama.—While I feel the last word has been said on this subject by Dr. Mayo, I want to ask him three questions: 1. To what he attributes his uncured cases of cholecystectomy? 2. What are the classical symptoms of chronic pancreatitis, if any, which demand surgical interference? 3. What conditions of the gall-bladder, not highly infectious, demand extirpation?

DR. W. P. CARR, Washington, D. C.—I wish to express my great pleasure in hearing Dr. Mayo's paper. His thought along the line of saving the gall-bladder has been right in line with my own ideas on this subject. I read a paper on this subject many years ago and I have never had any reason to take a different view from the one I then took. We ought to save the gall-bladder when it is unnecessary to take it out, for the reason he has given. In a number of cases in which I, fortunately, left the gall-bladder, I have had to operate again and do a cholecystenterostomy which did relieve the patient of symptoms. I have found it personally extremely difficult to tell whether the common duct is open or not. I have tried every way that I know to probe it, and to inject fluid through it, and to find out whether it was patulous or not, and I have not been able to do it. I have tried this on the cadaver a number of times, without success. It is more difficult on the cadaver because the ducts become hardened and are not as easily probed as in the live subject. But I know Dr. Halsted has had trouble, and has in some cases opened the duodenum to probe upward from below in trying to find out whether the common duct was patulous or not. I have worked unsuccessfully an hour or more on cadavers without finding the normal duodenal opening of the duct. So I think it is an impossibility in many cases to tell whether there is constriction at the lower end of the common duct or not. It is impossible to palpate it or probe it, and if we inject fluid, through the gall-bladder, we do not know whether it is passing up into the liver or going into the intestine. I have had four cases in succession in which the gall-bladder was greatly distended and was absolutely unable to determine what the cause of the obstruction was. Two did well with simple drainage; the other two had persistent biliary fistulas until I did cholecystenterostomy. I do not know what I would have done if I had not left the gall-bladder in these cases. I do not believe it is necessary to remove the infected gall-bladder when it is badly thickened and infected. I have left the gall-bladder in a number of cases of that kind, and found that after draining the inflammation subsided and they have done just as well as the cases that were not infected.

Dr. J. Garland Sherrill, Louisville, Kentucky.—I rise with great temerity to speak upon the subject after listening to a report of 5000 cases of operation, and still I believe the pendulum is swinging too far toward cholecystectomy, recognizing that infection is the primary cause of disease of the gall-bladder and of stones. This infection in the majority of cases gets in from the gut, notwithstanding the fact that distention of the gut tends to close the duct, as has been shown by Coffey. This infection may be of a very serious or mild type. Stones may form early in the infection or very slowly, but in the presence of infection we have no better method of dealing with it than draining the gall-bladder. If by removing the gall-bladder infection can be eliminated from the biliary passages, then I should say cholecystectomy would be the operation of choice. But we cannot say this, and the gall passage once contaminated is liable to become infected again, and if this occurs when the gall-bladder is absent, serious complications are liable to occur, involving both the pancreas and hepatic structures. Like Dr. Guerry, my personal experience is limited as compared with that of the Mayos, but in every instance where the gall-bladder function can be reëstablished an endeavor should be made to accomplish it. We have seen markedly thick and inflamed gall-bladders, and following drainage the symptoms subsided and the patients have gone through life in comparative health. Very few cases have come under my observation where I have had to operate a second time. I have had to operate to remove stones once or twice in cases operated on previously, but none of my cases required a second operation for stone, and in the majority cholecystostomy was done. One indication for cholecystectomy is obvious when the stone is impacted in the duct a sufficient time to cause ulceration and cicatrization in the cystic duct preventing drainage. If you leave the gall-bladder it fills up with mucus, but you can do a secondary operation as safely as primarily. There are a few cases in which there is no discharge of bile after you have removed the stones. The bile will not flow for three or four days but occurs; later the drainage will go on, and the function of the gall-bladder be reëstablished.

I believe the time will come when Dr. Mayo will go back to cholecystostomy again.

Dr. J. A. Crisler, Memphis, Tennessee.—I would like to ask Dr. Guerry or Dr. Mayo a question or two, as it seems to be a matter of quizzing these gentlemen. They will have a good many questions to answer. I want to ask whether they have made any effort to treat the gall-bladder antiseptically at the time of the operation, and subsequently during the drainage? Of course, we all know the urinary bladder can be cured of a great many infections by treatment, and I have not heard mentioned that these gentlemen have attempted to treat the gall-bladder.

Dr. Mayo tells us of certain forms of infection inherent in the mucosa of the gall-bladder and in the walls. We may imagine the same in the urinary bladder, and in the urinary bladder these infections can be cured by irrigations and treatments with proper antiseptic measures, both at the time of the operation and subsequently, as I mentioned during the period of drainage.

DR. THOMAS S. CULLEN, Baltimore, Maryland.—I am particularly glad that Dr. Mayo still has his gall-bladder and that Dr. Finney was good enough to leave mine in.

This subject of gall-bladder surgery has of late been very close to me and I would ask you to allow me for a moment to digress from the main topic and briefly refer to a valuable therapeutic agent in gall-stone colic.

Half a cupful of hot water containing a teaspoonful of Jamaica ginger and about 30 mm. of paregoric will frequently completely relieve the pain in less than five minutes and will overcome the pain when one-quarter grain of morphin accomplished nothing. When I took it the warmth seemed to at once cause eructation of gas and at the same time to relieve the spasm which seemed to exist.

DR. J. M. T. FINNEY, Baltimore, Maryland.—I am sorry I was not able to hear Dr. Guerry's paper.

The subject that has been brought before us by him and Dr. Mayo, is of the greatest interest to the profession. Personally, I do not know whether my experience differs from that of other surgeons or not, but certain it is that I have more trouble with operations upon the biliary tract than any other abdominal operations. That is, I have more cases that subsequently come back to me with a recurrence of their symptoms and say, "I was all right for a while, but—" and they will then tell you their troubles all over again with possibly some variations. That is my experience regardless of the fact whether I have simply drained the gall-bladder or whether I have taken it out. Now I drain the gall-bladder more often than I take it out, for the simple reason that I have never been able to bring myself to feel that it was good surgery to take out a gall-bladder that was not physiologically down and out. I have maintained for some time that the taking out of gall-bladders at the present time as done by some operators is just another one of those waves of surgical fadism—I was going to say—which every now and then sweep over the profession, such for instance as ovariotomy, stitching up kidneys, taking out colons, etc. I believe that before long, just as Dr. Sherrill has said, the pendulum is going to swing back, for the simple reason that, as I examine my cases and study my postoperative results and as I read the reports of cases of other surgeons I do not believe there is sufficient evidence to warrant the taking out of as many gall-bladders as are being taken out at the present time.

I have operated on five cases referred to me where the gall-bladder had been taken out, and where for some reason or other a stricture of the common duct subsequently developed. That to my mind is a condition which ought to make one pause and think. You may say that it is the fault of the surgeon, and not of the operation. True, but we are not all experts, and a good many unfortunate things will happen in spite of the greatest care, and sometimes even in the best of hands.

Then another thing is the fact that the taking out of the gall-bladder does not always relieve the symptoms.

I would like just here to ask Dr. Mayo whether he has ob-served a chronic diarrhea following the removal of the gall-bladder? I would like to know why that is. I have seen it a number of times—a chronic intractable diarrhea after the removal of the gall-bladder. I do not know why. I have no explanation whatsoever to offer.

As to the question of chronic pancreatitis, we hear so much about it. I would like to know what chronic pancreatitis really is. I do not know it when I see it. I may be stupid in not recognizing it. I do see cases that suggest the picture described as chronic pancreatitis. We not infrequently find enlarged lymphatic glands; we may find a swollen, thickened, nodular condition of the head of the pancreas, but I find that in other conditions just the same where there has not been a symptom referable to the pancreas.

Dr. William Mayo refers to that fact and others have spoken of it. You will find the pancreas in apparent health varying between such wide extremes that it is difficult to keep in one's mind the picture of what constitutes a normal pancreas. I do not know just what it is. I have never been able to satisfy myself.

Then, there are a lot of other conditions. Take the straw-berry gall-bladder for instance. I recently operated on one of these cases for Dr. Barker. The patient had a chronic osteo-arthritis. He had had his tonsils removed, his sinuses drained, and other things done except that he had not had his appendix taken out. At the request of Dr. Barker, I took a look into the abdomen to be sure whether he had any focus of infection there. He had had some symptoms suggestive of some trouble about his appendix, and we found a subacute appendicitis of moderate grade. I found what looked to me like a perfectly normal gall-bladder. There had been no symptoms referable to it. I operated solely at the earnest request of my medical friend. I am often struck with the fact that medical men who have none of the responsibility of the surgeon are far more bloodthirsty and radical at times than are the surgeons themselves. It reminds me of the small boy on the street corner when a dog fight is going on. He has no responsibility at all, and so he says, "Sic' em, sic' em." I opened the gall-bladder just to satisfy my medical colleague, and to my surprise found one of the most typical strawberry gall-bladders I have ever seen. We took cultures from the gall-bladder: I resected a portion of its wall to see if we could find anything by which we could explain its presence. It showed really nothing but the usual picture. What was the significance of the strawberry gall-bladder in that case? I do not know. I do not know what strawberry gall-bladder really means. Does it always mean the same thing? I would like to know.

There are a lot of things that I would like somebody to tell me in reference to this whole question of gall-bladder surgery, and, it seems to me, the more of it I do, the less I really know, because so often the thing that you are cocksure of, when you go on a little bit further, you will find you have been mistaken in.

The paper of Dr. Mayo was splendid. It furnishes a good deal of food for thought. We can learn a lot from the citation of cases, so carefully studied as his have been, and we ought, everyone of us, to report our cases along these lines, making note of our mistakes as well as our successes, and some time by and by, I believe the consensus of opinion will enable us to draw certain definite, well-founded conclusions, which I do not believe we are in a position, at the present time, to do.

DR. STUART McGUIRE, Richmond, Virginia.—I have been greatly interested in this discussion. As I sat and listened to the various speakers I felt they were saying for me what I would like to have said myself and often doing it better than I could have done.

There are just two points I would like to make: One is that cholecystectomy in the hands of the average surgeon is an operation which will undoubtedly be followed by more mortality and greater morbidity than cholecystostomy. Dr. Mayo with his wonderful ability and large experience is able to get ideal results from cholecystectomy, but I know if I attempted to do the operation as a routine practice I would get more deaths than I do now, and if the surgeons from the small towns who occasionally attend my clinic would imitate the practice there would be more funerals in Virginia than now occur. Not only is the immediate mortality of cholecystectomy higher than cholecystostomy, but injury to the common duct and other complications are more likely to follow. When I was at the Mayo Clinic last September the most difficult operations I saw done were by Dr. Wm. J. Mayo in his efforts to restore damaged common ducts the result of improperly performed cholecystectomies in the hands of other surgeons. Personally I never remove the gall-bladder except for definite indications, such as irremediable obstruction to the cystic duct, gangrene of the gall-bladder, or actual or potential cancer. I get very good results in the average case of gall-stones by cholecystostomy followed by medical treatment.

I recently read a paper, written by a physician, on the medical treatment of gall-stones. He said the first indication was to dissolve the gall-stones, and he admitted that this was impossible. He said the second indication was to facilitate the passage of the gall-stones, and he admitted that this also could not be done. He said the third indication was to relieve the cholecystitis, which he claimed could be done in the majority of cases by proper dietetic, hygienic and medicinal treatment. He claimed that many victims of cholecystitis attended by gall-stones could be transferred from gall-stone sufferers to gall-stone carriers. If the medical man before operation can relieve cholecystitis even with the presence of gall-stones, then the surgeon should be able to prevent cholecystitis after operation, the gall-stones having been removed.

I believe a large proportion of the apparent failures from the operation of cholecystostomy could be obviated by the careful postoperative and posthospital treatment of these patients.

Dr. John Wesley Long, Greensboro, North Carolina.—There is one observation I wish to make. Dr. Mayo's presentation of this subject and the discussion bring out the curious fact that the indications for doing cholecystectomy stand midway between the indications for doing cholecystostomy.

I take it that no one would think of doing cholecystectomy in a case of simple, uncomplicated gall-stones, where there is no evidence of the bladder itself being involved at the time. I refer to those cases where there probably has been a simple cholecystitis, which has long since disappeared. The presence of the gall-stones is the only evidence that there ever had been an infection. This class of cases cannot be ignored, since autopsies show that 90 per cent. of those who have gall-stones presented no symptoms during life. We frequently encounter this same class of cases in operating for other conditions. Suppose while doing an abdominal hysterectomy for fibroids one finds stones in the gall-bladder; would you say that cholecystectomy should be done, simply because of the presence of the stones? Nay, verily! Hence, I take the stand that the mere presence of stones does not justify doing cholecystectomy. We may confidently say then that stones without involvement of the gall-bladder stand at one end of the list of indications for operation, and calls for cholecystostomy and not cholecystectomy.

The other extreme of the array of indications for operation has been well brought out by Dr. Mayo, when he says that in certain cases where there are complications, such as severe infection, abscess, peritonitis, etc., it would be unwise to do cholecystectomy, but rather one should do a cholecystostomy and depend upon the future for cholecystectomy. Between these two extremes, I grant there are many cogent indications for doing cholecystectomy instead of cholecystostomy.

There is another class of cases that has not been referred to. Let me illustrate. Sometime ago I had occasion to operate on a woman who, fifteen years before, had had a typical attack of gall-stones and cholecystitis. She came very near dying. When I opened her abdomen fifteen years after the severe attack referred to I found that the gall-bladder had anastomosed itself to the stomach and ruptured into that viscus. The cavity of the gall-bladder had finally become obliterated. Nature had done a cholecystectomy in this case, but the common duct and all the hepatic ducts were filled with stones. This case, and there are doubtless many others like it, goes to show that the total obliteration of the gall-bladder, which is nature's way of doing a cholecystectomy, will not always prevent the subsequent formation of gall-stones.

Dr. A. J. Ochsner, Chicago, Illinois.—We have a condition in a certain class of cases which was described many years ago most perfectly by Rydygier. This condition is present because at some time there has been a destructive inflammation of the mucous lining of the gall-bladder, consequently the gall-bladder has shrunken, tightly grasping the gall-stones, which caused the trouble. In those cases there is no doubt about what should be done; the gall-bladder is a wreck and everybody will agree that it should be removed. My former assistant, Dr. Stanton, who followed all of my cases and those of his own to a certain date, has made this observation which I think is of importance. There was a time, when we first performed cholecystostomy, that we sutured the gall-bladder, which was tamponed with gauze, regularly to the peritoneum and the transversalis fascia. This was done invariably until the time came when there was a great stir and uproar against fastening things which normally were loose, and then we followed the plan of inserting a drainage tube and dropping the gall-bladder after cholecystostomy. Later on we found we had trouble, so we came back to the old method. In these follow-up cases, Dr. Stanton found that in cases in which we had used a drainage tube and had dropped the gall-bladder after cholecystostomy, there was trouble in a very large proportion of cases, while in those in which we had used gauze tampons and had suspended the gall-bladder, there was almost no postoperative trouble. Why? Simply because in cholecystitis, unless the gall-bladder had been destroyed by gangrene of the lining, the gall-bladder is not up under the liver, but it hangs suspended from its cystic duct so that it cannot drain. We know that in the human body, whenever a cavity cannot drain naturally, there will be trouble, no matter what cavity we may consider. As long as there is obstruction to the mechanical drainage the resulting stasis favors infection and we will have trouble. In making a cholecystostomy for whatever condition, for gall-stones or cholecystitis, if you drop the gall-bladder you increase the likelihood of obstruction because the upper end of the gall-bladder is certain to become adherent to the hepatic flexure of the colon in a manner to obstruct drainage through the cystic duct. The infection probably travels alongside, and not through the ducts. On the other hand, if you suspend the gall-bladder to the transversalis fascia and the peritoneum, it is in a normal position again in which sacculation and obstruction are not possible. In the class of cases that have been enumerated by Dr. Sherrill and Dr. Mayo, we have come to adopt the following rule: If there is obstruction to the cystic duct which is not due to position, we remove the gall-bladder. We regularly remove gall-bladders which are hopelessly diseased, also those which for any reason are not likely to drain well through the cystic duct following cholecystostomy, and also the short, thick gall-bladders whose contraction is due to chronic inflammation in the past. I believe that this element in the treatment of gall-bladder troubles is worthy of consideration, and that many gall-bladders which are now being removed would be better treated if tamponed with gauze and sutured to the peritoneum and transversalis fascia in the upper angle of the wound.

DR. LE GRAND GUERRY, Columbia, South Carolina (closing the discussion on his part).—I have been very much pleased with the discussion that has followed the reading of my paper, because I think it will be of great benefit to every one of us. It will serve as a crystallized sentiment or an expression of opinion from the Association as to what ought to be done.

Dr. Mayo and myself have been approaching this subject from different angles. In my paper I had solely to do with the question as indicated in the title, namely, "In Cases of Symptoms Without Gall-stones what Disposition Shall be made of the Gall-bladder?" We are not making any effort to discuss the causes of gall-stones themselves. Personally, our practice has been to remove the gall-bladder when it is hopelessly diseased palpably, or when its function is destroyed. A very favorable type of gall-bladder disease in my experience for the average or the rank and file of the profession is the case in which there are gall-stones and you do a cholecystostomy. These operations are followed by an exceedingly low mortality and by uniformly satisfactory functional results. The difficulty, as we have indicated in the paper and brought out in the discussion, comes in the group of 25 cases of symptoms without gall-stones that we do not cure. Statistics and the results prove that 75 per cent. remain well after cholecystostomy, but it is the 25 per cent. of the cases we are after. We should attempt to clear up this group of 25 per cent. throughout the length and breadth of the land, for although operated on early they are not permanently relieved.

DR. CHARLES H. MAYO, Rochester, Minnesota (closing).— I am glad we are all in such harmony. Dr. Sherrill thinks the gall-bladder ought to be saved, like Pandora's box, for the good of the nation, so that we may know where it is afterward. It may be a good thing for that. There are a lot of cases in which gall-stones are present without symptoms. We have found them when working in the pelvis, and they gave the patient very few, if any, symptoms of their presence. Such patients have never complained of colic nor anything of that kind.

In the last year we have had to operate on cases for recurrent stones in the gall-bladder. The stones could be felt, and when removed they were found to be different in color and appearance. I recall one patient for whom we removed gall-stones five years before, and another one seven years before, both of whom came back on account of recurrence of the gall-stones. In some of these cases years ago we could not recognize cholecystitis and could not find stones; but with increased experience and becoming more familiar with the literature we have been able to find them.

Dr. Finney knows very well what a strawberry gall-bladder is. He only says he does not to create a ruction.

It has been stated that the dangers of cholecystectomy are great, but they are less now than they were. If one eliminates a lot of work of years ago as a basis of our knowledge of that day and at that time, one will remember when we did cholecystectomies they were done on bad cases and we had a high mortality as a result. Years ago such operations were necessary considering the class of cases that came to us. We had bad cases of inflammation, of infection and pus to deal with.

With reference to infection and how it gets in, it comes up through the duodenum. There is a preconceived idea that if infection goes the other way or toward the liver the germs cannot be killed and they get into the bile if they can. It is very much like breathing bad air. Germs do not light on healthy mucous membrane and attack it from in front. We can fight things in front, and so the skin gets the upper hand. You do not have as much trouble if you have an infection upon your skin. The mucous membrane of the intestine is exposed all the time, and it is so prepared as to ward off attacks as much as possible, but if the attack is in the rear, or if a man stabs you in the back, the visceral circulation is affected, bacteria gain entrance to the blood and circulate about in the capillaries of the mucous membrane. These things can be reproduced in the lower animals.

In pyemia and septicemia we have bacteriemia. Bacteriemia occurs in typhoid fever. If one takes blood from the ear of a patient with pneumonia a culture can be made and the organisms of the disease produced. When the surface is attacked it will take care of itself. Don't worry about it; but the attack in the rear is like the Italian who stabs you in the back. We cannot take care of it. So we can produce all the things we have looked upon as local entities. Your sciatica, where is it? It is in the sheaths of the nerve.

Let us take ulcer of the stomach. 75 per cent. of animals will develop ulcer of the duodenum and ulcer of the stomach. Take out the sympathetic nerve origin and you produce stasis of circulation. You can get multiple ulcers of the stomach. Take out the adrenals and you will get multiple ulcers of the stomach. These things are being done over and over again. It is a question of anticipating it.

We all like the idea of bringing out the point as to the group of glands involved. What is pancreatitis? We have a type of real inflammation of the pancreas, and we have lymphadenoma. If you get smitten on your own work and think there is no room for improvement, then there is no use in talking about such cases as we have under discussion. The minute you are satisfied with your work, send out a letter to your old cases and see how many of them continue to remain well. By this means you will find your percentage of recoveries is not as great as you thought it was. Are we going to cease operating for appendicitis simply because somebody makes a mistake or because accidents have taken place? Not at all. Are we going to quit doing gastro-enterostomies because three or four patients come in every year who have not had the right kind of surgical work done? I do not think so.

SHIRRING THE ROUND LIGAMENTS

A NEW METHOD OF SHORTENING THE LIGAMENTS FOR RETRODISPLACEMENTS OF THE UTERUS

By John Wesley Long, M.D., F.A.C.S.
Greensboro, N. C.

Operations upon the round ligaments for the purpose of overcoming backward displacements of the fundus have developed much ingenuity and a great variety of methods. A multitude of men have contributed to this phase of pelvic surgery. The bare mention of a method, whether new or old, rarely fails to evoke an interminable discussion.

To this arraignment I plead guilty to the extent of having invented one operation for shortening the round ligaments some nine years ago and now come forward with a second.

Before the North Carolina Medical Society in 1907[1] I read a paper with the title "Preperitoneal Shortening of the Round Ligaments." The occasion and paper were rendered memorable by a rather spirited but good-natured discussion of the subject by that master of gynic surgery Dr. Howard A. Kelly and myself.

At the Atlanta meeting of this Association in 1913[2] I gave a brief description of the operation which I purpose describing more fully at this time.

The operation I have christened "Shirring the Round Liga-

[1] Tr. North Carolina Med. Soc., 1907, p. 168.
[2] Tr. Southern Surg. and Gynec. Assn., 1913, p. 85.

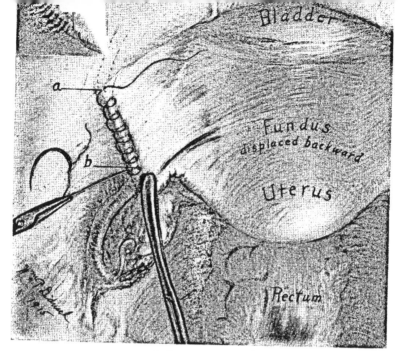

F<small>IG</small>. 1.—Shirring the round ligaments.

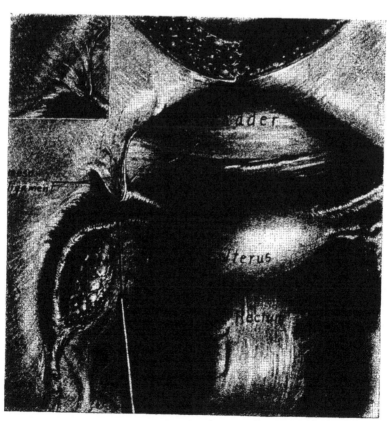

F<small>IG</small>. 2.—Shirred portion of ligament covered with mesoligament.

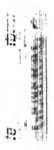

ments," since the designation describes to a nicety the procedure employed, as we shall see. The method is indicated only in those cases in which it is expedient to open the abdomen. For simplicity, ease of execution and efficiency it surpasses any operation for the purpose I ever tried or saw published.

I shall make no attempt to discuss the indications for shortening the round ligaments, or to enter into the relative merits of the many types of operations employed for this purpose. I leave those questions for a subsequent occasion.

The illustrations make plain the succeeding stages and immediate results of the operation.

The first step, after having opened the abdomen and exposed the parts, is to seize the round ligament about midway with forceps. The exact point at which to catch the ligament is determined by estimating the amount of slack to be taken out of the ligament. On making traction upon the distal portion of the ligament with the forceps from a half inch to an inch of the ligament will be pulled out of the inguinal canal. This is an essential part of the operation, as the sequel will show.

While tension is being kept up, a round needle, armed with linen or silk, is thrust through the ligament close to the pelvic brim just at its exit from the internal inguinal ring (a). The needle is again put through the ligament about a quarter of an inch farther toward the fundus. This is repeated again and again, until sufficient length of the ligament has been sutured to insure the proper degree of shortening. The last puncture of the needle is usually made through that portion of the ligament which is traumatized by the bite of the forceps.

By pulling ever so lightly upon the ends of the suture the ligament begins at once to "shirr," as a dressmaker would say. This is seen distinctly in the insert. Shirring the ligament necessarily shortens it. You will observe that the points indicated by (a) and (b), representing the extremes of the sutured portion of the ligament, approach each other.

When the knot is tied it hugs up closely against the internal inguinal ring. If, perchance, sufficient of the slack in the ligament has not been taken up to tilt the fundus forward, one or more sutures can be introduced through the ligament, traveling always toward the uterus. The same needle and suture are used throughout the entire operation.

The operation might well be stopped here. In fact I had performed it many times before noticing that after tying the knot, gentle traction upon the suture develops a tiny *mesoligament*. The base of this psuedomesentery springs from the pelvic wall. The major portion of it lies in front of the round ligament. This discovery gave me an idea, namely, that the peritoneal fold forming the mesoligament might be utilized as a cover for the shirred portion of the round ligament.

On trying out the suggestion I found it to be readily accomplished with most satisfactory results. Catching the edge of the little meso with forceps it is pulled inward over the shirred portion of the ligament. While the meso is held in this position the same needle we started out with, armed with the same suture still uncut, is thrust through the mesoligament from below upward and another knot tied. Could anything be simpler? A little skill displayed here will hide even the last knot. I asked the artist, Mr. Didusch, to let the knot show in the illustration so that its position might be seen. The shirred portion of the ligament is entirely hid from view, and, what is better, out of reach of a troublesome intestine seeking an adhesive alliance.

The operation as finished evinces a refinement of technic that appeals to the most esthetic surgeon. It is also so exceedingly simple that even a well-trained operating-room nurse could perform it, under the guidance of the surgeon of course.

I have employed the operation for three years or more. Having demonstrated to my own satisfaction both it's feasibility and efficiency, I feel, in the language of the newspaper, that it is time it should be "released for publication."

ULCER OF THE JEJUNUM, WITH
REPORT OF A CASE

By ROBERT C. BRYAN, M.D., F.A.C.S.

Richmond, Virginia

VAN ROOJEN has been able to collect from literature three cases of apparently undoubted peptic ulcers of the jejunum in whom no previous gastro-enterostomy had been performed.

He says: "The jejunal peptic ulcer is one which manifests itself in its outer appearance, its symptoms, as well as results, analogously to the peptic ulcer of the stomach, with the difference that while no tangible cause can, as a rule, be attributed for the development of the gastric variety of this ulcer, the jejunal is practically always a sequela of an antecedent gastro-enterostomy. I say practically always, in the literature on the subject, this relationship is considered a constant one. I know, however, of three cases of jejunal ulcer in which no antecedent gastro-enterostomy was performed." In 1861, that is twenty years before the first gastro-enterostomy was performed, Wagner reported such a case. Professor Rotgans while performing a gastro-enterostomy for a peptic ulcer of the stomach discovered during the operation a peptic ulcer of the upper part of the jejunum. Dr. Schoo, the pathologist at the Wilhelmina Hospital at Amsterdam, informed Van Roojen of having found two such spontaneous ulcers of the jejunum at autopsy.

That anatomical deviations and anomalies may be found in the upper abdomen are frequently observed. Normally the duodenum and the jejunum are continuous, the following differences may be noted: In the duodenum the glands of Brunner are found which penetrate the muscularis mucosa, their fundi lying in the submucosa. These glands are not found in the jejunum or in the ileum. They manufacture an akali juice which, with the glands of Lieberkühn that are found in the duodenum, along with the product of the pancreas, produces the succus entericus. The muscular coat of the duodenum is thicker than that of the jejunum and the normal habitat of germs are also different in these two segments of the gut. The most striking anatomical variation is the fixed position of the duodenum with its anterior mesentery and generous blood supply. The thin jejunum, on the other hand, enjoys a large excursion being fixed only at its proximal end, its minimum mobility is therefore greater than the maximum of the duodenum. It has a complete mesentery and is swung vertically.

The case to be reported is W. H. M., aged forty-eight years, white, inspector. Family history negative, but for one sister who died of cancer. Father alive at eighty. Usual mild diseases of childhood.

He had typhoid fever twenty-five years ago, and was confined to his bed several months. He was operated on for mastoiditis twenty-three years ago in New York, and has had continuous rubber drainage ever since, and is entirely deaf on the left side. His leg was broken fifteen years ago; good result. He had measles six years ago and was very ill, but there were no complications. He never drank or used tobacco. In the last four years he has had severe attacks of indigestion, with increasing frequency of late, characterized by violent cramp in the region of the stomach. He has always been a hearty eater and chronically constipated. Two years ago he had constant pain and nausea which continued for four months, and vomited constantly, but he never noticed any blood in the vomitus. He then consulted a physician, who said he had an ulcer of the stomach. He was now thoroughly incapacitated for work of any kind and lost considerable weight and strength. At this time he started washing out the stomach which always made him feel better. The washings were green with yellow mucus. The pain would come on from two and a half to three hours after eating. Recently, in the last few months, there had been persistent pain and nausea, but no vomiting, although there was a constant desire to eat or drink something, and he had noticed that he could not eat very much at a given time. For several years he had used strong liniments on the pit of his stomach. This with a hot-water bottle was his accustomed treatment. He did not believe in medicines and would not take them. The patient had been unable to do any regular work in the last three years, and consulted many physicians, who said he had cancer of the stomach, spasm of the pylorus, appendicitis, and ulcer of the stomach.

September 8, 1915, at 1 A.M., while employed as an inspector in a munition factory, he was suddenly seized with a most agonizing pain in the abdomen and groins. This pain was unlike any that he had ever had before. He was found about an hour later by some of his fellow-workmen in a collapsed condition and brought to Grace Hospital at 3 A.M., two hours after the sudden seizure.

When seen by the writer at 8 A.M., the patient was fairly comfortable, the pain had been controlled by morphin, the face was drawn and pale, and the extremities cold; pulse 104, temperature 96° F., respiration 22. There was persistent nausea and frequent attempts to vomit, but no eructation. An insatiable thirst was very distressing. The abdomen was board hard. There was no area of tenderness greater than another; a most annoying and painful priapism persisted throughout the day. The catheter gave two ounces of urine which was acid; 1030; moderate amount of albumin; occasional red blood cell; no pus; few hyaline and several fine granular casts; phosphates normal; no sugar;

no chlorides; indican, acetone, diazo, and urobilinogen negative. White blood cell count, 8400. Liver dulness absent; heart sounds distant but clear; respiration shallow. The picture was that of acute abdomen, and the diagnosis of probable perforation of ulcer of the stomach was made.

The patient positively refused operation, and only consented at 8 P.M., seventeen hours after the onset, with temperature 101° F., pulse 114, and respiration 38.

Ether anesthesia; right rectus incision. The peritoneal cavity was full of greenish fluid with flakes of lymph and food particles floating about in it. The stomach was atrophic, hard, bound down, pulled to the left and firm, the walls white and heavy, the omentum shrunken and thick. The duodenum was plastered down, the jejunal wall was likewise indurated, whitish and thickened, and on its anteior wall, about three inches from the duodenojejunal juncture, a round punched-out ulcer, the size of a cherry-stone, was found. The induration of the jejunum extended several inches below the point of perforation and tapered off gradually in the jejunal wall. The patient's condition was desperate on account of the great thickening, diminished lumen, and fixed position of the stomach, duodenum, and jejunum; no anastomosis could be made; purse string and invagination were impossible. A piece of omentum was plugged into the opening, and several retaining catgut sutures sewed over it; the belly was irrigated with warm saline. A large drainage tube was inserted and a stab wound made into the pelvis; the patient died the next morning at 10 o'clock. Autopsy was refused.

JEJUNAL ULCER FOLLOWING GASTRO-ENTEROSTOMY. In 1899 Braun first described this complication, and although the subject has since received considerable attention in Germany by Hahn, Kausch, Schwarz, and Korte, Keen's case in 1904 was the first described in English records. Mikulicz, Pinner, Tiegel, Mayo, Robson, von Haberer, Van Roojen, Paterson in his Hunterian lectures, and Gosset contributed the early literature on this topic. Extremely interesting experimental studies have also been carried out by Exalto, Katsenstein, Hotz, Kathe, and Wullenstein, and more recently by Soresi, of New York.

FREQUENCY. Statistics show that jejunal ulceration occurs in 1.5 per cent. of all gastro-enterostomies. Keen states that all of these cases were of the perforating character, and therefore were not recognized, causing death by abscess or in other ways in which adhesions and complications so obscured the parts that even an autopsy failed to reveal the true nature of the disease.

Mikulicz says that in 34 instances in which the location of the gastro-enterostomy anastomosis was mentioned, 25 times it occurred in the anterior and 6 times by the posterior method. In the posterior operations the jejunal opening is about nine inches distant from the beginning of the jejunum; in the anterior it is from sixteen to twenty inches distant from this point. It would appear, therefore, that the lower the point of anastomosis in the jejunum, the more susceptible the mucosa to the digestive action of the peptic juices.

1. The ulcer developed rapidly and perforated shortly after operation.

2. The ulcer developed in a few weeks or a month after operation, suggesting a recurrence of the former trouble.

3. The ulcer developed slowly and insidiously undergoing a subacute perforation.

4. The ulcer perforated into a hollow viscus.

ETIOLOGY. That ulcers of the intestine frequently occur has been well established; most of them are superficial, heal spontaneously, and consequently possess no surgical interest. As a rule they are merely the expression of a general disease such as gout, syphilis, scurvy, anthrax, leprosy, tuberculosis, dysentery, or erysipelas. Any form of intestinal ulcer may lead to perforation. The duodenal perforation following extensive burns has been frequently recorded.

Age. The age in jejunal ulcers following gastro-enterostomy does not seem to play an important rôle. Of the 146 cases collected by Schwarz, in 1914, the youngest patient was two months old, while the oldest had reached the age of seventy. The disease most frequently occurred between the ages of thirty and fifty.

Sex. It has been supposed that the predisposition of the male is perhaps due to the fact that men are most apt to be indiscreet about eating and drinking, especially alcoholic indulgences, and that their greater participation in the more strenuous demands of life likewise predispose them to this affection. Pinner would add to this excessive smoking.

Time. The jejunal ulcer develops most frequently within the first six months following the original gastro-enterostomy. Of the 146 cases above referred to, 50 developed within this period, 22 within the second half year, 23 within the second year, 20 between the second and fifth years, and 13 between the fifth and tenth years. According to Pearson, rough handling, marginal bruising, and excessive dragging on the parts, the use of blunt instruments in effecting the opening into the stomach and bowel, and the injudicious right application of clamps and forceps, hematoma, emboli, tension traction are the factors following gastro-enterostomy which do the mischief.

Next in importance is sepsis, either as the result of infection at the time of the operation or already existing in the diseased stomach. Insufficient blood supply resulting either from excessive tension of the sutures, or due to thrombosis in the vessels around the anastomotic opening.

The presence of a foreign body is a frequent cause, according to Pearson, of the gastro-jejunal variety of this complication, and the most frequent foreign body, as well as the most frequent source of irritation, is the prolonged retention of an unabsorbable inner suture.

Paterson offers the three following suggestions as the cause of jejunal ulcerations:

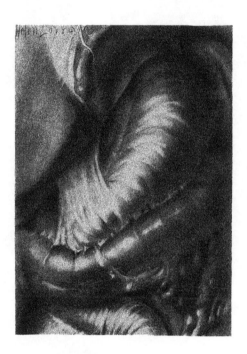

Fɪɢ. 1.—Stomach shows great thickening, walls white and heavy, organ markedly contracted and bound down to the left of the median line.

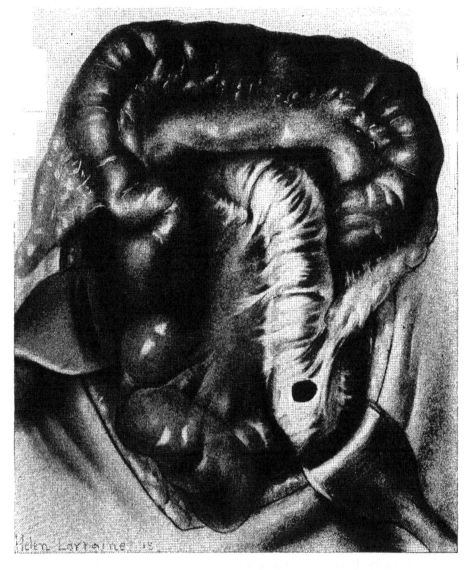

FIG. 2.—Jejunum greatly indurated, the mesentery shrunken, its walls white and hard. Perforation shows about 3 inches from the duodenojejunal juncture.

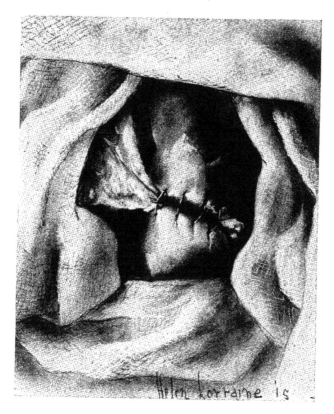

FIG. 3.—Illustrates a tab of omentum packed into the opening and secured by some retained catgut sutures.

1. That jejunal ulceration is due to circulatory disturbances in the attached jejunum.

2. That jejunal ulcer is an infective process.

3. That jejunal ulcer is due to the digestive action of gastric juice on mucous membrane accustomed to the presence of alkaline contents only. Paterson holds to the view that such ulcerations are toxic in origin, and states that "this toxic agent usually present is hydrochloric acid, but that other toxic agents may possibly be present and either may increase the effect of the other."

Thus a small percentage of free hydrochloric acid in the jejunum which by itself would not cause ulceration, in the presence of some other toxic agent, might produce ulceration. The circumstances under which free hydrochloric acid may be present in the jejunum are:

1. Hyperacidity of the gastric juice so that the bile and pancreatic juice are unable to neutralize completely all the acid entering the jejunum.

2. Normal percentage of hydrochloric acid in the gastric juice but excessive secretion so that the amount of hydrochloric acid discharged into the jejunum is greater than can be neutralized.

3. Diversion of the course of the bile and pancreatic juice so that the jejunum is exposed to the action of gastric fluids unmixed with the bile and pancreatic juice as in certain operations.

4. Normal acidity and normal amount of gastric secretion but incomplete neutralization in the jejunum, owing to temporary diminution of the flow of the bile and of the secretion of the pancreatic juice.

Moynihan is inclined to the idea that jejunal ulcers are always secondary to an infective process elsewhere, most likely in the abdomen.

Pinner in commenting upon the reported cases doubts from the available anatomical description if they were actually peptic ulcers.

From time to time various theories based upon anatomical, clinical and experimental considerations have been brought out, but ever since Tiegel expressed in 1904 his belief that the chief cause of these ulcers following gastro-enterostomy is to be found in the deleterious effect of the acid gastric juice upon the mucosa of the jejunum, a tissue not accustomed under normal conditions to this chemical agent, all authorities are inclined to concur in this opinion. Despite the fact that not an inconsiderable number of cases have been reported in whom the hydrochloric acid content of the gastric juice was normal or even subnormal.

Keen thinks that a mild form of sepsis leading to an excess of free HCl in the gastric juice, traumatism either by coarse food or through external injury, and interference with the circulation in the bowel, must be considered as possible causes.

Von Bergmann states that if the gastric juices pass directly into the jejunum, a typical gastric ulcer may be produced, the gastric juice being found to contain excess acid.

Oviatt, in the *American Practice of Surgery*, declares that ulcer of the jejunum has never been found following operation for pyloroplasty or gastroduodenostomy. In pyloroplasty and gastroduodenostomy the acid secretion is neutralized by mixing with the bile, pancreatic juice and succus entericus. Mikulicz reports a case of a child three months old in whom an ulcer formed following an operation for congenital stenosis of the pylorus. H. J. Paterson states that in most instances, hyperchlorhydria is due to insufficient use or inefficient working of the anatomic opening; also that arteriosclerosis of the bloodvessels of the mesentery, or kinking of these structures may interfere with the blood supply and so predispose to the formation of ulcer.

The above are some of the theoretical explanations of a condition which to the writer is apparently directly contingent upon an acid autodigestion, for ulceration lower down in the alimentary tube, following an entero-enterostomy or enterocolostomy is unknown; in other words, the acid chyme of the stomach is done away with in these anastomoses, as only alkaline products are found from the pyloric ring to the rectum.

EXPERIMENTAL. The theory of hyperacidulation is supported if not in its entirety certainly to a very large extent by some of the foremost surgeons. Schwarz dismisses the etiological consideration with the terse sentence, "Where the gastric juice has no access there is no peptic ulcer." It is further confirmed by some of the experimental work carried out by Katzenstein, Wullenstein, and Kathe who sutured into the stomach of the dog, loops of intestines and parts of other organs, and observed the deleterious effects of the gastric juice upon the living non-stomach tissue of this animal. They assume that the stomach mucosa secretes a neutralizing antiferment which renders this tissue immune to the effects of the gastric juice.

Katz and Exalto carried out similar experiments, and came to the conclusion that the disintegrating effects observed by the former investigators were due to interference with the blood supply of the invaginated part, and that whenever sufficient precautions were taken to avoid circulatory disturbance no digestive effects were observed. Whatever these experimental studies may mean, certain it is that the clinical facts point strongly to the correctness of the hydrochloric acid theory, for the complication follows much less frequently those operations which do not prevent the neutralizing alkaline fluids of the gall-bladder and pancreas from reaching the gastric juice and becoming mixed with it; in short, those operations which do not deprive the patient of this "inner drug-shop," as Roux aptly termed it.

Axel Key records but one case of ulceration of the jejunum following gastro-enterostomy for carcinoma of the stomach (*Nordisk Med. Archiv*, 1907, xl, 97). Rowlands was unable to find any such case. This apparently corroborates strongly the acid theory of jejunal ulcer formation.

Wilkie, in 1910, performed gastro-enterostomies of different types upon a number of cats, and later administered to these animals hydrochloric acid in various amounts and noted the effect of this upon the subsequent development of jejunal ulcer.

Exalto performed gastro-enterostomies in two series of dogs, seven in each series. In the first series he performed the ordinary anterior and posterior retrocolic gastro-enterostomies, while in the second series he used Roux's operation, in some anteriorly and in others posteriorly.

The dogs of the first series after uneventful recoveries from the operation, showed no subsequent involvement of the intestines, and in 3 of those which were killed, the autopsies showed no signs of ulcer formation in the jejunum. On the other hand, of the 7 dogs in the second series, 5 died of a perforative peritonitis due to a jejunal ulcer, and of the 2 others who were sacrificed only 1 was free from this complication.

It is rather interesting to note that in the specimens photographed and fully described of the jejunal ulcer following gastro-enterostomy which the writer has seen, the necrosed area was located opposite to the new hiatus or in other words, in the direction of the flow of the gastric contents.

LOCATION OF DUODENAL ULCERS. Moynihan divides the stomach from the duodenum by that important landmark, the pyloric vein. He says: "It runs generally a little to the gastric side of the pylorus, is constant, and its recognition allows one to see instantly where the stomach ends and the duodenum begins. It runs upward from the greater curvature, and is thick and short. If this landmark be taken as the beginning of the duodenum 95 per cent. of the total number of cases of ulcer lies within the first portion of the gut—that is, within one and a half inches of the pylorus."

Eustermann says that the average ratio of gastric to

duodenal ulcers is about 1 to 3. That is 75 per cent. of all ulcers are duodenal. Of 814 cases of duodenal ulcer, 77 per cent. were in males and 23 per cent. in females. Wilkie has explained this on an anatomical basis.

In Collins's series there were in the 262 cases 242 in the first part, 14 in the second, 3 in the third, and 3 in the fourth.

In Perry and Shaw's series of 149 cases there were 123 ulcers in the first part of the duodenum, 16 in the second, and 2 in the third and fourth. In 8 instances the ulcers were scattered.

Moynihan says: "The first part of the duodenum is especially prone to attack. It may be that against it the jet of chyme directly impinges as it is expelled through the pylorus."

In other words, after the neutralizing effect of the duodenal and pancreatic juice have become evident there is no ulcer formation.

Theoretically, then, if a severe acid chyme, not enjoying the beneficial effects of alkalinization, would be hurriedly emptied through the duodenum into the jejunum, it would appear from a review of the literature and experimental work that ulcer of the jejunum by this autodigestive process should take place. It has therefore occurred to the writer that the explanation of this necrosis rests not so much with an actual hyperacidity as it does with a prolonged and intermittent failure of proper alkalinization by the normal ferments which should be found present in the duodenum. A transient cholemia, interstitial pancreatitis, or duodenitis, constitutional diseases, psychic, neurotic, or hysterical influences may lessen or inhibit this alkaline product and thus permit the acid fluid to reach the jejunal membrane uncontrolled or modified by alkaline juices, ulcus jejuni would be all the more likely with this state of affairs, if associated with duodenal abnormalities such as shortening, anomalous blood supply, and an early or mesial duodenojejunal junction.

The writer's case of jejunal ulcer was associated with the pathological states of the stomach, duodenum, and jejunum already mentioned, apparently a cirrhosis of the stomach, linitis plastica—or the gastro-intestinal sclerostenosis of Krompecher.

In 1850 Glüge, of Germany, first described a case of complete cirrhosis of the stomach. Brant tells us of a case in which the lesion was found in the stomach and cecum. By these authors the disease was held to be benign. Krompecher holds that gastro-intestinal sclerostenosis is not a mere disease of the pylorus, but is found in the intestines and peritoneum, and that it is the result of a chronic venous edema, caused by cardiac insufficiency and arteriosclerosis, and that the pathological process bears a close relation to scleroderma.

Brinton states that with the great thickness the mucosa is often normal in appearance, "the secretary structures remaining substantially healthy."

Lyle in his article ("Linitis Plastica") states that "in the majority of cases, evidences of an associated subacute or chronic peritonitis are prominent, lymph on the coils of the intestines, fibrous adhesions, ascites, thickening and opacities of the lesser and greater omentum, white waxy-like plaques on the visceral and parietal peritoneum with thickening of the retroperitoneal tissue" (the retroperitoneal callus of Hanot and Gombault).

From the hurried operation and great haste made necessary by the condition of the patient, the writer would not care to venture an opinion whether this was a case of linitis plastica with a coincident jejunal ulceration, or whether it was primarily an ulcer formation with perforation, associated with many other old healed ulcers of the duodenum and stomach resulting in great induration and thickening.

The latter is probably the most tenable.

Diagnosis. There being no literature upon diagnosis, our investigations must be limited to or deduced from jejunal ulcers developing after a previous gastro-enterostomy.

Mayo-Robson says: "If after a period of good health subsequent to the operation of gastro-enterostomy a patient begins to complain of acidity, flatulence, and discomfort after meals, followed after a time by definite pains from an hour to two or three hours after food, and relieved temporarily after taking milk or some other light diet, or some form of alkali; if the pain occurs on the left side of the umbilicus and is associated with marked tenderness and rigidity of the left rectus the suspicion of ulcer of the jejunum will arise. Hematemesis or melena or even the presence of occult blood in the feces will make the diagnosis fairly certain; but if with all these symptoms a swollen and tender loop of bowel can be felt in the region of the anastomosis or below and to the left of the umbilicus the surgeon can no longer be in doubt as to the nature of the disorder."

Pearson, from whom we quote liberally, says: "Epigastric pain is the most constant symptom. Usually it bears no relation to the taking of food, but is dull, aching, or stabbing in character and more or less persistent. In some instances, however, it closely simulates the periodicity of ulcer pains, a meal affording initial relief followed after a definite interval of exacerbation. The pain is usually in the middle line or slightly to the left and above the umbilicus, and might strike through to the back when most acute. Epigastric distress, fulness, flatulence, and eructations of sour gas with acid fluid may occur. Vomiting is not frequent, hematemesis and melena are rare. Loss of weight will probably be observed, especially if the patient has enjoyed a period of good health before the onset of symptoms. Next to pain, epigastric tenderness is probably the most common sign. It closely corresponds in position to the pain, being more commonly to the left of the median line. A variable degree of muscular rigidity may be present."

Another objective sign which is very much stressed upon by Barsony in the *Wiener klinische Wochenschrift*

1914, is furnished by the roentgenological examination of the jejunum. He believes that an intense spotlike shadow which breaks through the filling in the jejunum and partly extends over the contour of this viscus, which furthermore remains uninfluenced by lavage, and the locality of which is tender to pressure, is characteristic of postoperative jejunal ulcer.

But these are the diagnostic measures worked out for that variety of jejunal ulcers which follow gastro-enterostomy.

With necrosis and mural disintegration the degree of pain is accurately adjusted to the proximity of the pathological process to the peritoneal investment, the writer would venture to state that in ulceration of the duodenum there is more pain and a longer course with the ulcer in the anterior or peritoneal wall than obtains upon the posterior or uncovered wall. This pain is aggravated by functional activity and, according to experiments, by the presence of hydrochloric acid. On the other hand it is controlled by rest and alkalies. This pain is to the left of the median line, at times referred to the back, is more localized in the upper abdomen and, like most pain in the small intestines, is temporarily bettered by a gentle pressure. It may radiate to the groins, along the spinal column, toward each renal fossa; in short, assumes the varied characteristics of location or intensity of the pain of a localized inflammation of the small intestines, which is constantly referred in its early development to an area about the umbilicus. This intermittent distress, whether it be the gone, empty, hunger pain of auto-acid-digestion or the severe colicky pain of peritonism, should not be immediately benefited by an intake of alkalies and food, as is evidenced in cases of ulcer of the stomach and first part of the duodenum, so that the relief will be delayed several hours at best.

Nor is the gastric finding significant of ulcer of the stomach or duodenum. Vomiting with melena is the rule, but hematemesis with melena should not obtain. The history, blood count, urinary findings, and emaciation should also follow the course of ulcer of the stomach and duodenum.

The writer's experience in surgery of the stomach and with one case of ulcer of the jejunum hardly justifies the presentation of a symposium of classical features which may be dignified with the title, "diagnosis of ulcer of the jejunum."

TREATMENT. Keen states that if more attention were to be given to oral sepsis and to the gastric condition of hyperchlorhydria relapse of ulcer might be prevented.

Apparently ulcer of the jejunum is found associated with other pathological states of the upper alimentary tract. Since so little is known and understood about primary ulcer of the jejunum, it may be stated that these associated conditions should be more readily translated and diagnosed by the routine laboratory procedures, and when so worked out and accounted for, the remaining untoward expressions may be laid at the door of a suspected ulcer of the jejunum.

Gastro-enterostomy being one of the causes of jejunal ulceration, one should hesitate to perform the operation for primary ulcer of the jejunum.

In appropriate cases, excision, resection, or enterectomy are apparently the operations of choice.

BIBLIOGRAPHY

Braun. Verhandlungen der deutschen Gesellschaft f. Chirurgie, 1899.

Tiègel, M. Ueber peptische Geschwüre des Jejunums nach Gastroenterostomy, Mitt. a.d. Grenzgeb. d. Med. u. Chir., Jena, 1904, xiii, 897–936.

Paterson. Ann. Surg., August, 1909.

Van Roojen, P. H. Ueber das Ulcus pepticum jejuni nach Gastroenterostomie, Arch. f. klin. Chir., Berlin, 1909, xci, 381–448.

Robson, A. W. M. Peptic Ulcer in the Jejunum, Med.-Chir. Tr. London, 1904, lxxxvii, 339–348.

Von Haberer. Ulcus pepticum jejuni, Deutsche med. Wchnschr., Berlin, 1913, xxxix, 724.

Pinner, A. W. Ueber die perforation des postoperativen Ulcus jejuni pepticum ins Kolon transversum, Berlin, 1912, E. Ebering, 31 p.

Gosset, A. L'ulcere peptique du jejunum, Presse méd., Paris, 1906, xiv, 525–527.

Schwarz, K. Beiträge zur Kasuistik und Chirurgischen Therapie des peptischen jejunalgeschwürs, Arch. f. klin. Chir., Berlin, 1914, civ, 694–732.

Exalto, J. Ulcus jejuni nach gastro-enterostomie, Mitt. a.d. Grenzgeb d. Med. u. Chir., Jena, 1911, xxiii, 13–41.

Katzenstein. Verhandl. d. deutscher Gesselsch. f. Chirurgie, 1906, i, 72.

Hotz. Mitteilungen a.d. Grenzgeb. der Med. u. Chir., 1905.

Kathe and Wullenstein. Quoted by Pinner.

Soresi, A. L. Secondary Ulcers of the Stomach and Jejunum, Ann. Surg., Philadelphia, 1915, lxi, 328–333.

Rowlands, R. P. Jejunal and Gastrojejunal Ulcers, Guy's Hosp. Gaz., London, 1913, xxvii, 149–154.

Key. Nord. Med. Archiv., 1907, I. Abth, Heft No. 5.

Pearson, W. Gastrojejunal Ulcer, with Report of a Case, Tr. Roy. Acad. Med., Ireland, Dublin, 1912, xxx, 192–212.

Mayo, W. J. Surgery, Gynecology and Obstetrics, 1910, 1912, xxx, p. 204.

Wilkie, D. P. D. Gastrojejunal and Jejunal Ulceration following Gastro-enterostomy, Edinburgh Med. Jour., 1910, new series, No. 5, pp. 316–327.

Mayo-Robson, A. W. British Med. Jour., January, 1912.

Barsony, T. Beiträge sur Diagnostik des postoperativen jejunalen und Anastomosenulkus, Wein. klin. Wchnschr., 1914, xxvii, 1059–1062.

Finney and Friedlander. Am. Jour. Med. Sc., October, 1915.

DISCUSSION

DR. A. J. OCHSNER, Chicago, Illinois.—This splendid paper deserves a thorough discussion. There is no doubt but what the acid theory of the production of jejunal ulcer is the correct one, for the reason that, from a clinical standpoint, we have found that in our clinic jejunal ulcer disappeared directly after we learned the fact that we must not permit the acid stomach contents to accumulate in the stomach after gastro-enterostomy. Dr. W. J. Mayo pointed out nearly twenty years ago that a viscious circle occurred at that time after gastro-enterostomy was made because of the fact that in trying to attach the jejunum to the lower part of the stomach, by the time you got through with the operation, the attachment was about the middle of the anterior surface of the stomach instead of the lowest point. We would have our opening an inch or more above the lowest portion of the stomach and would have all of the portion of the stomach below this opening for the accumulation of a lot of hydrochloric acid. The suggestion of Dr. Mayo was so reasonable that immediately we paid attention to it in our clinic, and from that time on we made our anastomosis at the very lowest point of the stomach. I made over two hundred of these anterior gastro-enterostomies—after the time Dr. Mayo had pointed out this fact, and we never had a jejunal ulcer after I did that; consequently, to my mind it was settled positively that there were no ulcers when you actually did succeed in catching the lowest point of the stomach. Although our reason for placing the gastro-enterostomy opening at the lowest point of the stomach was to prevent continued vomiting or a viscious circle, it had the effect of eliminating jejunal ulcer at the same time. Since that time we have had but very few cases of jejunal ulcer. In our operations for the relief of this condition, we have always found that there was a mechanical fault. We make the posterior gastro-enterostomy always now except in cases of cancer, involving the posterior wall of the stomach in which to relieve the pyloric obstruction. Since then, where we had jejunal ulcer, and we have had but a very small number of these, there was always some defect in the posterior gastro-enterostomy. There was some slight blunder at the time of the operation, so that it again was possible for the acid gastric juice to accumulate and be forced against the mucous lining of the jejunum in considerable quantity.

Some ten or twelve years ago we found that in a considerable number of cases there are larger transverse muscle fibers below the entrance of the common duct than there are above. You have the pyloric sphincter, and another sphincter just below the entrance of the common duct into the duodenum, so that in a normal patient the gastric juice is fairly well alkalinized before it passes out through the distal end of the duodenum and into the jejunum; consequently, under ordinary conditions there cannot be any real peptic ulcer of the jejunum provided the secretion of the pancreas and the liver are normal. There cannot be any real peptic ulcers in the jejunum where no gastro-enterostomy has been made.

We have had one case in which there was, however, a perforating jejunal ulcer in which the diagnosis was not made before the operation, but was made at the autopsy. The reason for the ulcer in that locality we have not been able to determine.

DR. F. W. McRAE, Atlanta, Georgia.—There is one point in reference to the diagnosis of perforation of these ulcers that Dr. Bryan mentioned which has interested me very much. So far as I have been able to follow the history of the cases of acute perforation of gastric or duodenal ulcer I have had come under my care, every one of them has fallen when perforation has occurred. That to me is a point I lay great stress on in determining that I have a case of perforation of a gastric or duodenal ulcer. These patients fall as if they were shot. I do not know whether that has been the experience of the other gentlemen or not.

DR. WILLIAM R. JACKSON, Mobile, Alabama.—There are two causes for such an ulcer. If hyperchlorhydria, or the presence of a superabundance of hydrochloric, lactic, or butyric acid in the stomach, passing into the duodenum or jejunum, were sufficient cause to produce circumscribed ulceration, why do we not have multiple or diffused ulcers? Therefore, there are other essential factors, namely, embolic infections that lower the vitality of the mucosa or submucosa, and give us a *locus minoris resistentiae*, and proteolysis takes place by the presence of the acids, and we have an ulcer.

THE ESTIMATION OF RESISTANCE PRIOR
TO SURGICAL OPERATION

By A. C. Scott, M.D.

Temple, Texas

———

By resistance we mean the ability of an organism to overcome the effects of disease, bacterial invasion, and toxic substance or injury, and it depends upon the capacity of each individual organ or tissue and all the organs and tissues collectively to respond to the increased demand upon them proportionate to such demand. Such increased activity is usually called compensation. When we undertake to foretell what an organ or tissue will do in a compensatory way, the complex character of our task at once becomes apparent.

It will not be practical within the scope of this paper to enter upon a detailed discussion of the various diseases, bacterial invasions, and toxic conditions which may be incidentally concerned while the organism is engaged in overcoming the effects of an injury resulting from a surgical operation, although a discussion of the latter necessarily involves frequent reference to them.

We have asked quite a number of surgeons the question regarding the facts upon which they determine a patient's powers of resistance prior to surgical operation, with special reference to the patient's ability to tolerate the proposed work, and it is really surprising to note how at variance their ideas are. One clinician of great prominence in the diagnostic field replied that "we depend upon our surgical judgment;" another said, "one's intuition must be his guide;" another that "the condition of the circulation should be one main dependance," etc. It seems that there are as many kinds of surgical judgment as there are surgeons.

The lack of uniformity of opinion clearly indicates that some more definite method of summarizing the facts concerned in the formation of surgical judgment should be worked out.

The chief temptation is to form an opinion upon a very limited number of clinical facts, such as heart action, facial expression and general appearance, renal function, hemoglobin, leukocytosis, etc., though often these things form only a small part of the data concerned in a safe conclusion.

It appears also that no one has given much well-defined attention to an effort at collecting all the pre-operative conditions upon which a surgeon bases his judgment as to whether or not a patient possesses proper resistance, and as far as I can learn, little effort has been made toward a collective consideration of each phase of operation which may be vitally concerned in outbalancing the weakened resistance of an individual.

Probably more definite study has been given recently to the matter of renal function as a guide to operation, and a prognostic sign in prostatic cases than to the condition or function of any other organ; and we now find W. F. Braasch, Louis Schmidt, A. J. Crowell and others proclaiming that the renal functional tests are only of relative value; that the clinical history and general condition of the patient's strength are of more intrinsic value in the proper estimation of resistance or in the formation of safe surgical judgment.

The surgeon of much experience depends upon his judgment which in a large percentage of cases proves to be sound, but unfortunately for himself and his patients, his judgment is too often based upon some single observation, or more often it is based upon a symptomatology which may ignore a number of elements which are deeply concerned in lowering the patient's resistance to a dangerous degree.

How often we have heard a surgeon say, "well, I wonder what killed that patient. I though he would surely make it through safely." Sometimes he will attempt to analyze the situation by saying, "she took the anesthetic all right, did not lose much blood, and there was very little manipulation of the intestines," etc. Not uncommonly a careful autopsy fails to reveal the exact cause of death.

There is now a growing tendency among some of our successful surgeons to assume an attitude of fearlessness because modern surgical methods have enabled them to operate upon such a large percentage of cases without fatality. Their phenomenal success should not, however, excuse them from blame in the occasional case where a little more care in preliminary investigation and a more definite grouping of data found would have altered their judgment and saved a life by causing a postponement, or possibly the selection of a different type of operation.

Many puzzling situations could be cleared up and an occasional disaster averted were we to systematically enter into our records something which tends to group and emphasize the various elements of lowered resistance and pit the net resistance remaining against the factors involved in each operation to be overcome, being mindful of the fact that in every surgical operation two forces are pitted against each other, one tending to destroy life, and the other engaged solely in an effort to save it.

For the purpose of illustration we will select three factors which may enter into an operation, any one of which might be severe enough to result fatally in a person possessing normal resistence. We refer to hemorrhage, trauma, and inhalation anesthesia, each of which have been measured experimentally. Other factors more difficult to measure are fear, pain, and muscular effort. The physiological effect of each of these factors is modified by the time consumed.

On the resistance side we have an unlimited number of factors, or elements concerned in lowering the standard.

It will be observed that they seldom appear singly and often many of them will be combined in a single individual. They may be roughly classified as follows: Constitutional weakness from inheritance and environment; previous debilitating diseases of any character; recent trauma by either injury or operation, starvation, drug habit, and psychic depression.

We have recently devised a plan in line with the idea of considering these factors collectively, and we have endeavored to give to them a percentage value which, of course, must for the present be somewhat arbitrarily placed, as are also the factors entering into the sum total of injury inflicted by operation. The inexact data drawn from physiological and surgical literature upon which these estimates have been partly made but illustrates again the absence of much exact information bearing directly upon the subject of resistance.

To simplify the problem, to place it more clearly before us, and to give us a working basis by which we may be better able to record the factors concerned in this important question, we have assumed that the maximum or ideal resistance is illustrated in a fully developed adult whose breeding, habits, and environment have been conductive to the acquisition of a complete, well-balanced, and functionally perfect organism.

We have diagrammatically represented this resistance by a perpendicular line forming the left side of a square marked 100 per cent. at the top. At a right angle to this line striking it at its base is another line marking the lower side of the square which is used to represent the destructive factors of an injury or operation. The fatal effect of an operation is represented as 100 per cent., terminating on the left when this line meets the zero point of the resistance line. The square is checked into small squares, altogether representing a large field which may be divided as shown later and taken to grossly represent the patient's chances for recovery. The two areas thus formed will be designated as safety and danger zones.

The simplest form of operation which may be fatal to one possessing normal resistance is that of blood letting. Haldene has recently shown that the total quantity of blood in a normal man is equivalent to practically 5 per cent. or one-twentieth of his weight; and it has been ascertained further that the sudden loss of approximately one-third of the total volume of blood is sufficient to result fatally. Assuming then that we have a normal individual weighing one hundred and fifty pounds and possessing seven and a half pounds of blood, representing 5 per cent. of his body weight, and we should suddenly abstract one-third of that amount, representing two and a half pounds, a fatal termination from such operation might be reasonably expected. We would represent such an operation factor by a red line showing 100 per cent. operation. If, however, but one and a quarter pounds of blood were abstracted which would represent but half per cent. of the former amount, a marked impression upon the patient's circulation might be reasonably expected, but so long as the patient possessed 100 per cent. resistance a fatal termination would not result. Let us now assume that a patient has a reduction of his hemoglobin to 50 per cent. which we will represent by a light-red line dropping from the 100 per cent. point down to the 50 per cent. level. When the two lines representing the factors of operation and lowered resistance intersect each other at the centre of the square, we will designate the two fields thus resulting as the danger zone and the safety zone, and it is at once seen that the danger zone is three times greater than the safety zone. It does not require much stretch of the imagination for a surgeon to appreciate the fact that this diagram represents an approximation to the truth, and we have to add but a small element to the lowered resistance, or another factor or two to the operation to bring about a dangerous situation.

With regard to the anesthesia factor we find that the Chloroform Commission of the British Medical Association together with the experiments of Embley, Paul Bert, and others, have shown rather conclusively that chloroform given in 2 per cent. vapor or less for a period of four to six hours was often sufficient to bring about fatal results.

As yet we have not such specific data relating to ether anesthesia, but we have chosen it for our illustration because it is the popular anesthetic in this country. Some of our most scientific anesthetists would lead us to believe that ether when properly administered, might be given indefinitely without bringing about a fatal termination; but, on the other hand, it is fair to assume from incidental observations upon dogs and from an abundance of clinical evidence that when ether is administered to a degree of full surgical anesthesia by the average hospital anesthetist, a patient with normal resistance would not likely survive longer than ten hours.

For the purpose of this discussion we will accept this as a basis, and call attention to the fact that ill effects of the anesthetic are rapidly multiplied as the patient's resistance is lowered from various causes. In fact, this applies to all the operation factors. As the resistance is progressively lowered each factor of the operation which tends toward fatality is increased in varying proportions as the fatal percentage is approached. Perhaps the most uniformly marked deleterious effect of each operation factor is to be observed in those cases whose resistance is decidedly lowered from some form of toxemia.

If ether anesthesia is maintained for a period of one hour (10 per cent. of the time required for a fatal issue) in a patient whose resistance is lowered only 10 per cent., it will be observed that the danger zone thus resulting is very small, while the safety zone is exceedingly large. If instead of these two small factors acting alone, we have a patient whose resistance is lowered by 30 per cent. as represented by loss of hemoglobin and 50 per cent. by an acute toxemia, the injurious effects of the anesthesia would not be limited to 10 per cent. as in the foregoing illustration, but would be increased at least 20 or 30 per cent. additional, and if this should be supplemented by the loss of one pound of blood, the danger zone would be so great that the safety zone would be virtually destroyed.

It has been shown experimentally that exposure of a considerable portion of the abdominal peritoneum accompanied by trauma, produced by frequent or continual traction upon the mesentery is sufficient to result fatally in from four to six hours. Thus for this study, we may take four hours of such exposure and trauma within the abdomen when acting alone to represent an operation factor of 100 per cent. If a patient has a large part of his intestines. and mesentery exposed and mauled about for an hour under ether anesthesia, these two operation factors acting jointly might very properly be placed at 50 per cent.; and if the patient has prior to operation lowered resistance from any cause of, say 50 per cent., it is at once seen that a proper estimate would be about the same.

Crile has admirably shown that pain and mental emotion represented in fear, anger or grief are capable of profoundly affecting the brain cells, thus contributing largely to the production of fatal shock. We do not know how long such agencies might be continued alone before a fatal result could be expected, but we do know that sudden fright may be so great as to result in immediate death. So while some of these factors always enter into the risk of an operation, it is more difficult to fix an approximate estimate of their influence in any given case.

Some of the above examples may at first appear unusual and exaggerated, but such extremes have been selected chiefly for purposes of illustration. It is indeed unfortunate that so many unwarranted deaths have occurred in our hospitals without proper reckoning having been made by which we might more accurately sum up the result, or estimate the influence of each element concerned in lowered resistance and each factor entering into the operation which contributed to the fatality.

The factors which clearly lower resistance have been briefly mentioned. At first it appears that no standard of measurement can be fixed for them and indeed it may be difficult to reach an exact percentage of influence exerted by each, for our main dependence must be placed in a mass of clinical evidence which has been poorly sorted and applied in a very haphazard fashion.

General reference having been made to the influences which bring about lowered resistance, we will now endeavor to treat specifically of a few things which may serve more or less as definite indexes of lowered resistance. They are to be found in the circulatory and respiratory systems, blood and urine, but much valuable information must be obtained by clinical observation of the destructive effects of certain diseases which we know play an important rôle in lowered resistance. Our time will permit only a brief discussion of a few of them.

Hemoglobin which bears a definite relation to the number of red blood cells and to the total volume of blood can be measured with some degree of accuracy and bears a fairly definite relation to the amount of resistance possessed by the individual. Since the blood is such a vital force the value of this index should not be underestimated. It, like many other influences, becomes of most value when reckoned with other influences with which it is most always associated.

High blood-pressure or hypertension is usually found in arteriosclerosis, acute and chronic nephritis, and toxic goitres. When not accompanied by aggravated toxemia in goitre or marked loss of kidney function it is not usually as significant of lowered resistance as hypotension. It has, however, been given much emphasis as a danger signal and, of course, should not be ignored, especially when it is above 200, but its importance hardly compares with that of hypotension. Hypotension may be either caused by or exaggerated by hemorrhage, shock and collapse. It is found in many of the wasting diseases, in acute and chronic infections, mitral stenosis, and tachycardia. It is common in diabetes and tuberculosis, and also in pneumonia after the first two or three days. When present from toxemia it may be considered a fair index to the amount of toxemia.

Hypotension, or at least, a marked falling off in blood-pressure, is noted late in cases of arteriosclerosis due to myocardial degeneration. It should then be considered as a very grave condition and it may be reasonable estimated that such patients have approximately 75 per cent. lowered resistance. Hypotension below 90 mm. of mercury from any cause should be considered as an index of grave lowered resistance and charted at not less than 60 per cent. or 80 per cent. loss.

Diabetes is a disease not infrequently found to coexist with some condition calling for surgical operation and it so frequently lowers the resistance to a dangerous degree that some surgeons are much disposed to refrain from any kind of major surgical operation when evidence of diabetes is found. Clinical and laboratory observations have shown that some diabetic patients tolerate operation very well, but when the total amount of sugar in twenty-four hours exceeds five grains, when 1.5 grams of ammonia are present, or more than a trace of diacetic acid is found, the patient's resistance is so low that any major surgical operation is very apt to prove fatal. Such lowered resistance might reasonably be placed down to the 20 per cent. level. The coexistance of nephritis with glycosuria has about the same effect in lowering the resistance even though the above findings are in much smaller percentages and a trace of diacetic acid not found. If only a trace of diacetic acid or less than one gram of ammonia are found in the absence of nephritis it would probably be proper to record the lowered resistance at about 50 per cent.

We have sufficient evidence to believe that a normal man who would abstain from all food a little more than forty days would die, and if he were to take neither food nor water his vital forces would give way completely at a much earlier .period. From this we may reasonably assume that any patient who has for any reason gone ten days without food ᴗor water has lost, at least, 25 per cent. of his resistance, before any consideration whatever is given to the ailment which participated in such starvation, and if he has had any febrile disturbance, toxemia, or vomiting and purging a 50 per cent. or 60 per cent. loss of resistance would not be unreasonable.

If, in pursuance of this study, we shall make a critical review of our fatal cases in which the histories, physiological and laboratory findings, together with the operation factors are all recorded upon the chart in accordance with the apparent importance of each factor as it impresses us, some surprising facts will be revealed. If nothing more it will serve to impress upon us how low the resistance may sometimes become without attracting serious notice and also what killing forces we are dealing with when we place a patient under full surgical anesthesia, then traumatize his tissues, bleed him and leave him in agonizing pain.

Fortunately as a result of a highly perfected technic in the administration of anesthesia, and an equally perfected surgical technic, the operation factors in the great majority of surgical operations has been reduced to a minimum. In the average modern surgical institution the resistance presented by the patient is the chief matter to be considered when operation is contemplated. With this fact properly before the surgeon's mind, he may govern the time, shape the character and limit the extent of operation accordingly.

Crile has shown that an acid condition of the blood lowers resistance; that a certain degree of blood acidity in incompatible with life and further that it is produced by those things which clinical evidence has abundantly shown are always indicators of lowered resistance, namely, muscular effort; emotional disturbances, such as fear or mental distress, infectious diseases, alcohol, inhalation anesthesias, starvation, diabetes, Bright's disease, etc. If the chemists and physiologists will now give us a method of ascertaining the percentages of acid in the blood, which is uncomplicated and practical enough for daily clinical use, we will predict a marked advance in the estimation of resistance which will be of inestimable value to the surgeon.

Some gross tests of resistance should not be overlooked. If the patient should be very young, or very old, clinical observation leads us to believe that in the average case an estimate of resistance reduction of about 25 per cent. is conservative. We also know clinically that a superabundance of fat is usually accompanied by a marked loss of resistance. The same applies to persons with very flabby muscular development. Many workers in physiological laboratories have learned to judge the resistance of animals by feeling their muscles. When the muscles are flabby and have a doughy feeling, they are most always recognized as animals of low resistance.

If either cardiac or renal disease give rise to edema a 40 per cent. reduction estimate would not be too much. Cardiac insufficiency is also recognized by presence of varying degrees of dyspnea upon exertion. If the dyspnea is well marked upon slight exertion a resistance reduction estimate of 60 per cent. would not be too much.

In no department of medicine is the team-work of an efficient staff of examiners and laboratory workers of more value than in the work of estimating a patient's resistance prior to contemplated surgical procedures. The importance of systematic examination for the purpose of noting the various things which may lower resistance is parallel to that made for diagnostic purposes and if our presentation of this subject shall even indirectly serve to emphasize this fact, we will feel that it has not been in vain.

While many of these percentage estimates are more or less arbitrarily placed and it may never be possible to deal extensively with exact figures in these computations, we feel confident that a large number of observations in which all of the known factors concerned in lost resistance are recorded and estimated together, adjustments leading to greater accuracy will naturally follow.

This paper should be considered largely suggestive and somewhat in the light of a preliminary report, for it is yet too crude and lacking in definite statistical data to be considered in any sense a finished product.

DISCUSSION

Dr. J. Shelton Horsley, Richmond, Va.—Dr. Scott has presented a subject that is of interest to us all. There is one point about the resistance of the patient that I wish to speak of. It is about that type of cases in which it is necessary to operate during shock. Of course, it is better, if it can be done, to wait until after the shock has passed; but there are certain instances, especially when shock is associated with hemorrhage, in which operation must be done during the state of shock. It is well known that patients who die from hemorrhage die more because of the quantity of fluid that is lost from the vascular system than because of the lack of hemoglobin. Our remedies heretofore have been salt solution given usually intravenously in emergencies, or transfusion of blood. Transfusion of blood is, of course, the most effective, but often a donor is not available, and the cases are usually urgent. Salt solution is rapidly extruded from the vascular system because no free water can stay long within the arteries and veins. Water in the blood is always combined with some colloid, and unless it is thus combined, salt solution, partly because of osmosis, is extruded into the tissues or thrown off through the kidneys and bowels with such rapidity that the blood-pressure soon falls again. Dr. James J. Hogan, of San Francisco, has worked along the line of introducing colloids and has devised a solution containing a colloid which when introduced into the blood current is not rapidly extruded. He uses a combination of gelatin and salts in about the proportion that the salts are used in normal saline solution. I have used Hogan's solution in four cases. They were all exceedingly desperate cases and each case eventually died. Two of them were septic, one who was leukemic suffered severe shock after childbirth, and the other was a case of intense traumatic shock. The immediate result was all that Hogan claimed and in two of the cases that were pulseless at the wrist and were apparently actually dying, the pulse came back within ten minutes, and these two patients lived about four days. Eventually, however, there seems to be some effect upon the kidneys, and while the immediate result in raising the blood-pressure is wonderful, it is possible that the late results may do away with its immediate advantages.

Dr. Robert T. Morris, New York City.—I want to impress a point made by Dr. Horsley. Man is a colloid machine, and his functions are colloid functions. Another point, knowing that resistance is lowered (this is a relative thing practically) or that it is not great, what are you going to do about it? Analyze the terms of that problem and act in accordance therewith.

Not long ago I amputated at the hip joint for diabetic gangrene in a patient who carried on a conversation with my assistants and looked about over the class while he was having an amputation at the hip joint. He was a large man, weighed two hundred pounds. Why was that? First, spinal anesthesia, second, cutting down quickly and injecting novocain into the sciatic nerve and the anterior crural group; then ligating the large vessels in advance, and following the Crile method of cutting off his noci-ceptor nerves with novocain. There we have three American surgeons represented: Corning, Cushing and Crile, in three of the greatest advances of the day—Cushing, blocking the large nerves; Crile, blocking the small nerves, and Corning, blocking the spinal centre.

Dr. Francis R. Hagner, Washington, D. C.—I want to say a few words about a group of cases in which we study resistance as carefully as in any branch of surgery, and I refer to prostatic surgery. The majority of patients with prostatic trouble are old, and we have to be very careful in handling them. When I was at the Garfield Hospital as a resident, at the Hopkins Hospital the mortality was 40 per cent. But there has been a great improvement in prostatic surgery. The reason for that is unquestionably by following out the work that the Doctor has shown here, but the careful preoperative and postoperative treatment of these cases, the taking care of shock, studying resistance in these cases before operation, studying the kidneys, the circulation, the hemoglobin, and other things that the essayist has mentioned. We should think also in these cases of the psychic side which has a good deal to do with it. I do not mean to be irreverant, but I feel that patients who are active in Christian work are very susceptible to psychic shock. We may do twenty-five prostatectomies without a death, and when we have such a group of cases we think we can operate on anything, and these patients will not die. On the other hand, we have a man who apparently is in excellent condition. His phthalein test and his hemoglobin and circulatory condition are in good shape. I had such a case recently. We did not find out until after the operation, that he had made up his mind he was going to die. After coming out of the anesthetic he did not vomit; whenever he would have the slightest pain, he would almost have a convulsion from fear. He lived two days. There was no hemorrhage in his case that could have caused death, and I am firmly of the belief that his psychical condition was the cause of his death so far as I can determine. We did not get any autopsy.

The patients that have been known for years to have large amounts of residual urine without infection are the cases that we fear most. As I see it, these clean bladder cases, with large amounts of residual urine, are the most fatal cases, because they have not acquired the resistance to infection, and they will die when we do not expect it. Whereas patients with foul bladders are more likely to recover from operation as they have an acquired resistance to infection.

Dr. Goodrich V. Rhodes, Cincinnati, Ohio.—I would like to ask Dr. Scott whether he has made any estimate of the presence or absence of eosinophiles in connection with his work.

Dr. W. P. Carr, Washington, D. C.—Dr. Scott has opened up a very interesting subject, and I think we are going to find that certain things may lower resistance in one direction and some in another. For instance, I think the things that lower resistance to infection ought to be looked for in a different way from those that lower resistance to the vital functions of life. I have noticed for many years that patients who have a soft buttery fat, and who are accustomed to an easy life, are very susceptible to infections; whereas, they can stand a great deal of infection, not having the vital resistance lowered so much, while, on the other hand, men who are sometimes strong, hearty, healthy, will resist infection very well, but they will not resist loss of blood or psychic shock.

I want to endorse what Dr. Hagner has said about the psychic element. I had a man recently operated on for cancer of the tongue, an operation under the chin, and had to drain the wound for a while. I never saw a man so afraid of dying, yet he was the son of a general noted for his bravery. After he got up and was going around he had a slight hemorrhage from the wound, about a teaspoonful, and he was so frightened that he would not go back to bed. He finally paid a nurse to watch him all night and to call a doctor if there was any more hemorrhage. I assured him that the wound would not bleed again. He had a slight hemorrhage however, a few days later and was so shocked that he went into collapse and died. The three hemorrhages would not amount to more than an ounce of blood. He died, I am sure, of fright.

DR. F. W. PARHAM, New Orleans, Louisiana.—I want to lay stress upon the point made by Dr. Morris and Dr. Horsley. I want to say a word in favor of spinal anesthesia in these cases of lowered resistance from any cause except serious heart trouble and especially in shock. My remarks have reference especially to the cases where we have got to operate in a state of shock.

Last June, at the meeting of the American Surgical Association, Dr. Bevan read a paper on anesthesia in which he said that in his opinion the time had come when spinal anesthesia should be dropped from surgery. That is not the opinion of a great many surgeons who have done a good deal of operating under spinal anesthesia and continue to do it in selected cases, and especially upon cases in great shock. While I do not use this method of anesthesia anything like as frequently as I did, I do still use it in some cases.

A gentleman living in Scranton, Pennsylvania, expressed the matter very well when he said in comparing the different anesthetics, that with chloroform he likened the patient to a man going on a trip; with chloroform he had his going ticket but no return ticket; with ether he had also his return, but there were many things that might hinder his return, obstructions in getting through the gate, or accidents of various sorts, but with spinal anesthesia he had not only a ticket both ways, but his return was insured against accidents. I believe this to be true of spinal anesthesia, properly conducted, and if we carry it out in such cases without lowering the head unnecessarily, I believe we can carry it out as a safe procedure, and we will be able to operate under certain conditions where it would be unsafe to use any general anesthetic. Local anesthesia with us is now taking the place of spinal anesthesia to a great extent, but there are still cases where spinal anesthesia reserves its rights to continue as one of the legitimate anesthetic methods.

Dr. John Wesley Long, Greensboro, North Carolina.—Just one word, Mr. President. Dr. Hagner in speaking of the fear of death recalls to my mind the fact that the Bible explains why people who are not Christian workers are not afraid to die, when it says, "The wicked have no bonds in their death!"

Dr. Hubert A. Royster, Raleigh, North Carolina.—I am afraid we are getting too near a thin border-line. I confess I am a materialist about the causes of death. If a man dies, he must die of something, and I would like to ask the gentlemen who recorded deaths from psychic causes, what they put on the death certificates. Certainly I know of no board of health that would accept a psychic death. A certain doctor in my city had a case of this kind, but he did not get there soon enough, so he placed as the cause of death, "Died without the aid of a physician."

What I want to impress most clearly in the discussion is that the human body is not a laboratory and the human stomach is not a test tube. An operation is not a mathematical problem. If we can figure upon every particular case and prevent danger before operation, there should be no deaths. Of course, Dr. Scott has come near it, and I think the things to which he has called our attention mean something. I have always had to look at these things carefully before I understood them. I want to say further, when you say a man dies because he has made up his mind to die, you are virtually saying that any human being can will himself to live or to die. If that were so, he would have to disturb the whole physiology of the universe and write it all over again. If a man could say, "I am going to die," then do so, we would have an easy means of suicide. The point is we cannot get too close to the material on the one hand, and too close to the psychical on the other. There is a border line of which we know absolutely nothing.

Dr. A. C. Scott, Temple, Texas (closing).—I appreciate very much the discussion that my paper has elicited. I would like to call your attention to the fact that I did not endeavor in this paper to deal with the treatment of lowered resistance, or with the question as to how we could handle a patient when we do ascertain the fact that he or she has a lowered resistance. As a matter of fact, we have only had time in this paper to touch a few important things. We did not realize until we got down to the study of the details that were concerned in this subject for the preparation of this paper what might be worked out of it. We did not realize to what extent we had been derelict ourselves in taking snap judgment on the matter of a patient's resistance.

If you will ask some of your friends on what they base their judgment in a given case, you will find that the man who is accustomed to working in the urological department of the clinic will say, "We base our judgment upon certain color tests, or certain blood-freezing tests," or something of that character. He will not go beyond that very much. If you ask some of the gynecologists about it, they will say something regarding the question as to whether the patient has had frequent or continuous hemorrhages, or something of that character.

Before I forget, I want to say I heartily approve of the statement made by Dr. Horsley regarding the importance of blood volume. That is of value only where we have had some very recent trauma, where we can get some idea of the amount of blood lost. There is no practical method of measuring the volume of circulating fluid, otherwise it would be a difficult thing to ascertain definitely about the volume of circulating blood in experimental lines of work.

As regards the psychic influence, I wish to say that I think Dr. Crile has shown in a very satisfactory manner that it is entirely possible to lower resistance very materially through some psychic influences. From a clinical standpoint, we have had occasion to observe that is true, and we have learned to handle certain patients on that basis because of the fact they are badly frightened; that they are in great danger to go right into the operating room. It is not an uncommon thing for a patient, when she starts for the hospital, to have some friend say, "Good-bye, I hope to meet you in heaven," or something to that effect. She starts off with that idea in her mind. By the time she gets to the ambulance she thinks it is a dead wagon.

When she arrives at the hospital and is placed in a room, someone comes along with a patient from the operating room who has perhaps had an ingrowing toe nail taken out and bawling to beat the band, and she thinks that poor fellow is dying. A little later on, when she sees someone taken from the operating room covered up, she perhaps exclaims, "There goes another one dead." Now, that patient is in a bad mental condition to undergo a surgical operation. If that patient should get about an ounce of castor oil, which is all she needs, and is operated the next morning, see what condition she is in for operation. Her resistance is lowered still more.

The things I have pointed out are essential and are of such importance that we ought to put them down in black and white, or have these items before our minds when we go to the operating room. We are accustomed, whenever we find a patient particularly frightened and worried over the matter of operation. to offer some excuse in order to get the patient in the hospital a few days. Such a patient must become hospitalized. She must be given time to become familiar with her surroundings, then she will lose that dread of operation she previously had. All these things ought to be considered in every one of these cases.

I regret we have not time to discuss the details, but there are too many items of interest to be discussed at this time.

PSEUDOMYXOMATOUS CYSTS OF THE APPENDIX AND RUPTURED PSEUDOMUCINOUS OVARIAN CYST

By FRED. WARREN BAILEY, M.D., F.A.C.S.

Saint Louis, Missouri

WITHIN the last few years there has been recorded in medical literature, a number of cases of cystic tumors of the appendix and ovary, pseudomucinous in character. Without doubt many such tumors have been removed and destroyed, unrecognized. As near as can be determined, less than one hundred such cases have been accurately described and as there still exists some doubt as to etiology, and considerable difficulty as to diagnosis, the addition of case reports, though not in themselves enlightening, may stimulate instructive discussion.

CASE I.—E. B., St. Louis, Mo., male, aged twenty-five years; electrician.

Family History. Negative.

Personal History. Usual diseases of childhood. Health normal in every respect until November, 1913, when at the age of twenty-four he developed acute appendicitis.

Operation performed within a few days followed by slow convalescence, sinus at site of incision persisting for several weeks. Finally healed, he returned to his work, but pain in right inguinal region continued with frequent exacerbations and reappearance of the sinus discharge at intervals. Constipation, anorexia, and postprandial nausea combined to reduce his weight and vitality and he applied for surgical attention.

Physical Examination. Fairly well-nourished man, with right rectus tonicity, and tenderness on pressure over entire right side of abdomen as high as costal arch, particularly severe over scar, where blind pocket of pus was preparing to escape. Temperature, 100° F.; pulse, 90; tongue heavily coated. Face and back well marked with acne eruption. As appendix was supposed to have been removed at previous operation, exploration for the purpose of obliterating the sinus and determining the reason for its persistence, was advised.

Operation. December 5, 1914, at St. John's Hospital.

Sinus was opened and a seropurulent exudate released, which contained several flakes of gelatinous appearing material. Abdomen was opened and a large omental tumor enclosing the cecum presented. Upon removing the omental sac, the colon was found constricted at three points by strong fibrous bands which radiated mesially from the right parietal wall across the cecum and ascending colon to disappear in a Jackson's veil on its inner surface.

When lifted, the cecum at its lower point presented a tumor the size of the distal phalanx of the thumb; traced up, postcecally, this proved to be a large appendix, distorted and doubled upon itself, and fixed by an exceptionally strong fibrous fold which crossed and constricted it just proximal to the distended tip. The bed in which the appendix rested was filled with a gelatinous substance to the amount of two ounces, and the distal loop of ileum which was attached to the appendix tip, was coated over with this same material all of which came away readily upon a saline sponge. The appendix was released and removed, the omental sac resected, and the cavity gently but thoroughly sponged free of its contents and treated with 3 per cent. iodin. The sinus was then dissected and the wound closed without drainage. The patient left the hospital on the fifteenth day and has since recovery enjoyed perfect health (over one year).

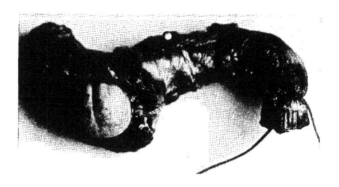

FIG. 1.—Specimen removed from Case I.

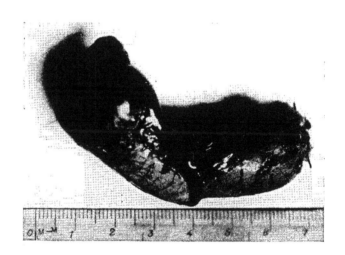

FIG. 2.—Specimen removed from Case II.

Pathological Report (Dr. Goerge Ives). "Gross description: The appendix is 6.3 cm. long; diameter near the distal end 1.3 cm., near the proximal end 1 cm. On the side of the mesenteriole is a smooth-walled tumor-like mass projecting from the appendix, it projects between the layers of the mesenteriole. The shape of the portion of the tumor exposed to view is hemispherical. The wall of the tumor is tense, but fluctuation is elicited. The tissue of the appendix adjacent to the tumor appears gelatinous.

"Upon dissection it was found that the so-called tumor is a cyst filled with gelatinous material. The lumen of the appendix is obliterated excepting for about 1 cm. near the tip. The patent portion of the lumen communicates by a narrow opening with the cyst.

"Microscopic: The muscular coats are thickened. The lumen is displaced by fibrous connective tissue, an abundance of fat, distended capillaries and areas of round-celled infiltration. No lymphoid tissue is observed. The lining of the cyst consists of mucous membrane similar to that of the appendix. The lining cells of the former, however, are markedly flattened.

"Diagnosis: Chronic appendicitis and pseudomyxomatous cyst of the appendix."

The primary operation, conducted by a very competent surgeon, evidently was limited to drainage of the abscess and disclosed no sign of pseudomucinous exudate; a mild type of chonic appendicitis, as the history indicates, followed this operation, and temperature, pain and increasing activity of the sinus denoted an acute exacerbation.

It would be interesting indeed to have undeniable evidence that the cyst represented in Fig. 1, had formed during the interval between the two operations. The nature of the sinus discharge, the contents of the peri-appendicular pocket, the local pseudomyxoma peritonei, and the pathologist's findings all indicate that the cyst was actively discharging its contents.

Recently published articles by Castle,[1] Phemister,[2] and E. G. Lewis,[3] have admirably presented the present-day knowledge of pseudomucinous cysts, and a repetition of the symptoms, etiology and pathology would be superfluous. There is no record of a preoperative diagnosis having been made.

The process of pseudomucinous cyst formation of the appendix is evidently slow. Two essential conditions are:

1. Gradual obliteration of a portion of the mucous tract by some agent.

2. Sterilization of the mucous lined tract distal to the obstruction.

The experiments conducted by Phemister and Dean Lewis, as well as our own observations, prove rather conclusively that any sudden blocking of the appendicular canal, even where care has been taken to avoid circulatory interference, results in gangrenous appendicitis.

The attempt to artificially produce such cysts will naturally fail until we can simulate in our experiments, the course followed by nature in the development of appendicitis obliterans, wherein the process is so slow that drainage into the cecum is not obstructed until the bacterial contents of the lumen are inactive.

While, theoretically, such a condition would be ideal for the formation of pseudomyxomatous cysts, we know the origin is not always so serene. In Case I of this report there existed distal to the cyst, 1 cm. of non-obliterated mucosa and a section of acutely inflamed mucosa between it and the valve of Gerlach. Fowler[4] reports a case with a cystic dilatation of the proximal end of the appendix. There is no doubt but that such cysts may develop in an appendix, gall-bladder or intestinal diverticulum that is subject to chronic inflammatory changes and it is also likely, as suggested by Phemister, that chonic hydrops or empyema of the appendix resulting from a proximal obliteration, may become sterile and displaced by the altered secretion and a pseudomucinous cyst result. Under normal conditions the secretion from the mucosa of the appendix is identical with that of the cecal mucosa, but the degeneration incident to the senile change which takes place in the isolated section, and the mucosal atrophy resulting from retention cyst pressure naturally alters the secretions, and the final contribution of the cell is pseudomucin.

Eden,[5] Wilson,[6] Rathe,[7] and the writer, each report a case of pseudomyxomatous appendix complicated by an ovarian cyst of large size. In all 4 cases, there had been a rupture of the ovarian cyst with resulting pseudomyxomata peritonei.

Author's case report is as follows:

CASE II.—Mrs. Mary E., Carrollton, Ill., aged fifty-two years; multipara.

Family History, negative.

Personal History. Usual diseases of childhood. Mother of several normal children. General health excellent until a few years ago, when she developed a right inguinal hernia and at about the same time a constant right inguinal tenderness. Severe back and pelvic pains were present at intervals. Gradual enlargement of the abdomen was noticed two years ago, with increasing bladder irritation and severe attacks of nausea which were controlled by relieving the obstinate constipation. Several weeks before coming to St. John's Hospital she suffered an acute pain in the pelvis. This was followed by general abdominal tenderness and her state of health declined rapidly until the present time.

Physical Examination. The patient is poorly nourished; appears to be sixty years of age. Skin sallow and lax, indicating considerable loss of flesh. Temperature and pulse normal. Heart, lungs, blood, feces and urine examinations, negative. Contour of abdomen normal except in right lower quadrant where a large inguinal hernia was present, and in left lower quadrant where a symmetrical enlargement extended across the median line. This was palpable as a softly resisting mass, regular in outline and evidently directed into the left pelvis. No distinctly tender points over abdomen except at McBurney's point, where a thickened mass, the size of an orange could be palpated.

Vaginal Examination. Relaxed outlet from old perineal tear. Bilateral laceration of cervix. Uterus normal size and freely movable, not attached to mass in left pelvic region. Cul-de-sac of Douglas filled with mass of doughy consistence. Right adnexa not palpable. Rectal examination, negative.

Operation. June 12, 1915. Ether anesthesia. Cervix and perineum repaired. Median incision revealed fundus of large tumor, leading down to site of left ovary. Posterior surface nodular but symmetrical, anterior surface broken just above its broad ligament attachment by a tear which admitted three fingers. The tumor was delivered quickly and with the left tube excised. The uterus and right adnexa were normal. The fluid contents of the tumor could easily, by light manipulation, be expelled through the rent in the sac, and had soiled the entire peritoneal cavity. In addition to the contents of the tumor, at least one liter was removed by hand from the pelvis and as much more by saline irrigation.

The small and large intestines, omentum, stomach, gallbladder and liver were covered with a glairy mucilaginous material, of varying thickness and the intestines resident in the lower half were agglutinated, and could be lifted from the pelvis *en masse.* These intestinal coils were gently separated to enable the saline to reach all parts of the cavity. On some loops of ileum, large masses the size of a pecan had attached themselves, but readily washed away. After persistent irrigation and gentle manipulation, the entire cavity was well cleansed, but the glairy coating on the visceral peritoneum could not be removed without severe trauma.

The cecum was elevated and an interesting appendix, (Fig. 2) removed. After noting that it was cystic, care was taken to observe that there was at the time no evidence of an active exudate from its lumen into the peritoneal cavity. There being no intra-abdominal complications at the hernial site, the abdomen was closed without drainage, leaving within about one liter of physiological saline.

The patient was sitting up in bed on the seventh day, and on the tenth day under local anesthesia, the hernia was repaired. The hernial sac had a capacity of about 40 c.c. and was entirely filled with pseudomucin, undisturbed by the abdominal irrigation.

She went home on July 11, thirty days from the date of entry.

Pathological Report (Dr. Ives). "Gross description: The specimen is a large appendix, 7 cm. long, in diameter fairly uniform. The greatest diameter is near the distal end where the measurement is 2.5 cm. The least diameter is near the centre where the measurement is 2 cm. The wall of the appendix is very thin, translucent, smooth and tense. Fluctuation is easily elicited. There is a small mass composed of gelatinous material attached to the surface near the tip. A platinum wire which was inserted into this mass passed into the lumen without resistance. This latter observation indicates that the wall had ruptured and that there had been an escape of contents.

"At the proximal end the appendix is constricted. Upon dissection it was determined that the lumen at this point was displaced by what appears to be dense fibrous tissue. The appendix is distended with gelatinous material. The latter varies somewhat in its appearance. Part of it is nearly transparent and part of it has a grayish appearance, due to a fine network. The microscopical differs in no way from Case I.

"Diagnosis: Ruptured pseudomucinous cyst of the appendix. The tumor is cystic and is apparently derived from an ovary. As some of the larger cysts had been ruptured and the contents had escaped, the exact dimensions of the tumor could not be determined, but its size was apparently about that of a man's head. The larger portion of the tumor is made up of a few large cysts, but there are many small cysts, some of which are minute.

"The surface of the tumor is smooth in parts and in other parts irregular. The latter condition is due to variations in the thickness of the fibrous tissue and to the presence of small cysts. The cyst wall is thin and the internal surface has practically the same appearance as the outer surface of the tumor.

"The cysts contain a clear, fairly thick, pale yellowish, gelatinous material. A small portion of the tumor consists of gelatinous material in a mesh-work of fibrous tissue without cyst formation.

"A Fallopian tube was removed with the tumor. This is normal in size. A portion of the peritoneum covering the tube and in its vicinity, is coated with gelatinous material.

"Diagnosis: Cystadenoma pseudomyxomatosum and pseudomyxomatous peritonitis."

Interesting features in this case are, the evidently primary involvement of both appendix and ovary (left); the mild display of symptoms accompanying the rupture of the ovarian cyst, and the complete dissemination over the peritoneal cavity and its contents following the liberation of pseudomucin. The fact that the patient still continues to improve in health, after ten month's time, encourages one to hope that with the removal of the primary feeding foci, nature, by the aid of a versatile peritoneum, will care for the remainder.

Unfortunately, the danger of malignancy is far greater in pseudomyxomata peritonei of ovarian origin, than from a cyst of the appendix. A determination of this distinction is beyond the intent of this report.

Enlightenment on the method of growth of pseudomyxomatous cysts, and so-called colloid ovarian cysts before rupture and after its departure from the mother-cyst and attachment to the peritoneal surface, would be a valuable contribution.

Is it due to proliferating epithelial cells, as found in colloid ovarian tumors, or is there possibly some organism to account for the growth that continues after dissemination?

From a case in the service of Drs. Brown and Engelbach at St. John's Hospital, the following observation was furnished by Dr. Ives.

"The specimen had been removed from a case of pseudomucinous peritonitis. Cultures were made from several of the tumor-like masses by spreading the gelatinous material over the surface of slant glucose-agar and Löffler's blood serum. In all of several tubes, a pure culture of yeast was obtained. The organisms occurred singly and united, several in a group. They were oval in shape. There were no thread forms as produced by the organism of blastomycosis on artificial media.

"The growth on agar spread over the surface; it had a dry appearance. The organism was anaërobic and fermented glucose with the production of gas."

Curtis,[8] also cites a case in which the yeast cell was observed in a pseudomucinous cyst of the appendix. There is no proof that the presence of yeast cells in these 2 cases was not purely accidental, but the demonstration justifies a more careful observation of such cysts in the future.

Ruptured ovarian cysts, of whatever character, are not without an element of serious danger, for in each such case there lies a potential malignancy. There is no record, to my knowledge, of true malignancy following a pseudomucinous cyst of the appendix, but from the plastic peritonitis and mechanical interference which follows such an extravasation, equally dangerous conditions may develop.

An early diagnosis would be of prime importance were it practical. Unless the disease has advanced to a stage where ascitic fluid can be drawn and pseudomucin found, an accurate diagnosis is hardly probable, for the symptoms differ in no way from those present in chronic appendicitis or ovarian tumor. Here again is demonstrated the value of early exploration in all obscure abdominal conditions, the logical result of a fair broad-minded coöperation between the internist and the surgeon.

REFERENCES

1. Castle. Annals of Surgery, May, 1915.
2. Phemister. Jour. Am. Med. Assn., May 29, 1915.
3. Lewis, E· G. Surg., Gyn. and Obs., 1914, xix.
4. Fowler. Treatise on Appendicitis, 1900, 95.
5. Eden. Lancet, 1912, ii, 1498.
6. Wilson. Lancet, 1912, ii, 1496.
7. Rathe. Monat. f. Geb. und Gyn., March, 1913.
8. Curtis. Ann. de l'Inst. Pasteur, 1896.

CONSERVATIVE PELVIC SURGERY: STATISTICS

By FLOYD W. McRAE, M.D., F.A.C.S.
Atlanta, Georgia

I AM sure that we are one in the opinion that marital felicity is the very foundation stone of our civilization; that intelligent propagation is the highest destiny of the race. Nature has decreed the perpetuation of the species at all hazards.

The influence of Battey, Tait and many others of the forceful early advocates of radical operations still permeates gynecological surgery. These great pioneers in this branch of surgery unwittingly put in operation practices that, in their cumulative destructive consequences, are simply appalling. Could we convoke in one great gathering the army of the marital unfit; could we flash upon the screen a grand panorama of the homes blighted, of the throngs of neurasthenics who fill the offices and sanatoria of the neurologists, treatment gynecologists, and general practitioners we should be shocked, I believe, into more consistent conservative pelvic surgery. We would then be willing in every case to take the time and pains necessary to preserve rather than remove ovaries, tubes, and uteri. It takes more time and patience to do conservative than it does to do radical surgery. The immediate results of conservative surgery are less satisfactory to both patient and surgeon than are the immediate results of radical operations. How different the picture presented after two, five, and ten years later. The first class are real wives, frequently happy mothers; the second class are unsexed creatures without interest in life—unhappy, devoid of the hope that makes life worth living to every woman.

Not all conservative operations are successful, nor are all radical operations surgical failures. But I have yet to see a young woman whose ovaries had been removed who, after several years, did not bemoan the day she fell under the knife of the destructive surgeon. All who consult me have only words of condemnation for the surgeon who did the work. I cannot believe that my experience is peculiar. These poor women are timid and reticent about their unhappy state, and one must be both tactful and sympathetic to draw them out.

I do not advocate attempts at conservation in late menstrual life, or after the menopause, when there is danger of malignancy. Conservatism here demands complete removal of all suspicious organs. In young women, however, the problems are quite different.

The real objects of gynecological surgery other than life-saving operations should be to fit women for wifehood, to preserve to them the possibilities of motherhood. Is it not worth, if need be, an extra half-hour of even the busiest surgeon's time? To me it seems abundantly to be.

Tuffier's results in ovarian transplantation have been very illuminating, but not sufficient to induce me to try his methods.

General peritonitis is an infrequent sequel of gonorrheal infection. Notwithstanding this fact, operations are advised and performed in the early stages of these specific pelvic inflammatory conditions and uteri, tubes, and ovaries ruthlessly sacrificed, thus sacrificing in large measure health and happiness. Many such cases get well without operation and subsequently bear children. Others may be relieved by simple vaginal puncture and drainage of abscesses.

B. Van Sweringen (*Conservation in Operations for Acute*

Inflammatory Pelvic Diseases): "It must be remembered that structures the seat of acute inflammation tend to more or less complete recovery. The edema disappears, the discharge lessens and finally disappears, and it is not every case that is left with the lumen of the tube strictured and occluded. Even in case they are so left, after the subsidence of the inflammation they may be inoffensive and symptomless. Ovaries which are found surrounded by exudate and adhesions may be liberated, the adhesions wiped off, retention cysts evacuated, and the ovary allowed to remain. Many of these will subsequently prove themselves capable of discharging ova.

"On the other hand, note the ultraconservative statements of Ashton (*Prac. Gyn.*, 513): 'The conservative modern treatment of infections, involving the uterine appendages and the pelvic structures, is a marked advance in the surgery of the female pelvis. The former practice of early operative interference in these cases not only was attended by a high mortality, but was also responsible for the unnecessary sacrifice of the organs of procreation. The treatment was based upon the following facts: That many patients recover their health, and the pelvic organs are spontaneously restored to a normal condition without the aid of operative measures.

"Ashton also says that even in the presence of gross lesions, as tubal or tuboövarian abscess, recovery has occurred, and he adds that this is especially true in septic infections which cause but little injury to the tubal mucosa, and very large pelvic exudates have been known to disappear in time without the aid of surgery.

"It is rather between these extremes that the author finds himself at this time, and does not recommend early operation in any pelvic infection. The danger is greater than if the body is allowed time to deal with the invading germ by establishing its own protecting mechanism.

"On the other hand, one should not allow a large pelvic

exudate or a tuboövarian abscess to remain until absorbed. That means chronic invalidism. But when once inside the abdomen for the purpose it is wrong to think that all pathology present must be removed by the knife. Ample provision for drainage and the ablation of the original focus will be sufficient and save many a tube and ovary which will result in much greater peace and happiness to the patient."

Wm. H. Humiston ("Conservative Operations on the Ovaries, Including a Report on 112 Cases," *Tr. Am. Assn. Obstr. and Gynec.*, 1912, xxv, 243) advocates conservative pelvic surgery, and reports 112 cases. Of this number 19 have given birth to 22 children. "If a similar percentage of pregnancies occurred in those patients not heard from it would increase the percentage to about 28. This, of course, is speculative and cannot be used. But in the 19 per cent. out of the 112 cases there is a showing, convincing to a judicial mind, that conservative operations are worthy of general adoption."

Dr. Albert Goldspohn, Chicago, discussing Dr. Humiston's paper, states: "The resection of ovaries is one of the best things that gynecologists do, that is, in the operations that are not for saving life. It is something that has interested me ever since August Martin, in Berlin, brought out his first publication on the subject. After that a surgeon in New York did the operation and published it. I was the next man who published anything on the subject west of New York. I have had many tussles in these years with men on that subject who, on account of a defective technic or bad judgment, had poor results. These were mostly general surgeons. What may be saved and what must be removed? They did not know, and they did not succeed; and others failed because they did not use the right technic. Furthermore, I have had tussles with visionary theorists who, by making a series of sections of some of these enlarged cystic follicles, would occasionally, not often, find a Graafian follicle in such cysts; and therefore this morbid physiology must overthrow and paralyze everything the gynecologist can do. They have said that it is a normal ovary; you must not touch it if it is six times its normal size, and it does not matter how much pain it may cause the patient. It is better to do nothing for her. There are that kind of men in the world. They do not succeed in gynecology, however."

Dr. Francis Reder, St. Louis, concurred in the conservative methods advocated and practised by Dr. Humiston, as did also Dr. Isidore Sanes, of Pittsburgh, and Dr. Hugo A. Pantzer, of Indianapolis, whose statements in reference to the number of pregnancies following these operations herewith quoted are well worthy of consideration: "The number of cases operated and followed by pregnancy that become known does not indicate the full percentage actually occurring. The full estimate of the gain by conservative methods should, moreover, include the cases not traceable after operation, and also cases that could conceive, but where conception is countermet by preventive measures. The latter class is large because of the fear of a pregnancy, and parturition is uncommonly heightened in the mind of those who have undergone operation for the relief of parturient injuries."

As shown by the above quotations from eminent gynecologists and surgeons, borne out by practically all the papers reported in the appended rather extensive comprehensive bibliography, it is made clear that gynecologists and surgeons are agreed on the principle of conservative pelvic surgery. Notwithstanding this, scores of ovaries, tubes, and uteri are being sacrificed daily by inexperienced and incompetent surgeons who operate early in the midst of acute pelvic infections, and who have not taken the time and trouble to study pelvic pathology and prepare themselves to do conservative work. I see a great many of these poor patients recently operated upon, or being operated on, in the various sanatoriums and hospitals in Atlanta. Many of them consult me afterward.

I have done conservative operations on 338 women. Of this number I have been able to get reports to date from only 191 (59 unmarried), 47 of whom have reported pregnancies. Practically all have gone to full term and been delivered of healthy children. One woman has had three children, another two, another has had three or more induced abortions. Another was delivered of a living child by Cesarean section on account of uremic convulsions. Both mother and child are now in good health. I have written the 198 cases that I have not kept in touch with, and hope to receive definite information from many of them to incorporate in this paper before publication. Of the 338 women, 17 have had subsequent operations done by me or other surgeons. I have only included in this record the women whose pelvic organs were left in a state compatible with possible future pregnancies. I do not include individuals whose tubes or uteri were removed or where partial hysterectomies were performed precluding pregnancy.

In my work I have resected cystic ovaries, preserving all healthy stroma, suturing accurately with fine catgut. I have endeavored to so separate adhesions, embedded ovaries, and tubes as to leave the least possible area of raw surface; hanging up prolapsed ovaries, plicating the ligaments, so readjusting uterus, tubes and ovaries as to approach as nearly as possible the normal arrangement. A very large majority of these women have been relieved of their suffering and restored to all the privileges and enjoyments of healthful womanhood.

I have brought this subject to you for discussion in the hope that you would place the stamp of your disapproval upon this class of surgery in such a forceful way as to call a halt and save innocent women from surgical destructionists.

Ovarian operations, 338 (191 followed up, 59 unmarried). Of the 191 heard from to date, 47 have been pregnant, some several times;-147 lost track of.

	Total.	Pregnancies
Both ovaries resected	120	11
One ovary and tube removed	75	10
One ovary removed, one resection . . .	20	5
One ovary resected	98	12
Ovary and tube removed, ovary and tube resected	6	1
One tube removed, one resected	2	1
Ovary removed, tube resected	11	4
Prolapsed tube, ovary and uterus suspended	5	2
Ovary removed, tube resected, myomectomy	2	1
	339	47

BIBLIOGRAPHY

Beyea, H. D. The Preservation of the Physiological Functions in the Treatment of Gynecological Diseases, Penna. Med. Jour., 1913–14, xvii, 655.

Prof. Beuttner (Geneva). The Transverse Cuneiform Excision of the Fundus Uteri as First Stage to the Extirpation of Bilateral Chronically Diseased Appendages, with Conservation of the Menstrual Function, Tr. Internat. Cong. Med., London, 1913–14, Obst. and Gyn. Sect., 131.

Vanverts, J. Conservative Surgery in Ovarian Cysts, Arch. mens. d'obstr. et gynec., Paris, 1913, iv, 359.

Jacobs. Some Observations on the Remote Results of Conservative Operations on the Adnexa, Bull. Soc. Gynec. et d'Obstet., Bruxelles, 1913, xxiv, 337.

Furber, E. P. A Plea for More Conservative Treatment of Uterine Appendages, Lancet, London, 1914, ii, 1273.

De Tarnowsky, G. Tubal Implantation, a New Conservative Operation for Sterilization of Women, Jour. Am. Med. Assn., 1913, lx, 1221.

Price, John W. Conservatism in Pelvic Surgery, Pediatrics, 1914, xxvi, 305.

McGehee, J. L. Conservative Operations on the Uterine Appendages, with Two Instances of Transmigration of the Ovum, Memphis Medical Monthly, 1913, xxxiii, 50.

Bonnard, L. Conservative Operations in Tuberculous Adnexa, Thèse, Paris, 1913.

McGlinn, J. A. Can Surgery be Eliminated in the Treatment of Fibroid Tumors of the Uterus? Gynec. Trans., 1914, xxxix, 165.

Van Sweringen, B. Conservation in Operations for Acute Inflammatory Pelvic Disease, Amer. Jour. Obst., 1913, lxviii, 872.

Falgowski. Ueber die Konservative Tendenz beider Operation des Uterus Myoms, Gynäk. Rundschau, 1914, viii, 351–354.

Bauer, B. A. Zur Konservativen Therapie der Adnexer Krankungen, Deutsch. med. Wchnschr., 1914, xl, 2069–2071.

Pilcher, L. S. The *I*mportance of Conserving a *P*ortion of the Ovary, Long Island Med. Jour., Brooklyn, 1913, vii, 426–430 (Discussion), 446–449.

Stone, I. S. The Conservative Treatment of Salpingitis by Uterine and Tubal Injections, Jour. Am. Med. Assn., 1913, lx, 656.

DISCUSSION

DR. ROBERT T. MORRIS, New York City.—During the past year I have tried to introduce a new idea experimentally in conservative surgery. If we call this (indicating) the uterus and these tubes (indicating), the tubes are removed, and the ovaries allowed to remain. In some cases you will find a little of the fimbriæ remaining. These have a separate secretion of their o'wn. If you cut off a bit of this fimbriated part and spread it out and graft a bit of the fimbriated extremity to the cornu of the uterus it may keep the lumen permanently.

DR. J. WESLEY BOVÉE, Washington, D. C.—I congratulate Dr. McRae upon the results which he calls successes, but I am sorry to say that I cannot duplicate them in my own work. I have become discouraged over conservative surgery; I have gotten to believe that conservative surgery lies in the direction of removal of diseased tissue. After having done a third and even fourth operation for the purpose of trying to conserve tissues, I have become very much demoralized. Tubal pregnancies have resulted in my conservative surgery on the tubes, and I have many cases in comparatively young women where I have had to do radical work after failure from attempts to preserve tubes and ovaries. I do not see the logic in the deduction of Dr. McRae that those women who have had secondary operations would probably have had secondary operations if they had radical operations at first. If we knew what these secondary operations were we might more definitely estimate the probability of secondary operations being called for.

I do not see the great distress of these patients mentioned by Dr. McRae following radical surgery, and I am not pleased with the work I do in resection of cystic ovaries. Many of these cases that I see after operation I find have adhesions along the line of suturing, in spite of the fact that I am trying to prevent them at the time of operation, and I use the galvano-cautery instead of sutures, so that while I desire to save the organs of these women, I have not the happy results that he has.

He has doubtless brought this subject before us with the hope that in the future we will do more conservative work. So far as the kind of surgery mentioned by him being done by incompetent men, I am in accord with his position; but if he comes to us and says we must condemn the larger part of the radical surgery done on the female reproductive organs by competent gynecologists, then I will have to disagree with him.

DR. ROBERT S. HILL, Montgomery, Alabama.—Generally speaking, I, like Dr. Bovée, have become somewhat discouraged in my efforts to do conservative surgery on the ovaries and tubes; on the other hand, I quite agree with Dr. McRae that these structures should not be needlessly sacrificed, and I am constrained to believe there are many needless operations done upon them. To my mind, if we are to serve the best interest of our patient, we must consider, in reaching a decision as to the extent of the operation to be done or the degree of conservatism to be adopted, individual conditions and environments. In a young woman without a family I would certainly carry my conservatism further than in an older woman with a family; and in a woman of the laboring class whose circumstances demand a quick return to her duties, I would be inclined to be more radical than in a woman whose pecuniary conditions relieve her of the necessity of personal effort.

There is another element that must be considered and that is the attitude of the family doctor toward the operative necessities. In the management of this class of patients we not infrequently have to reckon with a psychic condition brought about no more by the diseased organs than by the frequent and positive assurances of the family doctor, in whom the patient has every confidence that nothing less than a radical operation will give her relief. Now, if we cannot change the radical attitude of the doctor who is to care for the patient after she leaves the hospital, the cause of the psychic condition will not be fully removed and our conservative operation will very probably prove disappointing; the patient continuing the life of an invalid as long as she is under the care of that doctor, or until the radical operation is done. You may say we should be able to control the general practitioner in surgical matters. As a rule they will yield to our opinion, but not always.

Right here I want to refer to a case bearing upon this point and that shows how strong sometimes is the harmful influences that I am talking about. A woman was brought more than a hundred miles to the hospital. She came to have her ovaries removed, as her trouble had been diagnosed as ovarian disease. She was confined to her bed because of weakness from inability to retain nourishment. Her real condition was nausea from pregnancy. Her improvement was rapid, and in a short while she was up and going about. The change of environment, probably more than anything else, brought about the improvement. She returned home cheerful and happy. Her doctor called to see her and assured her that her improvement could only be temporary, as the diseased ovaries had not been removed, and insisted that, as we would not do the operation, that she permit him to do it. After two or three weeks of this harmful influence she allowed him to remove her ovaries, had a miscarriage and just did escape with her life.

I may also mention another case, the wife of a doctor from the northern part of the State. The husband made a diagnosis of cancer of the womb, and I could never get him away from his diagnosis, notwithstanding a satisfactory repair of the lacerated cervix. He returned home and she improved. In time she returned home to be greeted with an expressed fear by her husband that she had not been relieved. In about six months she came back to me much alarmed because "her husband had discovered a return of the disease." Examination revealed nothing, and after a week or ten days' assurances that she was all right she went home happy, only to have her happiness clouded by the inexplicable conduct of her husband, who had said "the horse was ten feet high" and wouldn't have it anything else. In time he took her to the late Dr. Douglass, of Nashville, but failing to find the cancer there he returned home. This poor woman spent two or three years, made miserable by fear and apprehension, coming every few months to me to receive assurances that she was cancer-free. Her husband dying several years ago, she is now in good health, enjoying life and has not felt it necessary to be examined by me since his death.

I am sure I did the right thing in each of these cases, yet I did not relieve either of them, because the trouble of each was a psychic condition brought about chiefly through the unchangeable, radical, surgical attitude of their respective attending physicians.

While, of course, I could never advocate an operation where no operation was needed simply because someone else thought it indicated, yet, if there is a diseased condition of the ovaries and tubes calling for operative intervention, I am convinced the interest of the patient would be better served by the surgeon's being a little radical, if he cannot bring the family doctor around to a proper coöperation in conservatism. We may indulge to our heart's content in well-rounded sentences expressive of beautiful and lofty sentiments of the surgeon's absolute responsibility and obligation to act independent of all influences save that of a consciousness of a correct and proper knowledge of the science and art of surgery; yet, I tell you our daily observation and experience forces upon us a recognition of the fact that the best interest of our patients is subserved only by a hearty "Yea," and an enthusiastic coöperation between the surgeon and family doctor. This being true, I say again, in deciding upon the degree of conservatism to be adopted, we must reckon with the attitude of the family physician.

DR. CHARLES M. ROSSER, Dallas, Texas.—No matter whether we are surgeons, scientists, or sociologists, or whether we are dealing with a proposition from the standpoint of the surgeon or family or individual patient, if the surgeon is going to operate with the idea of affording relief from complaints, he must do as radical work as he thinks necessary to begin with, and if he does so there is less likelihood of the patient complaining afterward. If radical work is not undertaken at first, many of these patients may have to submit to secondary operations sooner or later. Our idea should be about like this, that the least radical work should be done which promises rational and reasonable hope for relief, knowing we can always do a secondary operation, if necessary. If everything has been sacrificed in the beginning and the patient still complains we have nothing further to do.

Our ideas have come to us because we have not evolved our intellectuality along with our scientific successes. When the abdomen was hazardous to invade, the surgeon said, "I must do everything while I am in here, because I may never come back again." In our operative work we should strive to remove only those pathological conditions which will relieve patients of their distress and suffering. No surgeon would think of performing a high amputation when a low one would be sufficient.

No oculist would take out an eye if he thought he could afford the patient relief by non-operative measures. I think we should become idealists as scientists along with our sociological endeavors. I believe we should do just as little to a patient as we have hope of relief, knowing we can take care of the condition subsequently if we must.

DR. CHARLES R. ROBINS, Richmond, Virginia.—I am sure all of us are in favor of conservative pelvic surgery. The effects of radical surgery give us very definite ideas, and the only question I want to bring up is that in using the word conservative, what do we mean by conservative pelvic surgery? My own practice has been to conserve the menstrual cycle. That is what I always aim to do in a pelvic case in a young woman. I think all of us endeavor to preserve the menstrual cycle. We try to preserve the uterus and ovaries wherever it is possible to do so. If conservatism applies to the bearing of children, I would like to inquire from Dr. McRae what form of operation or treatment he applies to the tube in order that pregnancy may take place? I have been unable myself to do any operation on the tube that would permit of subsequent pregnancy. If we resect the tubes, I believe in the vast majority of cases they close over again, and the question is simply one of whether we are going to leave the tube alone or take it out. If we separate adhesions around the fimbriated extremity, nature can take care of the inflamed tube better than the surgeon can. As I have said, I would like to inquire what form of operation Dr. McRae does upon the tube in order to enable the woman to have children subsequently. I do not find in my own practice that operating on women so that they may have children is such a desideratum. A great many women come to me and ask to be "fixed" so they cannot have children. Now and then, I have a woman who comes to me who wants to have children. I have had this rather unique experience: I had one patient who came to my office and said, "Doctor, I have been married eleven years and I have become pregnant; is there anything you can do for me?" Such cases are hopeless. I cannot find a thing in the world the matter with them. Another patient came to my office, sat down in a chair, and began to cry. The first one cried, and the patient who followed her began to weep also, and I said. "What is the matter with you?" She replied "Doctor, I am afraid I ————."

DR. THOMAS S. CULLEN, Baltimore, Maryland.—In a dispensary experience extending over several years my views on conservatism became thoroughly crystallized. If we make a long incision, carefully pack the intestine off and get good exposure we can then usually dissect the pelvic structures free under sight instead of pulling or dragging them. Furthermore, if in suturing we use a very fine needle and fine catgut and employ continuous suture where possible we can accomplish a great deal. In any case where a slight infection might possibly exist a small pelvic drain brought out through the vagina is a great advantage. I think conservatism is here to stay.

DR. FLOYD W. McRAE, Atlanta, Georgia (closing).—The discussion has taken much the line I expected it to. The question of surgical judgment and wishes of the patient should be considered of very vital importance. However, surgical judgment varies with surgeons. Dr. Bovée would do radical surgery in cases in which I would possibly resort to more conservative measures. I feel that I can save structures that he would remove. I believe in removing palpably diseased structures that we have no reasonable hope will approach to an ultimately normal state after an operation. The women must be entirely different in the section of the country where Dr. Bovée operates from those in that part of the country where I operate, if he sees none of the distressing conditions following radical operations. I see these cases over and over again. I have seen them five, ten years after operation when you could not introduce a finger into the vagina, making the slighest attempt at an examination without causing bleeding and the most intense distress. I have had Dr. Sawyer, our leading lady gynecologist, keep track of a large series of cases. She sees more of these women than I do, and all of them have deplored the fact of having had a radical operation done. The neurologists and general practitioners in Atlanta have had the same experience with this class of patients. Personally, if I had a daughter who required operation, particularly in these days of clean surgery, I would rather have her operated on two or three times, if necessary, than to have her ovaries and uterus removed at the primary operation, thus removing everything that makes a woman and her life worth while. I don't mean simply bearing children. When you unsex a woman, she is no longer a real woman. Follow your cases for a few years after you have removed everything.

We need to consider the internal secretion as it is worth while.

As to Dr. Hill's case, we ought not to allow any family physician to induce us to do what we ought not do. Dr. Hill was right in not operating on that woman. If the family doctor took out her ovaries, he did so on his own responsibility, and not Dr. Hill's. I think most surgeons are willing and expect to shoulder their own responsibility.

With reference to the remarks made by Dr. Rosser, while we consider ourselves operators and scientists, yet we must likewise consider the sociological and psychic features of the conditions we have to contend with. When we do so, we will find ourselves saving more and more tissue; we will be doing more and more conservative work on the pelvic organs of women.

I want to leave the thought with you that there is the possibility of a future operation in connection with these cases, but we should leave them normal individuals as long as we possibly can. All of us may need operations. I have been put under anesthetics eleven times myself for operations, but I have not had any of my useful organs removed, and I do not regret the operations I have had done.

In answer to Dr. Robins's question, I have had absolutely no success in resecting large pus tubes and in trying to save pieces of them.

With reference to the breaking up of adhesions, Dr. Cullen has said that by breaking up adhesions and dissecting them off we open up the tubes; we will find the fimbriæ hugging the ovary and completely sealed. Oftentimes the ovaries are enlarged and cystic, and you can remove a portion of the ovary, cover over the raw surface, after breaking up adhesions, with fine needle and fine catgut, avoiding trauma and excessive manipulation.

As to the question of whether a woman shall have children or not, is not one for the doctor to decide. We have no right to say that this woman may have children, and that woman shall not have children, simply because she does or does not want them. That is not our responsibility. If we advise her that she cannot have children, then the responsibility is ours, and it is serious. But if she does not want to have children, in spite of our advice to have her live a normal life, and she does not have children, that is her responsibility. Most of this class of women will sooner or later need a surgeon, because they go along and do various things to prevent themselves from having children.

I am very much concerned about this question because I see these distressing cases over and over again. I am quite sure that most experienced surgeons and gynecologists would handle the same class of cases in much the same way. Dr. Cullen's experience and practice are almost indentical with mine. Finally we need to sound a warning to stay the hand of the embryo gynecologist, of the inexperienced surgeon.

FRACTURE OF THE NECK OF THE FEMUR

A STUDY OF THE TREATMENT AND END RESULTS IN FIFTY–FIVE CASES

By Alexius McGlannan, M.D.

Baltimore, Md.

The system of arches formed by the bone plates in the cancellous tissue of the neck of the femur makes an ideal arrangement for lightness of construction with a maximum of weight-bearing capacity. The interaction of the arches one on another is necessary for carrying the weight of the body and the strain of its movements in the erect posture. When the neck of the femur is broken, this mutual relation is disrupted and unless the arches are restored, in the process of healing, either neck will bend at the site of union of the fragments, or a greatly increased mass of bone must be formed to provide rigidity. Either alternative results in a permanent deformity.

Accurate apposition of the fragments therefore, becomes an essential in the treatment of this fracture, and sufficient time must be allowed for complete bone regeneration before weight is put on the united fracture if deformity is to be avoided.

The position of the separated fragments in the fracture is as follows: The shaft fragment is drawn up above and behind the head fragment, the trochanter is rotated backward carrying the foot into eversion, the lower end of the femur is drawn toward the middle line by the adductors.

The head remains fixed in the acetabulum and the broken end of this fragment is directed upward and slightly forward.

Practically always some portion of the periosteum remains attached to both fragments and when the fracture is in a suitable position on the neck a portion of the capsular ligament is likely to bridge the separation of the bone.

The positions described give the general direction of the fragments, the relative positions of which vary in degree with the seat of the fracture. Several classifications have been advised to separate these fractures into groups according to the position of the break. Kocher's classification into subcapital, fracture at the junction of the head and neck, intertrochanteric, along the line between the trochanters, and pertrochanteric, obliquely through the trochanters is used in our hospital records.

The blood supply of the neck of the femur is peculiar and the effect of a fracture on the circulation of the head fragment is an important factor in the healing of this lesion.

Lexer's study of the circulation in bones (*Archiv f. klin. Chirurg.*, 1904, lxxiii, 481) shows that the blood supply to the neck of the femur enters from four points. One, an epiphyseal artery at the insertion of the ligamentum teres, a second just at the line of junction of the head and neck on the upper surface, a third near the great trochanter, and a fourth, the largest of the group, a metaphyseal artery near the lesser trochanter. Lexer states that the blood supply is greatest in childhood, and that in adult life the most marked change is seen in the diaphyseal group of arteries supplying the shaft, which becomes smaller and smaller with advancing age. The narrowing of the other two groups in the region of the epiphysis is less distinct, while the arterial supply of the joint apparatus becomes much more marked.

All these arteries reach the bone by way of the periosteum and the capsule. The importance of any attached and untorn area of these membranes is at once apparent. The fracture must have a profound effect on the circulation of the head fragment, because whenever this fragment is exposed at operation for nonunion, the blood supply is diminished in proportion as the seat of fracture approaches the subcapital type.

Here again accurate approximation offers the best chance for good union, diminishing the need for new bone formation, and giving the best opportunity for improvement of the local circulation.

Reduction of this fracture is accomplished by downward traction, and internal rotation of the femur with the limb slightly flexed and widely abducted. The method of reduction and of fixation varies, with several authorities, but the essential principle is expressed above and has for its object the complete correction of the deformity caused by the position of the fragments.

Bardenhauer obtains gradual reduction by weight traction acting simultaneously in several directions. Slightly modified, this is the method of Maxwell and Ruth. Whitman reduces the fracture by manipulation under anesthesia, using the completely abducted sound hip as a lever for fixing the pelvis. While forcibly carrying the fractured limb to the limit of abduction he presses down on the trochanter and at the same time lifts it forward, so as to overcome the external rotation. Both hips are slightly flexed in wide abduction and a plaster cast is applied from the toes to the nipple line on the injured side and a short distance on the sound side in order to securely fix the pelvis. A pad is placed behind the trochanter to support it and thus secure inward rotation.

Much criticism has been made of Whitman's forced abduction and the method has been condemned on the ground that the wide abduction is not required for all types of these fractures and that overabduction would lead to malposition of the fragments. We have demonstrated at operation, with the fracture open, and on a postmortem specimen, that abduction is essential to apposition and that after this point has been reached further abduction does not disarrange the fragments, because the taut capsule and other soft parts carry both fragments together to the limit of movement. This is an important point, because while it is almost impossible to calculate the exact degree of abduction that will give the best apposition in any particular fracture, the knowledge that complete abduction will surely carry the fragments out together gives us a definite position in which to fix the injured limb.

Impaction is most often a penetration with crushing and little fixation. Except in the rarest of cases the bones are driven into one another with adduction of the limb. Union in this position therefore gives great deformity and is the cause of most of the disability incident to fracture of the neck of the femur. There is no doubt of this being the case in those individuals who are incapacitated although their fracture has united. Therefore impaction should be broken up by a gentle hingelike motion and the fragments be brought into apposition in abduction whenever there is hope of treating the patient.

The cases[1] now being reported were all treated on this general plan, but with several modifications of the details both as to reduction and fixation. The modifications may be grouped into six classes, and in this way the cases will be reported.

CLASS A. Reduction under anesthesia, fixation in abduction by means of lateral wire splints and interrupted plaster bandages.

[1] This paper is based on a study of 55 cases of fracture of the neck of the femur observed in St. Agnes' and Mercy Hospitals, Baltimore. Of the former group 10 were under the care of Dr. Bloodgood or were put up by the resident surgeons, all, however, at some time in the course of their treatment, came under my personal observation. Of the latter group, those cases occurring previous to 1913 were treated by me as associate surgeon on the service of Dr. C. F. Bevan. The later cases came to me when I succeeded him as chief of this service.

Two mattresses are placed on the bed over a special frame of slats to give rigidity. This frame should extend beyond the bed on either side, or a single bar about six feet long may be placed transversely to the long axis of the bed near the foot. To this the legs are bandaged to keep up the abduction. A bar placed between the knees fulfils the same purpose.

The first dressing is removed at the end of two weeks and subsequent dressings are made weekly. The knee on the sound side is left free at the end of two weeks, the sound leg at six weeks. In from seven to ten weeks all dressings are removed and the patient kept on crutches for at least three months longer.

This was our original fixation. In this way we treated 5 cases; 3 women and 2 men.

CLASS B. Reduction under anesthesia, fixation in heavy plaster of Paris cast extending from toe to nipple line on the fractured side and taking in the sound thigh for a short distance.

Twenty patients were treated by this method; 10 women, 9 men, and 1 boy sixteen years of age.

CLASS C. Adhesive plaster traction in two directions (abduction and inward rotation). Two patients were treated by this method; both fat women, severely handicapped.

CLASS D. Direct traction by means of ice tongs. This method was suggested to me by Dr. Ransohoff at the meeting of this Association two years ago. It has been used in three cases. In one case an impaction was separated under anesthesia preliminary to the traction. The ice tongs are clamped into the femur through a small wound on either side just above the condyles, and are held in place by a sterile roll of gauze which, winding around the thigh and the blades of the tongs, makes the dressing for the wounds. The traction cord is attached to the outer handle only and in this way the pull of the weight rotates the femur inward, in which direction it is assisted by a pad under the trochanter. The

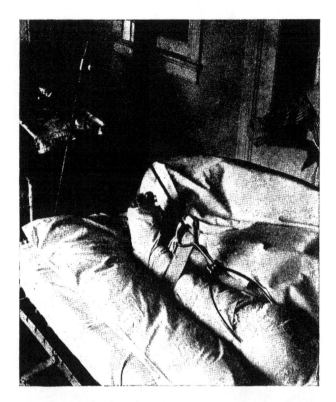

FIG. 1.—Ice-tongs extension. Shows the bandaged leg, and the ice-tongs covered in by the gauze dressing. The small board between the handles assists in maintaining inward rotation.

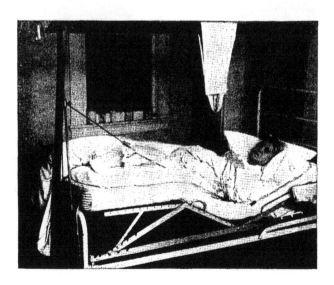

FIG. 2.—Ice-tongs extension. Shows the position of the patient on the Gatch bed, and the overhead beam with its soft bandage, by means of which the patient shifts her position (Case 29).

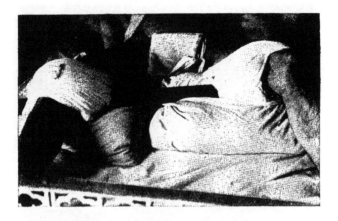

F<small>IG</small>. 3.—Tying out. Showing both knees made fast to the board spreader, after abduction. Fracture on the left side. The spreader also prevents rotation of the bandaged thighs.

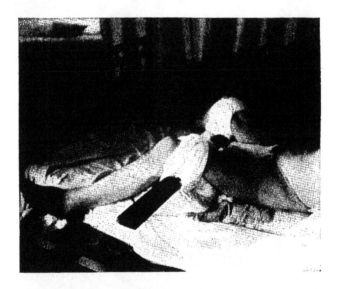

F<small>IG</small>. 4.—Tying out. View from the side. Note the sand-bag under the trochanter, correcting the outward rotation of the femur. The position of the foot is due to eversion below the knee. The cords fixing the spreader to the bed rail, and the pillows on the outrigger, under the foot, have been removed in order to make the picture clearer. (Photographs by Dr. E. I. Bartlett.)

patient is put on a Gatch bed, with the leg piece made horizontal and the foot of the bed is kept elevated, so that the upper portion of the body makes counterextension, even when the patient sits up in bed.

CLASS E. Nailing the fragments.

In one case of recent fracture we did an open operation, exposing the fracture, and fixing the fragments by means of a nail driven through the trochanter. In a second case a long drill was inserted through a small wound over the trochanter, and after the usual manipulations had been made, was driven through the reduced fragments into the head of the bone.

CLASS F. Loose fixation by tying out the knees to the bed rail.

The patient is put on a Gatch bed in a sitting position with a pillow behind the sacrum and the shoulders. The middle section of the bed is lifted so that the knees and hips are flexed to about 30 degrees and the foot section is raised so that it is nearly horizontal. A soft rope attached to an overhead beam, allows the patient to move about by grasping it in both hands.

A covered felt pad is fastened by adhesive plaster under the trochanter of the fractured side. The sound leg is abducted fully and is made fast to the side of the bed by a roll of gauze folded to make a soft bandage, which is first wrapped around the thigh above the condyles, just tight enough to avoid constriction. The thigh of the injured side is now rotated in and abducted as far as possible, and is then tied out as described. The foot of the bed is elevated, and the pillows are removed from behind the sacrum and the shoulders. As the weight of the trunk pulls away from the tied-out thighs, traction is made which gradually overcomes the shortening, and as the adductor muscles tire the abduction may be increased until finally after a few days both limbs are fully abducted. If the patient's general condition will permit, the reduction is done under general anesthesia and the limbs tied out in complete abduction at once.

RECENT FRACTURES

Number	Date of injury.	Age.	Sex.	Occupation.	Position of fracture.	Fixation.	Anesthetic.	Immediate result.	Time in bed.	Period of complete disability.	Period of partial disability.
1	Mar. 1907	67	M.	Hotel mgr.	Intertrochanteric	A	Ether	Union	63 days	77 days	3 months
2	Aug., 1907	71	F.	Religeuse	Subcapital	A	Ether	Union	70 "	154 "	4 months
3	Sept., 1907	65	F.	Housewife	Subcapital	A	Ether	Union	77 "	9 months	6 months
4	July, 1908	71	M.	Restaurateur	Impacted intertrochanteric	A	Ether	Union	70 "	130 days	4 months
5	Mar., 1909	68	F.	Cook	Intertrochanteric	A	None	Union	65 "	70 days +	
6	Jan., 1907	55	M.	Farmer	Impacted intertrochanteric	B	Chloroform	Union	63 "	154 days	3 months
7	Feb., 1908	16	M.	School-boy	Subcapital	B	Ether	Union	63 "	240 days	3 months
8	Jan., 1909	72	M.	Retired	Pertrochanteric	B	Ether	Union	89 "	243 days	1 year
9	Oct., 1909	74	F.	Housewife	Intertrochanteric	B	Chloroform	Union	65 "	80 days	3 months
10	Aug., 1910	46	M.	Motorman	Intertrochanteric	B	Chloroform	Union	78 "	117 days	4 months
11	Jan., 1911	59	F.	Housewife	Intertrochanteric	B	Ether	Union	72 "	7 days +	
12	July, 1911	49	F.	Housewife	Impacted intertrochanteric	B	Ether	Union	62 "		1 year +
13	Dec., 1911	60	F.	Housewife	Intertrochanteric	B	Ether	Union	80 "	1 year	4 months
14	Feb., 1912	50	F.	Housemaid	Impacted intertrochanteric	B	Ether	Union	70 "	115 days	5 months
15	May, 1912	60	F.	Seamstress	Impacted intertrochanteric	B	Ether	Union	64 "	80 days	7 months
16	Jan., 1912	45	M.	Tailor	Impacted subcapital	B	Gas	Union	60 "	95 days	
17	Feb., 1912	57	M.	Laborer	Intertrochanteric	B	Ether	Union	68 "	50 days +	
18	Feb., 1913	46	F.	Housewife	Intertrochanteric	B	Ether	Union	72 "		2 months
19	July, 1913	60	M.	Butcher	Intertrochanteric	B	Ether	Union	49 "	104 days	3 months
20	July, 1913	43	M.	Laborer	Pertrochanteric	B	Ether	Union	56 "	54 days	
21	Dec., 1914	42	M.	Laborer	Pertrochanteric	B	Ether	Union	42 "		4 months +
22	Nov., 1914	?	M.	Laborer	Pertrochanteric	B	Ether	Union	Not given		
23	Mar., 1915	65	F.	Housewife	Intertrochanteric	B	Gas	Union	42 "	111 days	
24	Sept., 1914	60	F.	Housewife	Intertrochanteric	B	Gas	Union	70 "	180 days	
25	Jan., 1908	71	F.	Housewife	Subcapital	C	Chloroform	Died	16 "		
26	June, 1913	70	F.	Housewife	Intertrochanteric	C	None	Non-union	59 "	2 years	1 year
27	Nov., 1913	72	F.	None	Intertrochanteric	D	Novocaine	Union	72 "	110 days	
28	May, 1914	76	F.	None	Impacted intertrochanteric	D	Gas	Died	92 "	not calculated	
29	Dec., 1914	69	F.	Nurse	Impacted intertrochanteric	D	Gas	Union	52 "		
30	Feb., 1915	60	F.	Housewife	Subcapital	D	Ether	Died	29 "	6 months	
31	Oct., 1909	56	F.	Housewife	Intertrochanteric	E	Gas	Died	80 "		1 year
32	Mar., 1915	56	M.	Hotel Mgr.	Intertrochanteric	E	Gas	Union	14 "		
33	Mar., 1915	60	M.	Market driver	Intertrochanteric	F	None	Union	50 "	52 days	7 weeks
34	June, 1915	70	M.	Driver	Impacted intertrochanteric	F	None	Union	48 "	4 months +	
35	Sept., 1915	69	F.	Housewife	Intertrochanteric	F	None	Union	38 "	1 month +	
36	Nov., 1915	71	M.	Farmer	Intertrochanteric	F	None	Union			

RECENT FRACTURES (CONTINUED)

Number.	Complication or handicap at time of injury.	Ultimate result, December, 1915.	Percentage of former wages earned after recovery.	Extent of permanent disability due to fracture.
1	None	Died 1913	100%	None
2	None	Living, well and active	Not affected	Slight stiffness of hip
3	None	Living, well and active	Not affected	1 c.m. measured shortening
4	Syphilis, arteriosclerosis	Died 1911	75%	1 c.m. measured shortening
5	Alcoholism	Lost after discharge from hospital		No note
6	None	Well and active	100%	2 c.m. measured shortening
7	None	Died 1912, pneumonia	Not affected	None
8	Chronic nephritis	Well and active	Not affected	None
9	Colles fracture	Died 1912	Not affected	None
10	Fracture clavicle and ribs	Wears rubber heel for shortening, Occasional pain	70%	2 c.m. short, limited motion
11	None	Lost after discharge from hospital		No note
12	None	Lost after discharge from hospital		No note
13	Fat and flabby, pressure ulcer	Well and active	Not affected	1 c.m. shortening, stiffness & edema
14	Pulmonary tuberculosis arrested	Well and active	100%	None
15	None	Well and active	100%	1½ c.m. shortening
16	None	Active, leg well abducted, no limp	80%	None
17	None	Lost after discharge from hospital		3 c.m. measured shortening
18	None	Lost after discharge from hospital		
19	Fracture of other hip, healed in adduction	On crutches because of old fracture	100%	None
20	None	Well and active	90%	None
21	None	Well and active		None
22	None	Lost after discharge from hospital	Not affected	
23	Arteriosclerosis	Walks on a cane, pain and stiffness		Stiffness of the hip
24	Mitral insufficiency	Died June, 1915, heart disease		Pain, helplessness
25	Alcoholism, nephritis, loss of control of bladder and rectum	Died three days after fixation, uremia	Not affected	
26	Chronic alcoholism	Died fifty-eight days, nephritis		
27	Left hemiplegia, incontinence of urine	Unable to walk or otherwise help herself		Total helplessness
28	Phlebitis and edema, ulcer of heel	Walks on a cane, has pain and edema		3 c.m. short, edema
29	Fracture tibia and fibula three months after discharge	On crutches because of complication		
30	Alcohol and drug addiction	Died twenty-nine days, uremia		
31	Obesity	Walks without apparatus, no shortening, stiffness of hip		
32	Fracture clavicle, B. P. 170, rales in chest	Died four days after operation of pulmonary edema		Rigid hip
33	Varicose veins, thrombophlebitis, ext. poplit. neuritis	Slight foot drop, limitation of hip movements		
34	Chronic interstitial nephritis	No pain or swelling, still on crutches	50%	
35	Fracture impacted in abduction	On crutches, no pain		None
36		Patient still under treatment		

OLD FRACTURES

Number.	Age of fracture.	Age of pt.	Sex.	Occupation.	Position of fracture.	Fixation.	Anesthesia.	Immediate result.	Time in bed.	Period of complete disability.	Period of partial disability.
37	1½ years	65	F.	Housekeeper	Subcapital	A	Ether	Firm hip	70 days	56 days	4 months
38	17 years	38	M.	Blacksmith	Subcapital	B	Ether	Abduction	42 days	3 months	4 months
39	3 years	52	M.	Carpenter	Intertrochanteric	B	Ether	Abduction, movable hip	91 days	4 months	4 months
40	2½ years	52	F.	Storekeeper	Subcapital	B	Ether	Abduction, fixed hip	45 days		
41	16 months	27	M.	Laborer	Commun. intertrochanteric	B	Ether	Non-union	70 days		
42	10 months	37	M.	Driver	Intertrochanteric	F	Ether	Union	48 days	2½ months	3 months
43	8 months	40	M.	Sailor	Subcapital	F	Gas and ether	Union	79 days	3 months	2 months

CASES NOT TREATED

Number.	Date of injury.	Age	Sex	Occupation.	Position of fracture.	Extent of Permanent disability due to fracture.	Ultimate result, December, 1915.
44	June, 1908	54	F.	Milliner	Subcapital	Died four days	Died four days, delirium tremens
45	Sept., 1908	83	F.	None		Complete	Living, gets about in wheel chair
46	Sept., 1908	59	M.	Merchant	Intertrochanteric	Died two days	Died two days, pulmonary edema
47	Dec., 1909	73	F.	None	Subcapital	Able to walk on crutches	Lost after discharged from hospital
48	July, 1910	74	F.	None	Intertrochanteric		Lost after discharged from hospital fourth day
49	Aug., 1910	69	F.	None	Impacted intertrochanteric	Died twenty-five days	Dead—edema of lungs
50	Dec., 1911	68	F.	Housewife	Impacted subcapital	Died twenty days	Dead—pneumonia
51	Old fracture	35	M.	Housewife	Intertrochanteric	Walked with a crutch	Unchanged
52	Jan., 1914	88	F.	None		Complete	Living, helpless
53	Oct., 1914	80	F.	None		Died three days	Died three days, shock
54	Old fracture	35	F.	Coat maker	Badly united intertrochanteric	Pain and limp, stiff hip	Unchanged
55	Sept., 1915	78	F.	None		Died ten days	Died, failing heart

The period of complete disability means the period in which the patient depends on assistance for ordinary movements, and does not include the time in bed. Partial disability indicates the additional period in which the patient is able to move about without crutches, but cannot resume work or former activities. All the patients in this series are white.

Extent of permanent disability due to fracture.	Percentage of former wages earned after recovery.	Ultimate result, December, 1915.	Operation.
5 c.m. shortening, stiff hip		Walks on crutches and high shoes, nearly helpless	Head of bone excised
Rigid hip	100%	Walks easily, is blacksmith to circus	Subtrochanteric osteotomy
2 c.m. shortening	Not obtained	1911, three years after operation at work	Freshening and nailing fragments
3 c.m. short. Limp	100%	1912, three years, died of intestinal obstruction	Subtrochanteric osteotomy
		1914, died, embolism after second fixation	Freshening fragments and animal bone peg
2 c.m. shortening	100%	½ inch lift on heel. At same work	Freshening fragments, tie out
Not estimated on account of an old fracture of shaft		Slight shortening, good motion. In Insane Asylum	Freshening fragments, autogenous bone peg

CASES NOT TREATED

Reason for non-treatment.

Delirium
Feebleness
Kidney
Restlessness,
Bronchitis,
Refused
Shock,
Refused
Feebleness, e

S Surg 24

By moving the various sections of the Gatch bed the position of the patient may be changed without damage to the fracture, and in this way the danger of hypostatic congestion be avoided. A slight movement of the fragments permitted seems to stimulate new bone formation.

Old fracture of the neck of the femur requires treatment on account of nonunion or because deformity interferes with locomotion. For nonunion the head may be excised and the neck fragment or trochanter placed in the acetabulum, or the ends of the fragments may be freshened and put in apposition for bony union. Direct fixation by means of a nail, an absorbable peg or an autogenous bone graft may be used to secure approximation and to stimulate bone formation.

When the fracture has united with deformity, subtrochanteric osteotomy is usually done. For the common deformity, adduction with outward rotation, a wedge-shaped piece of bone is removed from the outer and forward portion of the femur just below the trochanter and the bone is bent outward into abduction of about 20 degrees and twisted as far inward as is possible without making a complete fracture. Overcorrection of the adduction is the important object of the operation.

Twelve patients were not treated. Two young women declined operation for the relief of deformity following old fracture. One woman, aged seventy-four years, was taken home by her relative on the eighth day, after an unfavorable prognosis had been given. This patient as well as another woman who left the hospital unimproved ten weeks after the injury, cannot be traced. Two patients are known to be alive, one a man of eighty-eight years and the other a woman of ninety, one year and seven years after the injury.

All the usual contra-indications to elective operation apply in determining whether or not a patient should be treated for a fracture of the neck of the femur. Certain particular conditions have been noted in studying the fatal cases.

1. Circulatory. The presence of dilatation of the heart. intermittant or irregular pulse, and extremes of blood pressure are reasons for noninterference.

2. Pulmonary. Congestion of the lungs from any cause is a positive contra-indication to anesthesia and firm fixation dressing.

3. Renal. Most patients with a fractured neck of the femur have some kidney insufficiency. The phthalein test will indicate the vigor of the kidneys and be a guide for the inauguration of treatment. Uremia has a prominent place in the causes of death in the series.

4. Nervous. Lack of control of bladder and rectum is probably part of a general neurological breakdown. Restlessness, irritability and delirium may be uremic manifestations, or signs of alcohol and drug habits. If persistent these conditions indicate a fatal outcome and the patient should not be treated. Unconsciousness has the same significance.

The 55 cases of fracture of the neck of the femur here reported have been observed during the past eight years. Seven patients cannot be traced. Of the remainder 17 are now dead and 4 are helpless, either on crutches or in wheel chairs as a result of the fracture. There are 46 recent and nine old fractures in the series. Thirty-six recent cases were treated and 10 were not. Of these 36 cases 4 patients died during the treatment, 13 were completely cured, 8 partially cured. In 3 cases sufficient time has not passed since the fracture to allow an estimate to be made. One patient is unimproved, 1 patient was seriously incapacitated by pain until her death six months after she left the hospital. Six patients cannot be traced all of whom left the hospital in good condition apparently cured.

Of the 4 fatal cases, 1 patient developed uremic symptoms, restlessness and irritability, with occasional short periods of unconsciousness twelve days after the injury, and died on the fifty-eighth day. A second patient died three days after fixation. In this case the examination of the urine before anesthesia did not indicate a kidney insufficiency. The patient was vigorous in appearance, but she was unable to control the passage of urine and feces, almost constantly soiling the bed. The occurrence of this condition seems to indicate a fatal outcome. It was also present in three of the fatal untreated cases. The third patient died on the twenty-ninth day after a stormy illness. She was almost maniacal as a result of the use of alcohol and narcotics and finally died in uremia following two days of convulsions. The fourth patient died of edema of the lungs four days after fixation.

THE TREATMENT OF FRACTURES: WITH SPECIAL REFERENCE TO FRACTURES OF THE LONG BONES

By W. P. Carr, M.D., F.A.C.S.
Washington, D. C.

I present this subject because I believe we have retrograded of late in the treatment of fractures, instead of advancing, and I believe there is more confusion and difference of opinion upon this important subject than ever before.

I think it is my duty to surgery, and to our patients, to point out my reasons for this belief and to indicate what seems to me to be the remedy. I feel that with due modesty I can speak with some degree of authority upon this subject, because in the last twenty years, in my service at the Emergency Hospital in Washington, there have been treated more than 7000 fractures, of nearly every bone and variety. These fractures were treated by myself, or by my assistants, under my direction, by methods which experience has proven satisfactory and which we have improved and simplified from time to time. Our results have been good. In fractures of long bones not complicated by other serious injury or disease there have been no deaths, very few amputations, and in no single case has the end-result been unsatisfactory either to the patient or to ourselves. In every case an x-ray has been taken, *after* reduction and the application of a cast, and no case has been allowed to go out with serious anatomical defect, or functional disability. A good many have been discharged with slight anatomical imperfections not interfering with function. All such cases were told that by operation the anatomical imperfection could be remedied, but were advised against it and accepted our advice. Many patients have come into the hospital with compound fractures, often comminuted, inground with dirt, complicated by loss of skin and mangled muscles, not infrequently already suppurating or showing signs of infection. But even in these cases by proper cleansing, suitable fixation, absolute rest, the use of morphine, wet antiseptic dressings, appropriate vaccines, antitetanus serum and skin grafting, we have been able to prevent infection, or to tide over the acute stage, avoid amputation and secure a perfect or at least satisfactory result.

In this way I think we have saved many limbs that would ordinarily have been amputated. We have had excellent opportunity to compare our end-results with those of other surgeons using other methods, both in the same hospital, under similar conditions and in other hospitals and private practice, and we have been forced to the conclusion that some methods and teachings in common use today, not only in our city, but all over the world, are bad in principle and are causing more bad end-results than we were seeing twenty years ago. We have within the last two years seen a number of amputations for non-union or infection following open operation when in our judgment such operation was unnecessary and ill advised. We have seen limbs amputated when we were sure they could have been safely saved, and we have been called upon to correct many bad end-results due, in our opinion, entirely to faulty teaching and methods, sanctioned by one or other high authority, and in common use today. We are forced to the conclusion that many surgeons are too prone to amputate, too ready to operate, and too apt to use a faulty method of operating.

No one thing, I think, has contributed more to this condition than the teaching of Mr. Lane and Mr. Milne of

England, and the use of Lane's plate and other methods of rigid fixation. In one year fifty-four Lane plates were applied in the Emergency Hospital with the result that thirty of them had to be removed for one cause or another, mostly non-union without apparent infection. There was one death from infection and two amputations in this series, one for non-union, one for infection. None of these plates were applied by myself. I have never used one, nor ever seen an indication for its use. They were applied by a half a dozen of our best surgeons—in other lines of work at least. I have written two previous papers protesting against the use of the plates, and pointing out the numerous bad results I have seen from them, and I am glad to say that our fellow members, Drs. Trout, Albie and others have ably seconded my efforts in this direction, but the plates are still in every-day use.

We have seen wires put through and through the ends of broken bones, and wrapped round and round the bone with disastrous results when it was absolutely useless and unnecessary. We believe that it is bad surgery to operate when it is not necessary and worse still to use a method that has been followed, all over the country, by a train of such results as delayed union, non-union, suppuration, amputation and even death. A careful examination of the literature of the past two years will show, not a few, but hundreds of such disastrous results from the use of Lane plates, Milne's bands, improper wiring and the use of various large foreign bodies with the erroneous idea of maintaining rigid fixation and *alignment*. These reports come, not from a single locality, but from all over the country, and the majority of the worst cases have not been reported and never will be.

The methods of Albie and Trout of using autogenous bone plates are excellent for secondary operations for non-union or loss of bone, but are not often necessary in recent fractures.

There will always be deaths following serious fractures in persons who are diseased. Age of itself does not affect the prognosis in any way. Just as good and prompt union occurs in men over ninety as in young men, provided they are not victims of nephritis, angina, excessive arterioclerosis, or other advanced diseases. The prognosis is grave, even in young persons, with diabetes, delirium tremens, advanced nephritis, epilepsy, or cardiac disease; and in all persons nearing the end from any disease the shock of a serious fracture may bring about a fatal termination.

But in such case death should not be attributed to the fracture, which only hastens the inevitable end, and is not the real cause. Extensive complicating injury or hemorrhage may also prove fatal.

Leaving out such cases, in fairly normal individuals, in all classes and kinds of fractures the prognosis for life is good, and the final result should be complete restoration of function, without noticeable deformity, provided we can exclude infection, which is the thing most of all to be feared in compound fractures and to a less degree in open treatment.

Most surgeons do not like to admit even a remote probability of infection in fractures not compound and not already infected when seen, and are inclined to consider it a reflection upon the technic when it follows operation in clean cases. It does occur, however, and is not extremely rare even in the hands of the most careful. It is not always the fault of the operater. The mangled tissue and blood clots around the broken bone form a splendid nidus for germ growth, and in such a culture medium even the staphylococcus epidermidis, which is usually harmless, may cause serious trouble, and lead to secondary infection with more dangerous organisms. These skin germs cannot be absolutely excluded. Unavoidable infection may also occur from the blood of the patient. Abscesses are not very rarely deep in the muscles, brain and other organs, that are hard to account for except by infection through the blood. A few pathogenic organisms are not infrequently found in the blood of apparently healthy individuals and we are now finding streptococci every day in the blood of patients not very ill from chronic arthritis. Such organisms rarely cause suppuration in simple fractures; but when the additional traumatism of an operation is added, especially if a slight contamination with skin germs takes place, the result may be disastrous. The insertion of a foreign body for rigid fixation adds much to the danger of infection, which may occur weeks, months, or even years after the operation, as we have frequently seen. Such bodies always cause delayed union, even when no apparent infection occurs, and often cause non-union without suppuration.

There is a certain amount of risk in the open treatment of fractures that is unavoidable and no operation should be done unless really necessary. Experience has shown us that it seldom is necessary in fractures that are not compound. We make it a rule always to attempt reduction immediately upon the patient's admission—the sooner the better—and an *x*-ray picture is taken *after* a cast has been applied—*not before*. Then if the skiagram shows it necessary we operate. But with a good knowledge of applied anatomy and a little experience it is remarkable how few cases will need operation, or even a readjustment of the cast, even in comminuted fractures. We admit that operation is necessary in some cases but it can be just as well done at the end of a week, and we believe that the attempt should always be made first to adjust the fragments and apply a plaster cast. Try it and see how often you will succeed, even in comminuted fractures and those around joints. And remember, that when the anatomical position is not perfect, so long as it does not interfere with function, or render an articular surface uneven, or produce notable deformity, it is usually better to leave it than to risk interference. It is wonderful how nature will mould together a bunch of comminuted fragments or round off projecting points in the course of a few months.

The following facts and laws of nature should never be forgotten:

1. *Continued Pressure upon Bone Causes its Rapid Absorption.* This is well illustrated in many thoracic aneurisms where simple pressure of the growing sac causes absorption and complete disappearance of large portions of rib, sternum, or even vertebræ.

Bony irregularities, interfering with the movement of joints, may also be readily absorbed by keeping constant pressure upon them for a few weeks. It is easy to straighten a flexed and partially ankylosed knee when the ankylosis is due to bony irregularities of the joint surfaces, and not to fusion of the bones or to shortened or fixed tendons. It can be done by simply straightening the knee, as much as possible without pain, and applying a plaster cast. In a week's time the cast is removed and the joint readily gives several degrees more because the constant pressure of opposing surfaces has caused absorption. The process is then repeated and in a few weeks a right-angled knee may be made perfectly straight. I have done it in a number of cases both with the knee-, ankle- and elbow-joints.

Plates, nails and screws also cause rapid absorption of bone upon which they press, if there is a continuous tension upon them. Consequently such appliances cannot be depended upon to keep fractured long bones in alignment; and though they may prevent shortening, this can be better done in other ways.

2. *It is Impossible to Hold Down a Fragment of Bone, Tending to Ride Upward from Muscular Action, by Putting Compresses Over It.* The result will be absorption of tissues over the fragment and ulceration through the skin. Care must also be taken not to put undue pressure upon bony prominences or ulceration will result.

3. *Any Incision Through Muscle Playing Over a Bone, Down to the Bone, May Produce Scar Tissue Binding the Muscle to the Bone at that Point, and Interfering More or*

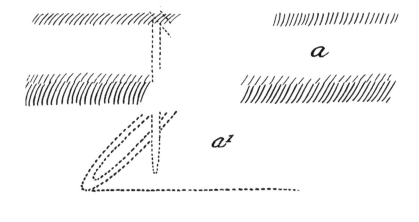

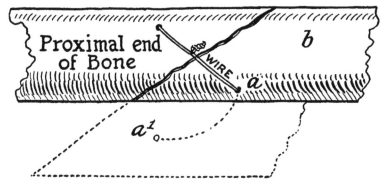

Proximal end
of Bone

WIRE

FIG. 1.—Right and wrong way to wire bones.

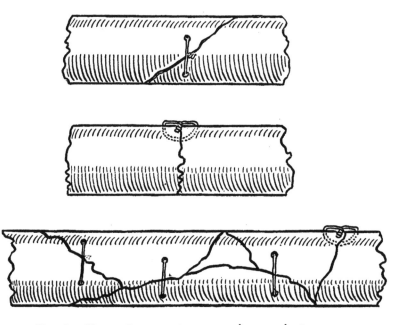

FIG. 2.—Shows the correct way to wire certain fractures.

Less Seriously with Motion. I have seen a stiff knee result more than once from incision through the rectus femoris, made on account of fracture in the middle third of the femur; and once broke the patella in trying to flex such a knee under ether. These were cases of primary union with no evidence of infection. When infection occurs the scar will of course be heavier still. Incision for fracture of the femur should therefore be made to one side of the rectus femoris, between it and the vastus externus preferably, or through the short fibers of the vastus externus or internus.

4. *Continued Irritation of Muscles and Tendons at the Seat of a Fracture Often Produces Thickening and Contraction of These Muscles, or Tendons, and Such Contractions May Seriously Impair the Motion of a Joint.* But, unless there has been an inflammatory welding of the tendons, the contractions will yield, in time, to ordinary use; and I believe it is only when *infection* has occurred that permanent welding results, except in fractures of the wrist where the tendons pass through long synovial tubes.

5. *Infection at the Site of Fracture Nearly Always Interferes Seriously With Union,* and even when good union occurs, may cause stiffness of a limb by fusion of muscle and tendon in a manner than can never be remedied.

6. Mangled and lacerated wounds are far more liable to infection than clean-cut incisions. Dirt and other foreign bodies also contribute to infection. Gunshot wounds for this reason are, according to Dr. Le Garde, a thousand times more liable to infection than clean incisions.

7. *Cutting off the Blood Supply of a Part of the Periosteum by Pressure is Equivalent in Effect to Removal of this Periosteum.*

8. *Large Foreign Bodies Imbedded in Bone Frequently Cause, Without Apparent Infection, a Rarefying Osteitis* not only in their immediate vicinity but often extending to the whole end of a broken bone, producing a conical point that will not unite with the other fragment.

This is particularly true of screws and of wires passed entirely through the medullary canal, or deeply into it.

These laws are as fixed and immutable as the laws of the Medes and Persians and the ignoring of some of them has led to pernicious methods of treating fractures that have come into common use under the sanction of high authority. If these laws are true it is self-evident that short fragments may be held in place by wiring. No appliance, however, should ever be fastened directly to the ends of a broken long bone with the *purpose of keeping the fragment in alignment; but only to prevent shortening*. The *alignment* must be maintained by splints, casts, or extension—never by metal plates, or any appliance encircling the bone, nor by wires passed through and through the broken ends. The Lane plate breaks three of the fundamental laws that should govern the treatment of fractures. (1) It causes continuous pressure of screws upon portions of the bone where absorption is undesirable; (2) it is a large foreign body causing, in at least 33 per cent. of cases, a rarefying osteitis resulting in delayed union, or non-union; (3) it destroys by pressure a considerable portion of the periosteum.

These results are *not* dependent upon *infection*. They occur in wounds healing by primary union as well as where infection and suppuration result. When both bones of the forearm or leg are broken, and a Lane plate is applied to one bone, but not to the other, it often happens that the bone to which the plate is applied fails to unite, while good union occurs in the other. This proves that the non-union is not due to infection, nor to any general or local condition of the patient—but to the plate itself and the screws used to attach it.

I shall mention briefly some of the methods that we have found simple, efficient, and safe: Pott's fractures, Colle's or Barton's fractures come in nearly every day. They are put up at once in plaster over glazed cotton. Anesthetic is seldom found necessary and many of them are reduced and put up by the internes. They are x-rayed the next day and it is rarely found necessary to make any change.

I know of no unsatisfactory result. In a good many cases slight anatomical imperfections have been allowed to go uncorrected, but never an obvious deformity or one that could interfere with function. The cast never extends beyond the metacarpals and there are no stiff fingers. For most fractures of the femur we use extension by means of the weight and pulley until muscular contraction is thoroughly overcome. In nearly every case all shortening and all perceptible deformity can, and *should* be overcome if extension be correctly applied within 36 hours after the injury. The sooner it is done the better. After two weeks when a muscular contraction has been well overcome, a cast extending from the toes to the nipple line is safe, and usually proves a relief to the patient. We find it easy to tell by measurement and palpation whether the bones are in good position. If, after a week's trial, good position cannot be maintained in this way, or by some modification of it, we may then operate to better advantage than at first. The patient loses no time for the preparation for union has been going on during this week, and the tissues are in better condition for operation than at first. We admit that operation is sometimes necessary in fractures near the lesser trochanter, in the lower fourth of the bone, or when the ends of fragments have caught and held in displacement by muscles, but such cases are rather rare.

In fractures of other long bones we use plaster almost exclusively with very satisfactory results. By studying the action of muscles upon the fragments, and putting the limb in position to relax such muscles as tend to displace them, much may be accomplished. I am afraid this is becoming a lost art through too much dependence upon the x-ray. I cannot go into details now, but would refer to Gray's Anatomy where, under the head of Surgical Anatomy, this subject is most clearly illustrated. In applying casts

we are careful to secure reliable extension and counterextension when it is needed, and careful to prevent rotation. In
fractures of the upper arm we have devised a method of our
own that has given great satisfaction. A plaster cast is put
around the chest and shoulders and another around the arm
and elbow with the elbow flexed at a right angle. These
casts are allowed to harden. The arm is then raised nearly
to a right angle to the body, brought a little forward, the
fragments reduced by strong traction and manipulation,
and held in position by traction while the gap is filled in
between the plaster jacket and the cast on the forearm.
Traction is continued until the plaster hardens. Such a cast
may usually be applied without an anesthetic, with little
pain, and is very comfortable and convenient, although
it does not look so. We have avoided operation by using
this jacket cast in may cases. We find, also, that it is often
necessary to fix the joint above the seat of a fracture to
prevent muscular action on the upper fragment, and to
prevent rotation of the whole cast and, with it, rotation of
the lower fragments. This is particularly true in fractures
of both bones of the leg. Unless the cast be made to extend
well above the knee the foot will rotate outward, the upper
part of the cast slipping around the smooth rounded calf
and upper leg. I have seen a number of cases, where the
pain was very great from this cause, made immediately
comfortable by extending the cast snugly around and above
the knee. When it does become necessary to operate we
have found wiring the most satisfactory method in nearly
all cases. When properly done, even in comminuted fractures, a single small wire loop is usually all that is required.
It is not necessary, nor advisable, to wire every small fragment, nor even large ones unless some muscular attachment
is pulling them out of place. I have seldom used two wire
loops and never more than three in any fracture. These
wire loops should never pass through the medullary canal
nor deeply into it. The only purpose of the wiring is to pre-

vent over-riding and shortening. or the tilting of some short fragment out of position by muscular action. The *purpose* of wiring is never to prevent angular deformity, nor rotation, though it often does prevent or limit the latter. Angular deformity and rotation can be perfectly controlled by a cast, splints, or extension. Properly done, it is easier and quicker to wire any given fracture than to apply to it a Lane plate; and the same result is obtained in a far safer way, with equal certainty by correct wiring. One or two wire loops, properly applied, will do all the Lane plate can reasonably be expected to do, and do it without danger of delayed or non-union, with much less danger of infection, and without danger of any serious remote trouble. I have never seen delayed union, nor any serious trouble result from one or two wire loops.

Most surgeons, I am sure, do not understand the simple mechanical principles involved in the wiring of bones. Many have told me that this was their reason for using plates. My best assistant could never understand this simple thing until I made a set of wooden models of fractures and showed him with them the right and wrong way of wiring. Before that was done he insisted that he could not get wire to hold the fragments, and persisted in using Lane plates, contrary to my wishes, and knowing even then the bad results so often following their use. He tried the plan of using them temporarily, taking them off after two weeks is several cases. One of these cases failed to unite. After six months of non-union I used Albee's method of bone grafting with good results. This assistant, now my associate, after learning the simplicity of wiring and becoming expert at it, has become enthusiastic about it and no longer feels tempted to use a plate.

I think most surgeons who use plates and other methods do so because they do not thoroughly understand wiring. I have personally converted a score or more. Compound fractures are given immediate treatment. Anesthetic is often necessary for thorough cleansing and repair. Benzine is used to clean the skin and the wound is freely swabbed with iodin 3.5 per cent. Badly mangled or dirt-inground tissues or skin are cut away cleanly with knife or scissors. Then, after a second iodin painting a small loop of wire is usually applied to insure against shortening or over-riding. This can usually be done with no further traumatism except the boring of two little holes. It takes but five minutes, and I have never seen it do harm. A few plain catgut ligatures or sutures may be needed to oppose muscles or stop bleeding. As little catgut as possible is used, often none, and the wound is closed with silkworm. No drainage is used. But sometimes packing part of the wound with iodoform gauze is necessary to control bleeding from some deep cavity when it would take much time and additional traumatism to tie the bleeding or oozing vessels. A cast is then applied and a window cut nearly through. Gauze packing is removed in 24 or 48 hours through the window. Morphine is given freely when needed for pain, for the first 24 or 48 hours. An immunizing dose of tetanus antitoxin is given as soon as possible. Few cases treated this way suppurate. But should infection occur a stitch is removed and the pus or secretion of the wound examined and an appropriate vaccine given. The stock staphylococcus vaccine is usually effective and prompt in action. Mixed infections and streptococcic infections generally require autogenous vaccines. In some cases we have made a culture from the wound at the primary operation, saving much time, but this cannot be done in routine. When there is much loss of skin, or a large open wound, heavy iron strips are moulded to fit and incorporated in the cast so that it can be cut away from the wound to allow wet dressings without interfering with the immovability of the fragments. Some of our good results in such cases we attribute to dressing with gauze wet in a 1 per cent. solution of potassium permanganate. Wounds heal under it more rapidly than I have ever seen them heal under any other dressing. Skin especially grows over raw surfaces with remarkable rapidity, and has the appearance and soft feel of normal skin which it more especially resembles in every way than it does ordinary scar tissue. This was first pointed out by Dr. Daniel C. Craig, of Washington, D. C., and has been confirmed by numerous assistants in the Emergency Hospital and Dispensary. Dr. Lewis, the present Superintendent of the Hospital, is an enthusiastic advocate of the permanganate solution and has also called my attention to the fact that few compound fractures become infected when tetantus antitoxin is used. Even when they are ground in dirt and grease and have been exposed for hours before coming to the Hospital the tetanus antitoxin seems to prevent infection. All such cases are of course cleansed and disinfected with iodin, but the percentage of infection has been notably lessened since we begun the use of the antitoxin.

DISCUSSION ON THE PAPERS OF DRS. McGLANNAN AND CARR

DR. CHARLES M. ROSSER, Dallas, Texas.—I believe in many respects the subject that has been presented is of more practical value and importance than any other we have had under consideration at this meeting of the Association: (1) As matters should be, the result to the patient; (2) as we must conceive, the results vary with the work of the individual operator; (3) in many instances we must not forget the medico-legal aspects which grow out of accidents.

I believe we have drifted very far from some of the safer ideas due to the work which the x-ray has done for us. Dr. Carr mentioned very properly that the x-ray is of value, and he likewise called attention to the fact that very properly the functional result should be considered. Possibly more importance should be attached to that phase of the subject than to the anatomical results. But the medico-legal aspect of this subject of treatment of fractures comes to us at once, that the x-ray will be the final arbiter in determining what these results are. If a patient is informed at the beginning that there will be some anatomical failure, but that, in all probability, the functional and physiological results will be entirely satisfactory, I believe we may follow our procedure to some extent by the concurrence of the patient in our suggestion.

The cases referred to by Dr. McGlannan are those which occur so often in the aged, and for that reason we must look upon fractures of the femur with some degree of difference as compared with the average fracture. We must not lose sight of the fact that the aged patient must be treated from the standpoint of debility, and that the length of their disability, the length of time in bed, is a very important factor in determining their recovery. For that reason, I believe we should practice the open operation in fractures in the aged more frequently than fractures occurring in young people. I believe they should be allowed more liberty after fixation by some medical means. The practice which I myself have followed—and I probably have observed a larger number of these injuries than any other class calling for surgery—has been from that standpoint. I have not had any serious results from the use of the nail in fractures of the neck of the femur. I have had good results. It has extended to patients as old as I would expect to have union at all.

There is another class of cases in which we must have mechanical help; I mean help from the open operation. For instance, take a case of non-union or improper union, and I think they present a class of cases in which we are more apt to employ the Lane plate and such contrivances with advantage to the patient. I will cite one case, that of a doctor, a well-developed, muscular man, who three months before had fallen, or rather an automobile fell upon his shoulder, fracturing the lower end of the humerus, driving the shaft into the axilla, and the two fragments were fixed by a large amount of callus. X-ray examination showed this condition of three months' duration. An open operation was done for its relief, chiseling away the callus until with Gigli saw the upper end of the lower fragment could be taken away. The head of the bone was displaced entirely, laid out in salt solution, freshened properly, and with the use of three small wire nails placed in anatomical relation again, replaced into the glenoid cavity, and patient after three months' disability was able to drive his automobile and take care of his work.

I am sure I know of no method other than the distinctly mechanical type which would have given such a result in this case.

Dr. BATTLE MALONE, Memphis, Tennessee.—Referring to the treatment of fractures of the femoral neck, I wish to offer a suggestion, not with any idea of criticising the methods of Dr. McGlannan, because his results have been excellent, very much above the average, but in the treatment of these fractures in old people, I would simply suggest the use of the Hodgen splint. In younger people we have a choice of methods; the Whitman or operative methods are all right, but in old people we have got to make them comfortable; we have to treat the patient as much as the fracture, and by putting these patients up in a Hodgen's splint they are made comfortable from the outset, allowed to sit up in bed from the time it is applied, and while I have not been using this splint very long, the success of its use in my hands has been such that I have been very much gratified.

I had an old man the past summer, aged seventy-seven years, with an intertrochanteric fracture, who was very emaciated and feeble. The case was complicated by the fact that he had prostatic obstruction. We were enabled to put him up in a Hodgen's splint and got a perfect result. There was good bony union, and now he is up and about town.

I believe in old people we will find by using the Hodgen's splint we can give them more comfort than by any of the more severe methods suggested.

Dr. C. E. CALDWELL, Cincinnati, Ohio.—I know that this subject always provokes a good deal of discussion, and one of the greatest functions of a society of this sort is to mold public opinion throughout the country and to offer suggestions to the profession at large in the treatment of fractures. I think we should stand unalterably for conservatism in the treatment of fractures. I feel that a position to the contrary is encouraging a great deal of meddlesome surgery in fracture work, and as Dr. Carr has so aptly said, a great many of these cases will never come to our notice. I have had one or two experiences myself that I would not like to publish. I should feel humiliated if I had to publish these cases without publishing others to substantiate perhaps the views I hold with regard to conservatism.

In fractures of the neck of the femur I am unalterably opposed to the attempt of breaking up impactions of the femoral neck, unless it be that the position of the ligament and impaction is such as to interfere with locomotion thereafter.

There is one form of fracture that has come to my notice

more frequently than I supposed was present, and that is a fracture that goes through here (intercondylar—indicating on blackboard) with impaction, when the fractured lesser trochanter is greatly displaced by contraction of the iliopsoas.

I have a number of x-ray pictures of cases showing that the lesser trochanter has been split off and dislocated. Obviously, such a case would not be benefited by any attempt to break up the impaction and treat the case in abduction. From correspondence with Whitman, he took exception to some statements regarding impaction made at a meeting at Buffalo last spring. He rejects the idea of the term impaction altogether, and moreover, I cannot exactly understand his point of view. He puts his so-called impacted fractures up in extreme abduction and then contends that he does not get any breaking up of the impaction. That I cannot understand because when you have impaction, you have traumatic coxa vara to a certain extent, and if you put such a fracture up in extreme abduction, you put the greater trochanter in a position where you have breaking up of the impaction, whether he accepts the term impaction or not.

I am thoroughly in accord with Dr. Carr that the majority of cases of fracture can be satisfactorily treated as regards functional results by conservative methods, and by traction and extension with a great deal of weight, as much weight as the patient can stand. Patients stand thirty pounds of weight and bear it well. It needs to be used only a short time to overcome muscular resistance. After that, if the fragments are in apposition let well enough alone. I have seen cases that did not promise well, but after several weeks of extension, different results were shown by the x-ray than they had shown in the beginning.

There is a certain class of cases of compound fractures that we are operating on where we find we cannot get proper apposition of the fragments, because we are doing the patient good by opening up freely and getting more opportunity for drainage if infection is present. You will not hurt these cases. In a number of instances I have been opening up the lower part of the tibia and adjusting the fragments, and by means of wire or chromicized gut replacing the fragments and holding them there until you get the cast on.

Fractures of the lower end of the femur are the ones that cause most apprehension by reason of the obliquity of the lower fragment; we have a tendency to backward tilting of the lower fragment, which, in this locality, means danger of impinging upon the sciatic nerve, with subsequent sciatica. In one case the sciatica lasted for many years. These fractures I have found are best treated in this way: The patient is put upon a double inclined plane, and traction is made in two directions; in other words, traction is made in the line of the femur, and traction is made in the line of the tibia; the plane runs over the foot of the bed, and the functional results and apposition in these cases have been fairly good.

DR. HUGH H. TROUT, Roanoke, Virginia.—Not only has there been too much done, but too much said on the question of treatment of ununited fractures. Personally, I said too much about a year ago when I stated that I was much opposed to the Lane plate because of some experimental work showing the harm from its use as regards osteogenesis and the great damage done in the presence of infection; and at the same time pointed out the advantages of the autogenous graft under similar circumstances. Shortly after the publication of the paper in the *Annals of Surgery*, I received letters from all over the United States regarding autogenous plates in the presence of infection; and from these letters one would be led to believe we were advocating infection as some sort of a stimulus to osteogenesis, when in reality, all we said was that a certain percentage of grafts "took" in spite, and not because of infection. We must be careful what we say about autogenous plates or anything else in fractures, or we will be misunderstood; and for that reason I am sorry Dr. Turck was not here to read his paper on "Regeneration of Bone in the Presence of Infection," because it is a dangerous title to turn loose on the public.

DR. ALBERT H. FREIBERG, Cincinnati, Ohio.—I dislike very much adding to the discussion on this subject even though it is so extremely interesting and always is the moment it is brought before a surgical body.

I have listened to these papers with a great deal of interest and with profit. I think Dr. Carr is extremely sensible, and I find myself in a position of being able to endorse what he says, as a rule. There is one thing he has advocated today concerning which I am at a loss to understand. While we are all familiar with the uncertainties that are attached to the readings of x-ray plates in fracture work or any other work, I am unable to understand why he should reject the use of the x-ray plate before setting a fracture. I would endorse heartily the view that the x-ray should be used after the fracture has been adjusted but why it should not be used to give the fullest possible information before the fracture is adjusted, is a thing I do not understand. I fail to see any disadvantage which would be attached to that.

Another thing which it might be well to impress upon us occasionally in connection with fractures is this, that accurate apposition does not necessarily imply that union will take place either in the usual time or a considerable time beyond that. In the first place, many of us have had the experience of finding non-union following the application of a Lane plate, or followed by prompt union after the Lane plate was removed; whereas at the operation nothing else was done at the site of fracture.

I have had experience in removing Lane plates in two instances, in which the plates had been applied by others, and in which non-union was present, and my activity consisted simply in cutting down on the plate and removing it and applying splints and union followed promptly. The x-rays in these cases, as well as the conditions at the site of fracture at the time of operation, showed that apposition was satisfactory.

Furthermore, I have a very distinct picture in my mind of a case which I treated quite recently in connection with Dr. Kelly across the river, a woman, seventy-six years of age, with intracapsular fracture of the femur, in whom we had about an inch of shortening, and in whose case without the use of an anesthetic we felt we had accomplished quite excellent reposition of the fragments, or as well as we could if we had used an anesthetic. The patient was extremely intractable. After eight weeks, an x-ray was made again with the patient lying in bed, with weight and pulley, and extension still on, and a splint applied to the limb. We found reposition by the x-ray was remarkable, so that the radiographer scarcely had words with which to express his admiration. We felt justified in this case in removing traction at the end of that time, since it was applied much longer than we were accustomed to do it. Within two weeks after traction was removed, the patient still being in bed, we had an inch of shortening. We have not taken an x-ray since then, so that I do not know the condition at the site of fracture. The x-ray shows us beyond peradventure that the fractured surfaces were in apposition, and I feel likewise from a clinical examination they did not remain in apposition nor did they heal in apposition.

Dr. James E. Moore, Minneapolis, Minnesota.—I am pleased to have heard these two papers on fractures, because while I am not treating fractures as I did at one time, I have the supervision of many men and trying to instruct the rising generation how to treat fractures.

I have been very much pleased with Dr. McGlannan's paper because it shows a distinct advance in this, that he approaches the subject of fractures of the neck of the femur the same as we would fractures in any other part of the body, readjusting these fragments and getting what we should expect, union. Up to within a few years the average text-book stated that these cases were considered hopeless. It was all our fault, as we know. We did not know how to readjust the fragments. We find now that if we put them in proper position and hold them there, by the various methods we will get union in about as large a percentage of fractures of the neck of the femur as in fractures of the shaft of the femur.

There is one additional feature Dr. Rosser brought out, namely, we have a lot of aged people to deal with, but we only have to consider them in the matter of treatment of the patient, and not the treatment of the fracture, because non-union in fracture occurs in middle-aged people as well as in old people.

With reference to the operative treatment of fracture, I have observed a great deal more of it than I have done, but it is my intention and function to say to the members of my staff these cases should be operated and those should not, so that in the end my experience is large. We are drifting away from the application of foreign bodies in the holding of fragments. They are less frequently used in our clinic than they were some time ago, for the reasons brought out in this discussion. We find that while these mechanical appliances, particularly the Lane plate, will hold fragments in admirable position, they oftentimes interfere with bony union. I feel the time is at hand, when if we are obliged to use any mechanical device it will be the bone transplant.

Dr. Charles R. Robins, Richmond, Virginia.—I want to call attention to one point in the treatment of fractures where we have to operate. One great difficulty with most fractures is we do not get them properly reduced. There is some interposition of tissue or something that prevents them from being reduced, and notwithstanding our best efforts at manipulation the fracture is not properly reduced.

I always make it a rule to get an x-ray after the fracture has been reduced, or after an attempt has been made to reduce it to see what we have got. I have found in a few cases, after getting an x-ray, that the fracture has not been properly reduced, and then making the open operation I am able to so adjust the fragments that they will stay adjusted without the use of any mechanical appliance whatever. I believe that is true in a very large number of fractures, and in examining these fractures, even an oblique fracture which the books describe, we never find a perfectly smooth oblique fracture. There is some interdigitation at some point or another, and if we can get these little pieces properly adjusted and then hold them by proper splints, or whatever we may use, the fracture will stay reduced. I have had opportunity to do this in fractures of the surgical neck of the humerus, where I have not been able to get reduction previous to incision, after which I got reduction and have had the fragments remain reduced without the use of any plates or any foreign body whatever, and I called attention to that fact some time ago by saying that in doing the open operation we can secure absolute adjustment of the fragments so that they will stay in position without using any foreign body whatever.

DR. WILLIAM R. JACKSON, Mobile, Alabama.—One advantage of the open operation is in those cases where the x-ray does not show us the interposition of fragments of aponeurotic tissue. In nearly all of these cases we have got perfect co-aptation, and later on we do not get union. and the pseudo-arthrosis is due to the interposition of aponeurotic tissue, and those are the cases that later cause us to do the open operation.

With reference to fracture of the neck of the femur, the best possible way in the majority of cases is to put these limbs in apposition and apply traction, abduction and elevation,—elevate the foot of the patient twelve or fourteen inches above the bed, not in the extreme abduction but moderately so, the same as a Travois splint would produce. Dr. Murphy uses that in the absence of any other treatment, and traction is applied of from twenty-five to thirty pounds at first. If we fail, in intracapsular fractures to get co-aptation, we will get pseudo-arthrosis, which is almost as good as the origninal articulation.

DR. ROBERT T. MORRIS, New York City.—If Dr. Carr has 7000 grateful patients it is a matter of applied psychology. I do not trust to that, but I have a blank printed, stating the nature of the fracture, the proposed plan of treatment, and the anticipated results, including shortening or non-union, so far as one's conscience will allow, A patient cannot object to each item of statement. All that you gain beyond that is velvet. This has protected me against suits in three or four cases. My only suit was one for $15,000.00 for not taking out an appendix. At times I believe in introducing rigid fixation, or more frequently than some surgeons do.

As to the use of Lane plates, I have given them up. I use instruments for taking out some that others have put in.

The Bier method of employing a blood clot has not been referred to. I still have confidence in that as one of the resources in secondary operation after the first non-union.

I have seen one case—the first one I have ever seen, yet they must occur occasionally—of muscle exhaustion from tiring. This case was seen in New York. The patient had a double sciatica. I went over every possible cause in that case and found she had fallen a year ago, went about on crutches for a while, then walking with a cane afterward. An x-ray showed she had an impacted fracture of the neck of the femur. We got a tired reaction of the muscles on that side, and she had undoubtedly exhausted the muscles from muscle spasm, and a year subsequently she came in for treatment of the muscles. There was a tiring out of innervation of the muscles on that side, and a reflex from a segment of the cord, the efferent impulse involving the sciatic nerves of both legs.

Dr. Joseph C. Bloodgood, Baltimore, Maryland.—I cannot understand the tremendous difference of opinion not only here but everywhere in regard to the treatment of fractures. It may be based on this. When I came to the Johns Hopkins Hospital all fractures of the neck of the femur were treated in the best manner by traction, and we were impressed with our splendid results in the treatment of fractures of the neck of the femur. When the Whitman treatment came out, I did not see why we should adopt it. I have found out the condition of patients treated by traction and abduction and all the methods at that time used for traction. I wrote and had seen almost all of the patients, and I think it was about 1898 and 1899 after the hospital had been opened almost ten years, and the results as they came back years afterwards were appalling. That was before the days of the x-ray, and all we had was our record of measurements and shortening. They went out on crutches, and some came back within the next few months. Some of them kept off crutches and began to walk. Two types developed. One was non-union, which was not great in number, and in the second true traumatic coca vara deformity. The results for two or three years after fracture were different from the results when they left the hospital.

We took up abduction later and Dr. McGlannan has reported practically all of his cases. I only had a few cases and I know he looked after most of them. These cases have been followed. Dr. McGlannan should pass not on the condition of the patient leaving the hospital but on the present condition. I have had experience in both. In my mind there is absolutely no question but that the results in abduction are better than by the methods of traction Dr. Halsted employed. I know Dr. Halsted pretty well and the care we gave these cases, and I believe they got about as good treatment as any.

Another point: From the beginning of the literature on fracture of the neck of the femur we have been told not to break up impaction but I have not been able to find any surgeon who has ever broken up impaction once to find what happened. It did not make any difference in our cases whether we broke up impaction or not if we put the fracture up in abduction afterward. Dr. Murphy says that of all fractures in the world in which absolute fixation is necessary, it is a fracture of the neck of the femur. Dr. McGlannan has demonstrated that of all fractures in the world the absolute fixation in fractures of the femur is not necessary. We do not get absolute fixation in abduction in the Loos method. If we get apposition, if we maintain the fragments fairly accurately, we get union. We ought to get good results in fracture of the neck of the femur, but unless statements are based upon the examination of the patients two years afterwards, I do not think it is fair to compare them with the results of Whitman and Dr. McGlannan.

Personally, I do not believe it is necessary to nail a fracture of the neck of the femur, whether fresh, old, or ununited. Dr. McGlannan has demonstrated cases in which fresh impaction was broken up, and cases in which the impaction was not broken up, old and ununited, but in the old and ununited, if the ends are freshened and brought into apposition, nailing is unnecessary. There was only one case where a nail was not driven into the fracture at all, and the result was perfect.

I would like to put this thought on record: I think it is a mistake to speak of the Lane plate. It is the same plate that was used in 1885, and the buried screw belongs to Halsted. He buried the screw in 1892; I know it because I handed him the screws he buried.

A great deal is said and has been said against the use of the Lane plate that has nothing to do with the plate or with the screw. If a fracture comes to you with non-union or bad union and has a Lane plate in it, you blame the Lane plate. If a case comes to with the same condition without a Lane plate, you never say anything about it. I know one case of fracture of the tibia came to me with non-union without the Lane plate. I reoperated and put in a Lane plate and it united. The next case of non-union came in with a plate, I operated, did not put in a Lane plate, and it united. Union is delayed sometimes for some cause we do not understand. If you put on a Lane plate early you may blame the Lane plate. If you believe that the Lane plate develops callus, you will get a good result. Non-union, in many cases where there is perfect apposition has nothing to do with the Lane plate. The rarefaction of bone about the screw has nothing to do with non-union.

Two articles have appeared by German surgeons recently giving their experiences in the war. One of them has used the Lane plate and says the results are absolutely perfect, but he believes in the autogenous graft, but he has not had any case. The other says the Lane plate is useless and the autogenous graft is the only thing, but he did not use any Lane plates, and the great probabilites are that most fractures, if properly treated, would unite very well without the Lane plate or without the autogenous graft.

DR. A. C. SCOTT, Temple, Texas.—Much of what has been said goes to prove that none of us know very much about fractures. I used to think I knew all there was known about fractures; that I knew exactly how to put up each kind of fracture, and that my results were better than those of anyone else, but after fooling with them for almost a quarter of a century, I have come to the conclusion that I do not know very much about the subject after all.

The real fact is, I have taken the floor gentlemen, to mention one point, and that is, we as surgeons ought to encourage somebody in our part of the country to make a specialty of treating fractures. I do not believe that every surgeon who wrestles with gall-bladders and appendices, with chest and brain operations, and all these things, should undertake to

do this work. It is work of a peculiar character; it requires
a lot of mechanical ingenuity; it requires a lot of care; it requires
so many things that are not possessed by the average everyday
surgeon, and the Texas members will perhaps recall that I
have on a number of occasions stated that if any man in my
part of the state would limit his work to the treatment of fractures, I will guarantee to send him every case that comes under
my observation, because I feel the man who will go to work
and devote his entire time to it, will come nearer making a
success in the majority of cases than the man who does a little
of this and a little of that and of everything else.

DR. ROBERT CAROTHERS, Cincinnati, Ohio.—I am sorry
I did not hear the two papers on fractures, and I hesitate to
discuss them because of not having heard them. However,
I do not want to let this subject go by without saying a word
or two from my own experience. In the last few years I have
seen cases of fractures of the thigh of all kinds, and especially
fractures of the neck of the thigh.

There are several things I have observed, and one of them is
that it is very essential to get these patients out of bed as early
as possible. In the past five years I do not think I have kept
a patient with a fracture of the leg in bed more than four weeks.
I have always felt that if we could see these fractures in an hour
or two after they have been sustained, and put the fragments
in apposition, that would be the thing to do. Once in a while
we see them early and treat them early. It is not muscular
contraction in the first four weeks that makes shortening; it is
a clot of blood around the fracture and into muscular tissue, and
something must give way for that clot, and it is the fracture
that gives way and the fragments ride one on the other and that
is what makes the shortening. If you put weight and pulley
on them until you are green in the face, you only annoy the
patient. If you wait six or eight days, depending upon the case,
you can with very great ease pull the fracture into place. I
had this very thoroughly demonstrated to me in two cases.

About three years ago a young woman came to me with scoliosis. She did not have scoliosis when sitting down, but when
she stood up she had it. Upon further investigation of the
case I found that one leg was an inch and a half longer than the
other. She wanted the longer leg shortened. We considered
the matter very carefully and seriously and decided on operation. I took an inch and a quarter of thigh bone from the

longer leg. The fracture was absolutely transverse and smooth and was apposed without plating. She was then put in a plaster Spica and it was supposed that muscular action would hold the fragments in apposition. Such, however, was not the case and it required the weight of her body through the spica onto the foot to create apposition of the fragments. Repair occurred in a few weeks. She is now normal with union and no scoliosis. Both were of the same length.

I had another case which is not so illustrative of this point as the first one, but the second case helps to prove the first one, that it is not the muscle that contracts. There does come a time when the muscle does contract, and that is six or eight weeks after fracture, the time when the fracture wants to get away. The patient wants to be sent to the gymnasium or to a masseur to stop the contraction of the muscle and get it to move, and that is where the general surgeon makes a mistake. He keeps these patients up too long.

Dr. ALEXIUS McGLANNAN, Baltimore, (closing the discussion on his part).—This loose fixation we have looked upon as a method of choice because it is simple to carry out, and it is applicable to many more patients than any other method of fixation. Almost any of our patients can be treated by this method if they are not too feeble to stand treatment or too feeble to get out of bed. The patient who cannot stand rest in bed with this loose fixation would not stand a general anesthetic and a cutting operation for fixation of a fracture of the neck of the femur. A patient who is too feeble to stand this sort of treatment would not stand fixation with plaster of Paris. He could not carry the plaster of Paris cast.

The use of the Hodgen's splint as a method of treatment is well known. It is like Smith's anterior splint, it is a very valuable means of treating a fracture, but we believe that tying out the knees in abduction is simpler, is more easily applied, and is less troublesome to the patient.

What is meant by impaction is difficult to define. Stimpson looks on it as a crushing rather than a driving in of the fragments. Some driving in of the fragments does take place, and we break it up. Non-union of a fracture of the neck does not cripple the patient as much as union in adduction, and union is not guaranteed by the impaction.

I should like to say a word or two about Dr. Carr's paper before I sit down, particularly about fracture of the upper end of the humerus, and would simply remind those who have forgotten it of the great value of Middledorf's triangle, and its modification, Von Hacker's triangle, in the treatment of these fractures of the upper end of the humerus. It is lighter than plaster of Paris, can be measured with the unbroken arm, so that you get the length of humerus, making the two arms symmetrical in length, and it can be applied with more ease than plaster of Paris.

DR. W. P. CARR, Washington, D. C. (closing).—There are a few important points I would like to bring out. Age has little or nothing to do with union of bone. I have cases of just as good union in men over ninety as in young men. It is a question of condition of the patients and whether they are diseased, not a question of age.

As to the Hodgen's splint, I have used it, and sometimes it works to good advantage.

The question has been asked why I do not take an x-ray of the fracture before setting it. In many cases the fracture is so simple that I do not need to do it. I have no objection to taking an x-ray before the fracture is set, but it is much more important to take it after putting the fracture in fixation.

There is a group of young surgeons in this country who have the idea that all fractures ought to be operated on, and many of them are operating on every fracture as a routine treatment. I think we ought to teach these young men that it is unnecessary to resort to operative treatment in the great majority of fractures. It is our duty to spread that doctrine. When we have to operate, I think it is ignorance of how to wire a bone that has led to the use of so many complicated things for the fixation of bones. The average man will wire a fracture across at right angles to the line of fracture; some of the text-books tell us to put the wire at right angles to the fracture. This is wrong. What will happen? The wire loop will swing around, the bone will shorten and the muscular contraction will gradually make the overlapping worse.

I have seen but one case of non-union in a fracture not operated on, and this was a simple fracture. I believe non-union is nearly always due to interference of some kind. If we use this common soft wire (iron wire) that we buy in any hardware store, it will not break. We get absorption sometimes around the wire, and in some few cases of compound fracture the wire loop comes out with a ring of bone around it; but this does not interfere with the union. With multiple fractures running in various directions, it only takes a few short wire loops properly placed to hold several fragments together. It is unnecessary to wire every fragment, unless there is some muscle pulling it out of place. All we need to do is to overcome muscular contraction. In spite of what Dr. Carothers has said, muscular contraction is the important thing, and he must have had an unusual case where he could cut out a piece of bone and did not have contraction of the limb, because we know that in most fractures there is almost immediate overriding of the bone. In the first two hours, we may take the hand and pull the fragments into place. It may not require more than a few pounds of pull. If we pull it down and keep it down, we will not have any trouble with it. But after thirty-six hours it is difficult to get the shortening reduced. Several days after fracture of the femur I have found it necessary to use an extension table and much force to get the leg pulled down.

There are many other things I would like to talk about, but the main thing is, let us teach the younger men that it is unnecessary to operate on most fractures. And when it is necessary to operate they should try to use some simple method to prevent shortening and not try to fix the bone in alignment. We should preserve alignment and prevent rotation by the use of a cast or by extension. But to be effective the cast must be properly applied.

Many surgeons in treating fractures of both bones of the leg carry the cast only to the knee. The result is the foot turns around and the cast with it, and there is nothing to prevent rotation. If we carry the cast above the knee, with the knee slightly flexed, these patients are made more comfortable and rotation prevented.

SUBCUTANEOUS DERMIC FISTULA IN THE
TREATMENT OF ASCITES

By Walter C. G. Kirchner, A.B., M.D., F.A.C.S.

St. Louis Mo.

The object of this paper is to call attention to a method of treating ascites by an operation which is comparatively simple, and which, I believe, has not been tried to any considerable extent in this country. Any operation that will assist in relieving the distressing conditions which are produced by the accumulation of ascitic fluid is always welcome and, indeed, no single operative procedure suffices in all cases. It is apparent that the various underlying causes of ascites must receive appropriate treatment, as well as the methods employed in removing the accumulation of fluid.

In the treatment of ascites we have recourse to the various methods of elimination through the bowel and kidneys, to tapping the abdominal cavity, to the establishment of collateral circulation by such procedures as are employed in the Talma operation, to the return of the ascitic fluid directly into the veins, to operations on the veins as represented by Eck's fistula, and to the various means that have been devised for drainage into the subcutaneous tissue.

By the withdrawal of fluid by tapping, it is evident that we deprive the system of a certain quantity of albuminous and, in a measure, of nutritious substances, and these elements are conserved by those methods which seek to eliminate the fluid through the normal organs of excretion. By means of subcutaneous drainage then, we may lessen a certain amount of the waste that would occur if tapping were merely resorted to. In those cases where tapping must of necessity be resorted to, it may be interesting to note that Osten[1] inserted a tube in the abdomen arranged in such a manner that the patient could draw off the fluid whenever it became necessary. Rosenstein[2] by an ingenious method constructed a valve in the bladder and succeeded in draining off the ascitic fluid by this means. Believing in the theory of autotherapy in cases of cirrhosis with ascites, Vitry[3], by injecting subcutaneously 10 c.c. of ascitic fluid on alternate days, succeeded in curing his cases, which during the treatment showed increased urination. The Talma operation, the use of Eck's fistula, the employment of the saphenous vein in direct drainage into the circulation, the operation of Kumaris[4], in which rather extensive areas of peritoneum are resected, are all of value, but they cannot always, for obvious reasons, be employed in the cases at hand.

The methods of subcutaneous drainage are comparatively simple. The earlier experimenters used threads or similar material which lead from the peritoneal cavity into the subcutaneous tissues. Tavel[5] used a glass spool to drain the fluid into the subcutaneous spaces. Perinoff[6] used a silver tube, and Franke[7] a silver wire in the form of a letter H for the same purpose. Henschen[8] employed thin rubber tubing and Schepelmann[9], with the same idea of subcutaneous drainage in mind, used a section of varicose vein hardened in formaldehyde solution. In general it may be said that a number of the methods of continuous drainage are of value in that excellent results were obtained. However, in all of the methods just mentioned, some foreign substance was employed, and to overcome this, and to simplify the procedure Oberst[10], September 1914, devised a method by which he used a flap of skin which, by its insertion in the peritoneal cavity, provided continuous subcutaneous drainage.

S Surg   26

My own experience with operations for ascites associated with cirrhosis of the liver, and in which procedures of the type of the Talma operation were undertaken, agrees with that of other operators in that a cure is established in certain cases; but when the Talma operation fails, or when it is only partially successful, or when, for special reasons, it cannot or should not be employed, we must resort to some other means of relieving the ascites, and this may often be accomplished by the method of subcutaneous drainage.

Having in mind the principle of Oberst's operation, I proceeded in the following manner:

The patient is prepared as for a laparotomy, and the operation is carried out under local anesthesia. An elliptical incision, four or five inches in length, is made through the skin and subcutaneous tissues at the lower portion of the abdomen, across the median line, and about half-way between the umbilicus and the pubes, and thus, as shown in Fig. 1, owing to the abdominal distension, a tongue-shaped island of skin is produced. One-half of this skin, for example the right half, is made free and is divested of its subcutaneous tissue, thus forming a free flap; the left half, being allowed to remain attached, then serves as a pedicle. The fibres of the muscular structures having been separated, say those of the rectus muscle, the peritoneal cavity is next entered with a trocar and the ascitic fluid is gradually drained away. The peritoneum is then slit open sufficiently large to admit the free end of the flap to be inserted. If the omentum is likely to obstruct the peritoneal opening, it should be pushed aside and sutured. By means of sutures, placed at either side of the free margin of the flap and through one side of the peritoneum, the flap after being inserted in the peritoneal cavity is securely fastened, and the free end of the flap is thus retained in the peritoneal cavity (Fig. 2). The cut edges of the peritoneum, at the upper and lower angles, are then approximated, and sutured in such a manner as to secure the posi-

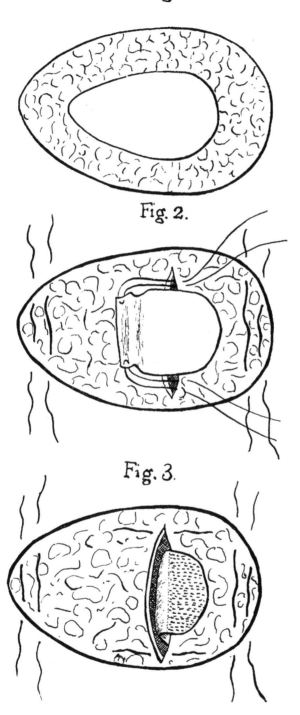

Fig. 1.

Fig. 2.

Fig. 3.

tion of the flap in abdominal cavity. The epidermal layer of the skin of the pedicle portion is then shaved off, and by means of interrupted sutures or clips, the cut margins of the skin are approximated and the flap, being buried, affords opportunity for subcutaneous drainage (Fig. 3). The resulting scar is represented by a transverse line.

In Oberst's original recommendation the skin of the pedicle portion of the flap was left intact. But in one case, following this suggestion, I found that the subcutaneous drainage and the lack of adhesion caused the pedicle to force its way through the wound and to come to the surface. I therefore resorted to the denudation of the skin of this portion of the flap, and firm union resulted, permitting the flap to remain buried (Fig. 3).

During the past year I have had occasion to try this operation on four cases of ascites. In all of the cases there was some benefit, even if only temporary. One case which had a previous Talma operation showed improvement for a time, but later died as a result of the heart complication. In two other cases the ascites later returned. A successful result was obtained in a patient who had an alcoholic cirrhosis of the liver with ascites.

Following all of the operations there was edema of the lower abdomen, and in the more favorable cases there was increased urination. It seems, therefore, that the good results depend greatly upon the integrity of the kidneys and their ability to eliminate properly. The simplicity and adaptability of the operation just outlined lends itself to those cases of ascites associated with weakened conditions of the patient, and to ascites following cancer, tuberculosis and other causes. In cirrhosis of the liver the best results may be expected when the Talma operation is combined with some operation affording subcutaneous drainage. In selected cases the operation may be given a trial. It apparently does no harm, and may be the means of accomplishing good in cases that are not amenable to the more hazardous and complicated operations.

REFERENCES

1. Osten. Zur Dauerdrainage bei Ascites, Therapie der Gegenwart, November, 1913.
2. Rosenstein, P. Autodrainage of Ascites into the Bladder, Zentralblatt f. Chirurgie, February, 1914.
3. Vitry, G., and Sizary, A. Autotherapy of Chirrhosis with Ascites, Revue de Médecine, Paris, February, 1913.
4. Kumaris, J. Treatment of Ascites, Zentralblatt f. Chirurgie December, 1913.
5. Tavel, E. Subcutaneous Drainage of Ascites, Correspondenz-blatt f. Schweizer Aerzte, August 10, 1911, No. 23.
6. Perinoff. Permanent Dráinage of Ascitic Fluid into Subcutaneous Cellular Tissue, Archives Générales de Chirurgie, November, 1913.
7. Franke, F. Versuche mit Dauerdrainage bei Ascites, Archiv f. klinische Chirurgie, 1912, xcviii.
8. Henschen, K. Condom for Draining Ascites, Centralblatt f. Chirurgie, January, 1913.
9. Schepelmann, E. Virchows Archiv, November, 1913.
10. Oberst, A. Zur Dauerdrainage bei Ascites, Zentralblatt f. Chirurgie, September 12, 1914, No. 37, p. 1465.

DISCUSSION

DR. C. E. CALDWELL, Cincinnati, Ohio.—I have been much interested in this case of ascites related by the essayist. I did the Talma operation without any ultimate success on a number of occasions. In one case, however, having despaired of any results, the woman filling up rapidly with fluid, I opened her up and drained the gall-bladder, and much to my astonishment, with drainage of the gall-bladder, the ascites disappeared. She lived a number of weeks, but she was pretty well exhausted, and I just offer this as an individual experience of the results of drainage of the gall-bladder in cases of this kind. It is my only experience, and my excuse for offering it is to elicit some experience from some other members of the Association in that respect, whether they have in these cases drained the gall-bladder, and whether they have obtained any results from such treatment.

DR. F. W. PARHAM, New Orleans, Louisiana.—I remember some years ago the subject was brought up in a discussion before this Association in a paper by Dr. Maurice Richardson, in which he reported a case, stating he had been impressed with the possibilities of surgery in cirrhosis of the liver. In the discussion that followed the reading of the paper, Dr. Matas, I remember, called attention to the Naroth operation which we have been following now for some years, where it was considered likely that any operation will do good in an ascites due to cirrhosis. This is a very simple procedure; it can be done under local anesthesia without any difficulty, and simply consists of taking the omentum and suturing it somewhere in the abdominal wall, and in the course of a few weeks it will be noticed that the veins at that point enlarge materially, and it is evident from the disappearance or non-recurrence of the fluid that a distinct improvement has been produced. I call attention to this method again because it is one of the simple procedures which can be carried out where the Talma and other extensive operations would not be suited to certain cases.

Dr. J. Shelton Horsley, Richmond, Virginia.—Dr. Kirchner's paper is very interesting, but I would like to ask if he expects the absorption of ascitic fluid to take place through the lymphatics solely, or if there is no provision for absorption by the veins, as in the Talma operation? The method of draining hydrocephalus into the lymphatics has been unsuccessful because in the course of time connective tissue forms along the drainage tract and blocks off the lymphatics and the pressure required to force fluid into them is too great. Theoretically, it would seem that a somewhat similar condition would obtain in the abdomen.

Dr. William R. Jackson, Mobile, Alabama.—Ascites is not due always, or in the majority of cases, to cirrhosis of the liver or to venous obstruction. Clinical observation teaches that ascites is due to a certain obstruction in the circulation somewhere in the peritoneum. We see it from miliary tuberculosis of the peritoneum very often; we see it in papillomatous disease of the ovary, carcinoma of the ovary produces an enormous ascites. The Talma operation works very well if it is a venous obstruction, but I imagine this operation that has been described equalizes the transudate or lymph and is applicable to almost any condition causing it.

Dr. Walter C. G. Kirchner, St. Louis, Missouri (closing).—Dr. Jackson has brought out the point of the paper. There are other causes, besides obstruction to the circulation, that produce ascites, and it is to meet such cases that an operation of this type has been devised.

I shall try to answer some of the questions that were asked, and to clear up some of the points that were brought out in the paper. The technic of the operation is very simple. Under local anesthesia, an elliptical incision is made, and the subcutaneous tissue, owing to the abdominal distension, separates in this fashion (indicating), so that we have this island of skin. One-half of this island of skin is loosened up, and the subcutaneous tissue removed. The cavity having been opened, sutures are placed at either corner of this flap, and this tongue shaped arrangement is put into the peritoneal cavity, where it is retained by suturing. These sutures (indicating) represent the method of closing the wound. The skin margins being approximated, there is then a single line of sutures, and the flap and pedicle are thus buried. We know that only like tissues will unite, and the skin being tucked into the peritoneal cavity prevents adhesions, and a patient subcutaneous opening is left. In a measure the buried pedicle acts as a foreign body, and this is well illustrated in one case in which the pedicle portion came through the healed wound as any foreign body would. Therefore, to prevent this, I modified the technic in that I denuded this pedicle by shaving off the epidermis, and the procedure resulted in firm adhesions.

There is still left the channel from the subcutaneous tissue into the peritoneal cavity through which peritoneal fluid may enter the subcutaneous tissue. In other words, the patient is giving himself what might be called "internal hypodermoclysis." It is to meet those cases of cirrhosis of the liver that are severe, and other cases in which there is ascites, that the operation that I have described has been devised, and the procedure being so simple, and one in which foreign bodies are avoided, I desired to call this method to the attention of the members of the Association.

DR. WATTS.—How long did you make the flap?

DR. KIRCHNER.—Four or five inches long.

DR. WATTS.—How wide?

DR. KIRCHNER.—About two fingers wide.

DR. WATTS.—How long does it drain?

DR. KIRCHNER.—In one case it is still draining after perhaps six months. After an operation of that type the lower abdomen becomes edematous. We get a favorable result if the patient's vital power is not too low, and when the kidneys are still functioning properly. There is then considerable increase in the urinary output, and it is probable that through this means excessive fluid is eliminated.

GIANT URETERAL CALCULUS; ANOMALOUS DEVELOPMENT OF THE GENITO-URINARY TRACT

By Irvin Abell, A.M., M.D., F.A.C.S.
Louisville, Kentucky

The following two recently observed cases seem to possess sufficient interest to warrant detailed report; the first, because of the size of the ureteral calculus which was removed; the second, on account of the anomalous development of the genito-urinary tract.

CASE 1.—F. E. B., male, white; aged thirty-two years; occupation, linotype operator. Date of first observation, August 17, 1915. The patient presented a negative personal history as regards any acute severe illness and also venereal infection. He applied to his physician for relief of "pain in his back," which had then been present for about ten days. He stated that he had first noted pain in the left lumbar region at the age of eighteen, that it had recurred at frequent intervals during the next three or four years, the attacks then becoming more irregular. At the age of twenty-eight pain of similar character was noted in the right lumbar region. Since then the attacks have appeared on the average of once per month. The pain has never been sufficiently severe to require the administration of an opiate to secure relief, and until the present attack had not persisted longer than one or two days. Relief was usually obtained by rest in bed, supplemented by a hot bath or the application of a hot water-bottle. He also stated that, excepting in the last attack, relief from pain was always secured by indulgence in sexual intercourse. Between attacks the urinary frequency was four to five times daily; during an attack once to twice daily. Blood had been noted in the urine on a number of occasions. The present attack of pain began ten days previously, and had continued without remission.

Examination. Patient rather thin, but well developed and muscular; pulse, 100, temperature 100.2° F., heart and lungs normal; right kidney easily palpable, enlarged and quite tender, apparently being as large as a medium-sized grapefruit. The left kidney was not palpable, and there was no tenderness on that side. The urine was muddy in color, acid in reaction, specific gravity 1020; it contained a marked trace of albumin, occasional blood- and pus-cells, calcium oxalate crystals, amorphous phosphates, a moderate number of bacteria.

Cystoscopy revealed a practically normal bladder. The left ureteral orifice was normal in appearance and easily admitted the catheter which was introduced without difficulty into the renal pelvis. The orifice of the right ureter was edematous, and 2.5 cm. from the entrance the catheter encountered an obstruction imparting a sensation like that obtained by contact of the sound with a calculus. Urine from the left kidney showed absence of albumin and pus, the presence of an occasional blood-cell. The blood-count was normal.

Radiography revealed the presence of two calculi, one in the pelvic portion of each ureter. The one in the left ureter was of moderate size, while that in the right ureter practically extended from the sacro-iliac joint to the meatus. Diagnosis: bilateral ureteral calculi with the right-sided hydronephrosis.

Operation, August 19, 1915. Gridiron incisions were made upon both sides, each being enlarged downward by incising the rectus sheath. The peritoneum was displaced mesially, and the ureters approached extraperitoneally. Considerable fibrolipomatous thickening was found about the right ureter, and it was separated with difficulty from

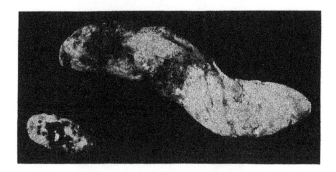

FIG. 1.—Calculi, actual size, Case 1; larger one 7.5 cm. in length, 7 cm. in circumference, weight 24 gms.

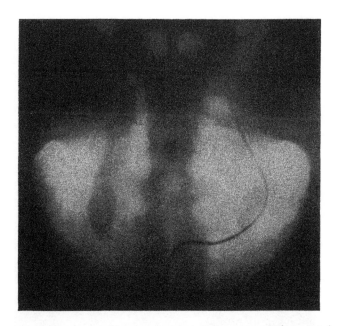

FIG. 2.—Skiagram of Case 1 showing large stone filling pelvic portion of right ureter; catheter in left ureter with stone in pelvic portion of ureter.

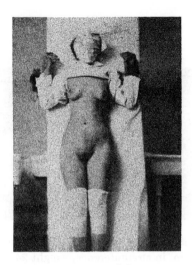

Fig. 3.—Case 2. Well-developed feminine figure; absence of vagina, uterus, tubes, and ovaries; single kidney located in pelvis.

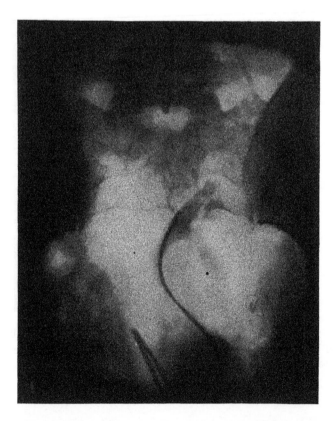

Fig. 4.—Pyelogram. Kidney in front and to left of sacrum; hilum looking internally, convex border externally.

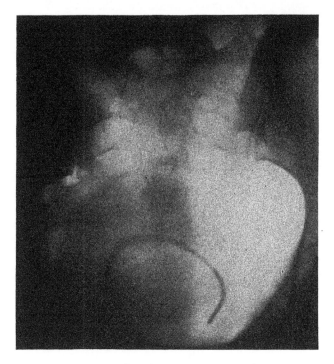

Fɪɢ. 5.—Cystogram, showing interference by kidney with normal rounded outline in distention.

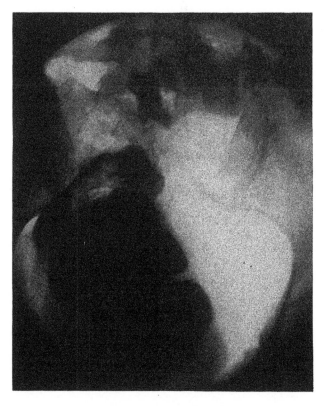

Fɪɢ. 6.—Showing rectum traversing right side of pelvis, Case 2.

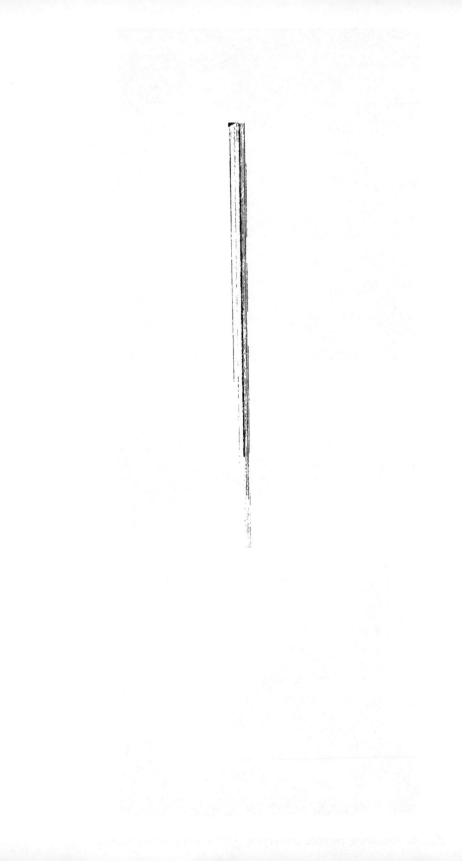

the surrounding structures. It was incised at a point cor-responding to the brim of the pelvis, and the calculus removed by traction. A similar procedure was employed upon the left side, both ureteral incisions being closed by interrupted sutures of catgut. Each external wound was drained with a small strip of rubber sheeting.

The postoperative history was uneventful, the patient returning to his work at the end of the third week. The calculus removed from the right ureter was oblong in shape, with a distinct beak or curve at either extremity; it meas-ured 7.5 cm. in length, 7 cm. in circumference at its largest part and weighed 24 gms. The left stone was more ovoid and weighed 2 gms. The small calculus was composed of carbonate of calcium, the larger one was phosphatic in character.

The points of interest aside from the size of the calculus are bilateral pelvic ureteral calculi, an absence of colic indi-cating ureteral descent, the symptoms being due to urinary retention with hydro-ureter and hydronephrosis; the pos-sibilities of intra-ureteral calculous growth on lodged nuclei of renal origin, an absence of bladder frequency or pain with practically normal appearance of mucosa, and the fibrolipo-matous thickening around the pelvic portion of right ureter comparable to the induration observed in the fatty capsule of the kidney in calculous disease of long standing.

Desguin describes a male aged thirty-four years who had suffered from paroxysms of abdominal pain since his fourth year. The patient was observed in an acute attack, and the diagnosis was between appendicitis and ureteral calculus. Abdominal incision to right of the rectus muscle; right ureteral calculus removed, irregularly triangular in shape, 26 by 23 mm., and weighing 10 gms.

Baker refers to a male aged twenty-four years, by whom he was consulted because of supposed prostatic disease, which improved under appropriate treatment, although pus in the urine persisted. An attack of ureteral colic two months later was attributed to extension of infection, but radiography revealed a concretion just above the vesico-ureteral orifice. A ureteral calculus weighing 94 grains was removed by operation.

Parker performed suprapubic cystotomy and removed a ureteral calculus weighing over three-fourths of an ounce. The patient had complained of no urinary symptoms at any time, the inconvenience suffered being referred entirely to the rectum through which the calculus was originally felt.

Bovée removed an unusually large ureteral calculus by transperitoneal ureter-lithotomy. The stone measured 2.75 by 1.75 by 1.15 inches and weighed 1310 grains. It was kidney-shaped, one extremity larger than the other, grayish in color, with rough surfaces.

Two cases of giant calculi are reported by Buerger: (a) A male aged twenty-six years presenting indefinite symptoms. Enormous ureteral calculus; hydro-ureter, ureteritis ureteral stenosis; hydronephrosis. Calculus more than four inches in length, with a bulbous extremity pointing downward at level of the spine of the ischium. The shape was sinuous, varying from 6 mm. to about 1 cm. in diameter. (b) A male aged fifty-five years; urinary symptoms ten years duration. Enormous ureteral calculus; hydro-ureter hydronephrosis. Calculus irregularly ovoid with one pointed extremity, measuring 2.125 inches in length by 1.125 inches in width at its superior pole.

Specklin describes a male, aged forty-eight years, from whom an enormous left ureteral calculus was removed. Urinary symptoms of many years duration. Nephrectomy and ureterectomy. Curved or "elbow-shaped" calculus weighed 51 gms., 11 cm. long from end to end, total length along outer curve 12 cm., knob-like projection in upper portion of middle third. In the literature he was able to find the following ureteral concretions of similar size: Fedcroff, length, 19 cm., weight, 52 gms.; Rovsing, length, 18 cm., width of a bean; Israel, two cases (a) length 13 cm., circumference, 9 cm., weight, 54.4 gms.; (b) length,

17 cm., circumference, 9 cm.; Pozzi, weight, 34.5 gms.; Lloyd, length, 52 inches, circumference, 22 inches.

In a case recorded by Morris the calculus was nearly six inches in length; in one of Gibson's cases the stone was half an inch in diameter and nearly round.

CASE 2.—P. G., female, white, aged nineteen years. Date of first observation, September 3, 1915. The patient had been married three years, but had never been pregnant, nor had she ever menstruated. There was no history of acute illness until the present. Ten days previously she had an attack of acute pain in the lower abdomen accompanied by nausea and vomiting. The abdomen became distended and tender, the temperature varying from 101° to 103.5° F., pulse 110 to 120. The lesion was regarded by the attending physician as appendicitis. At the end of a week the symptoms had practically subsided, and she was able to leave her bed.

On September 2 the patient experienced another attack of acute abdominal pain which was also accompanied by nausea and vomiting, and she was admitted to the St. Joseph Infirmary, September 3, with a pulse of 120 and temperature of 103° F. Her abdomen was found markedly distended and exquisite tenderness was elicited over the lower zone. While her figure was typically feminine, with well-developed mammæ and wide pelvis, examination showed absence of the vagina, although the external genitals were normal in appearance. The urethra admitted the index finger, the tip entering the bladder sphincter with difficulty. Rectal examination revealed an exquisitely tender pelvic mass located chiefly on the left side. The urine was acid in reaction, there was a trace of albumin, slight sediment, a few blood-cells, many pus-cells, and rod-shaped bacilli. The blood-count showed hemoglobin, 90 per cent., white cells, 30,500, with polynuclear neutrophile, 82 per cent.

From the history and the clinical findings, the most probable explanation of the pelvic mass was thought to be retained and infected menstrual secretion. Acting upon this hypothesis the abdomen was opened in the median line, and the tumor found to be a pelvic kidney situated in front and to the left of the sacro-iliac synchondrosis. Examination of both lumbar regions revealed no evidence of a second kidney. No uterus, tubes, ovaries, nor remnants of the same, could be detected. It was evident from the operative findings that the lesion was a pyelitis in the single pelvic kidney. The subsequent treatment consisted of the ordinary measures employed in such cases.

Three weeks later catheterized specimens of urine from the ureter and the bladder were found negative upon culture. Radiography after injecting the bladder and kidney with collargol showed the renal pelvis practically normal in size and shape, with one ureter which was between three and four inches in length. The ureter entered the bladder in the usual situation. No evidence of a right ureteral orifice could be found. A cystogram with the bladder in moderate distention showed that it pressed upon the kidney and that the latter produced a change in the contour as evidenced by variation in the normal rounded outline. The rectum was situated in the right side of the pelvis, and after being filled with barium was readily observed in the x-ray plate. Subsequent reports indicate that there has been no recurrence of the pyelitis.

Anders claims that congenital absence of the kidney is an exceedingly rare anomaly, and cites one case of this character. By averaging available figures, in 92,690 autopsies, the expectation of congenital single kidney was one in 1817. Since the publication of Moore's compilation (1898) he had found in the literature 60 cases of single kidney, which in addition to the 225 cases previously collected by Ballowitz and Moore, made a total of 285. In the personal observation cited, the left kidney, renal artery, vein, ureter, and suprarenal body were absent. He suggests that unquestionably nephrolithiasis is attended with peculiar danger to life in cases of single kidney where the ureter is occluded by calculi. It is important to remember that the vesico-ureteral orifice is generally absent on the side of the missing kidney. Cystoscopy should be supplemented by ureteral catheterization where two ureteral orifices exist, since in a small percentage of cases of congenital kidney a rudimentary ureter is present. The importance of a single kidney, from a surgical standpoint, can scarcely be overemphasized. According to Anders, advanced lesions of chronic nephritis were found in thirty-two of the fatal cases, or 42.3 per cent.; undoubtedly either acute or chronic nephritis in cases of renal agenesis gives a less hopeful outlook than when developing under normal conditions, *i. e.*, bilaterally.

Mayo states that a single kidney occurs more frequently in males, whereas the so-called horseshoe kidney is encountered oftener in females. Among thirty-six cases of gross renal and ureteral anomalies observed in the Mayo clinic during a period of five years, twelve were of the horseshoe variety and six of the single type.

Thomas reports a case of pelvic kidney in a married woman, aged thirty-two years, diagnosed prior to operation for pelvic diseases. The vagina was about an inch in depth, and no uterus as discoverable upon palpation. The patient had never menstruated, but suffered ovarian pain every two months. A rounded, tender mass the size of an orange was detected in the left fossa. There had been frequent attacks of urinary frequency during the last year. The patient complained of abdominal pain, especially on the left side. Cystoscopy showed the urethra and bladder normal. Left ureteral catheter arrested 2.25 inches from bladder; right side apparently normal; urine from both sides practically the same. Radiography after double injection of colloidal silver showed pelvis of hydronephrotic kidney low in left bony pelvis. The ureter was 3.5 to 4.5 inches in length.

Cullen mentions a girl, aged seventeen years, who had never menstruated. Inspection revealed absence of the vagina; rectal examination disclosed a hard, irregular mass filling right half of pelvis, thought to be uterus with retained menstrual fluid. Celiotomy: right pelvic kidney, uterus, and left kidney absent; prolapse of tubes and ovaries in inguinal regions.

Bissell reports the successful reimplantation of a right pelvic kidney in a female aged forty-one years. When observed the patient was about eight months advanced in uterogestation; premature labor was induced, and after some delay an asphyxiated child delivered. One month later the pelvic kidney was reimplanted in its normal situation.

During routine examination of the body of a male, aged thirty years, who died of valvular cardiac disease, Ward found no trace of the right kidney. The left kidney was twice ordinary size, with normal pelvis and ureter.

At autopsy upon the body of a female, aged thirty-eight years, who died following a protracted debauch, Glazebrook found a single right kidney. There were two pelves and a single bifurcated ureter. The left kidney and ureter were absent. The right ureter below the bifurcation was normal in size and communicated with the bladder in the proper situation.

Stengel observed at autopsy a single kidney with two ureters, and suggested that the surgeon in such a case after using the catheter might be deceived in thinking there were two kidneys and undertake an operation, thus the only kidney might be removed. In fact, a case of this character was operated upon by Polk of New York (1882), the pelvic mass removed being the right kidney. The patient lived thirteen days with complete anuria, and at autopsy it was found that this was the only kidney.

Mayer and Nelkin cite a case in which there occurred suparietal traumatic rupture of a solitary right kidney. No evidence of the left kidney could be found, although there were two ureters opening into the bladder in the normal situations. The patient died thirty-six hours after operation. Necropsy revealed congenital absence of left kidney; traumatic rupture of right kidney; retroperitoneal hematoma; acute nephritis; kidney infarcts.

Secher describes the necropsy findings in a child without left kidney or ureter, the suprarenal gland being unusually large; the genital organs were also asymmetrical. He states that while about three hundred cases of single kidney have been reported in the literature of the world, these figures are misleading since distinction between total aplasia and atrophy is not always clear. The kidney was single in .7 of 8150 cadavers examined, *i. e.*, once in every 1164 cases. According to the records the anomaly occurs twice as frequently in males as in females, and the left kidney is usually missing. The abdominal vessels and genital organs ordinarily display more or less deformity in such cases.

REFERENCES

GIANT CALCULUS

Baker.   Jour. Am. Med. Assn., 1912, May 11.
Bovee.   Washington M. Ann., 1905, September.
Buerger.   N. Y. M. J., 1914, December 5.
Desguin.   Cited in Medicine, 1899, September.
Federoff.   Cited by Specklin, loc. cit.
Gibbon.   Surg. Gynec. and Obst., 1908, vi, 483.
Israel.   Cited by Specklin, loc. cit.
Lloyd.   Cited by Specklin, loc. cit.
Morris.   Cited by Gibbon, loc. cit.
Parker.   Brit. Med. Jour., 1906, July 21.
Pozzi.   Cited by Specklin, loc. cit.
Rovsing.   Cited by Specklin, loc. cit.
Specklin.   Am. Jour. Urol., 1915, July.

PELVIC KIDNEY

Anders.   N. Y. Med. Jour., 1910, March 12.
Bissell.   Surg., Gynec. and Obst., 1910, xi, 66.
Cullen.   Surg., Gynec. and Obst., 1910, xi, 73.
Glazebrook.   N. Y. Med. Jour., 1905, July 22.
Mayer-Nelkin.   Jour. Am. Med. Assn., October 14, 1911.
Mayo.   International Abs. Surg., April, 1913.
Polk.   Cited by Cullen, loc. cit.
Secher.   Quoted in Jour. Am. Med. Assn., February 27, 1915.
Stengel.   N. Y. Med. Jour., 1910, March 12.
Thomas.   Am. Jour. Urol., 1914, February.
Ward.   Brit. Med Jour , 1908, April 28.

DISCUSSION

DR. THOMAS S. CULLEN, Baltimore, Md.—In connection
with Dr. Abell's paper I would like to mention a case of unilateral pelvic kidney, reported by Dr. William Polk of New
York. After Dr. Polk had removed this kidney it was found
that it was the only one she had. The patient lived if I remember
right for thirteen days. Later Dr. Polk published this case in
order that other surgeons might not be in the future place
in such an uncomfortable position. It is a pleasure to be a
member of a society which has men of such candid and sterling
qualities enrolled in its membership.

DR. FRANK D. SMYTHE, Memphis.—I was very much interested in the case reported by Dr. Abell and congratulate him
upon the fortunate outcome of his case.

I am anxious to know from the Fellows just what their
experience has been in suturing of ureteral slits, made for the
purpose of removing stones, especially small stones.

My present custom is to remove the stone, insert a tube for
drainage and make no attempt to suture the slit. On two
occasions I sutured the ureter. The suturing was difficult to
do and the results not satisfactory—that is, leakage occurred.
So the effort to do more than extract the stone and provide for
drainage was abandoned. Since adopting that plan the cases
operated upon have gotten along nicely.

The amount of urine escaping through the tube is considerable for a few days but by the end of the week, and sometimes
before, it has ceased altogether.

Experience has convinced me that patients thus treated
have done better and suffered less than those where an attempt
was made to suture the slit. And I think the danger from
stricture under the do-nothing plan is decidedly less than
where suturing of the slit is done after removal of the stone,
especially the small ones. In operating for large stones the
technic should be modified to meet the indications.

During the performance of a pelvic or abdominal operation,
should the ureter suffer injury or be severed, it should at once
be sutured or anastomosed. In ureteral cases high up my preference is to let it alone.

I would like to hear from some of the Fellows who have had
experience in this kind of work as to their views and their

method of dealing with slits in the ureter after stone has been removed.

DR. JAMES E. MOORE, Minneapolis, Minnesota.—In reference to the point just made by Dr. Smythe, I might say that years ago, when I did my first operation for stone in the ureter, I was very careful to close a minute opening in the ureter. I found, however, I had some dribbling of urine from my wound, and it was necessary to prepare for that by introducing a tube from the surface down to the point of operation. In later years I have grown more indifferent to the suture, and now do not suture, and my patients have done just as well and the operation has been done in a shorter time. There is no advantage in the ordinary case by suturing an opening in the ureter.

DR. IRVIN ABELL, Louisville, Kentucky (closing).—In answer to Dr. Smythe, I will say that in the fourteen cases of pelvic ureteral stones I have had occasion to operate on, the ureteral incisions have all been sutured with interrupted catgut sutures, and the majority of them have shown no external drainage of urine.

DR. SMYTHE.—Mine always drained urine.

ADENOMYOMA OF THE ROUND LIGAMENT AND INCARCERATED OMENTUM IN AN INGUINAL HERNIA, TOGETHER FORMING ONE TUMOR

By THOMAS S. CULLEN, M.B., F.A.C.S.

Baltimore, Maryland

FOR many years isolated cases of adenomyoma of the uterus have been recorded, but it was not until the epoch-making monograph on the subject published by von Recklinghausen that we were given a thoroughly comprehensive picture of this condition. In March, 1895, I reported my first case of adenomyoma of the uterus, before the Johns Hopkins Medical Society, since then I have been much interested in adenomyomata.[1]

In 1896 it fell to my lot to record the first case of adenomyoma of the round ligament. At this time I sent Professor von Recklinghausen a slide from the round-ligament tumor and when writing me a short time later he said that he had shown my section before the Naturforscher Versammlung

---

[1] Cullen, Thomas S., Adenomyoma of the Round Ligament, Johns Hopkins Hosp. Bull., 1896, May and June, Nos., 62 and 63; Adenomyoma uteri diffusum benignum, Johns Hopkins Hosp. Reports, 1896, vi; Further Remarks on Adenomyoma of the Round Ligament, Johns Hopkins Hosp. Bull., 1898, No. 87 (June); Adenomyoma des Uterus, Verlag von August Hirschwald, Berlin, 1903; Adenomyoma of the Uterus, 1908; Adenomyoma of the Uterus, Jour. Am. Med. Assn., 1908, January, i, 107; Umbilical Tumors Containing Uterine Mucosa or Remnants of Mueller's Ducts, Surg., Gynec. and Obst., May, 1912, p. 479; Adenomyoma of the Rectovaginal Septum, Jour. Am. Med. Assn., 1914, lxii, 835.

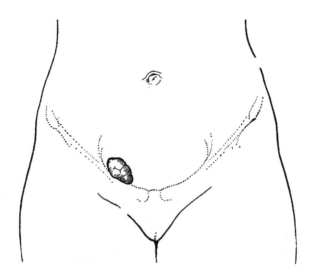

Fig. 1.—Adenomyoma of the round ligament and incarcerated omentum contained in an inguinal hernia, together forming one nodule. Gyn.-Path. No. 19,018. The nodule lay a little above Poupart's ligament. It was 4 cm. long, 2 cm. broad, and somewhat lobulated. It was perceptibly larger at each menstrual period. At operation the upper part of the tumor was found to be very dense and intimately blended with the fascia. It contained cyst spaces, some of which were filled with chocolate-colored fluid. The lower portion of the nodule consisted of omentum which had emerged at or near the internal inguinal ring. The histological appearances are shown in Figs. 2, 3, and 4.

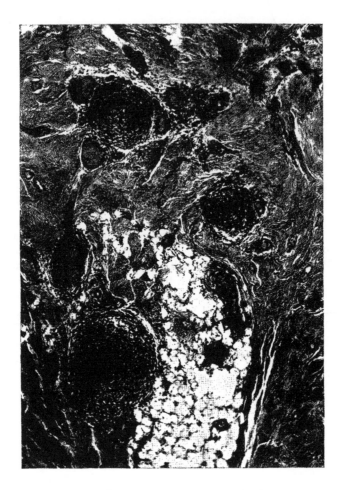

F<small>IG</small>. 2.—Apparently discrete myomatous nodules in an adenomyoma of the round ligament. Gyn.-Path. No. 19,018. The greater part of the specimen stains diffusely. It consists chiefly of fibrous tissue and contains non-striped muscle. It will be noted that the adipose tissue at the bottom is being irregularly replaced by fibrous tissue. There are three distinct areas that have a whorled appearance. They form a rough triangle in the picture. These areas are very cellular, and closely resemble young myomata. They may possibly, however, be very cellular areas of the characteristic stroma that usually surrounds uterine glands.

at their Frankfurt meeting. Since that time quite a number of adenomyomata of the round ligament have been detected. When analyzing the umbilical tumors recorded in the literature, I encountered quite a number that had been variously diagnosed. These tumors were found only in women, tended to swell at the menstrual period, and occasionally discharged a little blood at the period. On section some of them contained small spaces filled with old blood. These tumors proved to be adenomyomata of the umbilicus. To Goddard belongs the credit for first properly interpreting these tumors.

More recently adenomyoma of the rectovaginal septum has been noted. Cuthbert, Lockyer and Jessup have each recorded two cases and I have had four. In 1899 my colleague, Dr. William W. Russell,[1] reported a case in which a large amount of uterine mucosa was found in the hilum of the ovary. In this instance, however, no myoma existed.

From the foregoing it will be seen that we may find adenomyoma in the uterus, round ligaments, rectovaginal septum, or in small umbilical tumors.

Nearly three years ago I encountered another adenomyoma of the round ligament. Of this case I herewith give a brief report:

Mrs. J. Q. J., aged forty-three years, was referred to me by Dr. N. C. Trout, of Fairfield, Pa., and admitted to the Church Home and Infirmary March 6, 1913. She had complained of a lump in her groin for several years. This was very firm and appeared to be cystic. It was about 4 cm. long, 2 cm. broad, and somewhat lobulated (Fig. 1). She also complained of pain in the appendix region.

Operation. I first made a median incision and found the rectum firmly adherent to the left ovary over a considerable area. The adhesions were gradually loosened and the raw area on the bowel was closed. The lumen was not injured.

[1] Russell, William W., Aberrant Portions of the Muellerian Duct Found in an Ovary, Johns Hopkins Hosp. Bull., 1899, x, 8.

I then examined the omentum and found that it passed down through a hernial opening near the right internal inguinal ring and then directly out into the adipose tissue of the anterior abdominal wall. The omentum was cut off at the internal ring, tied, and pushed out of the way. The extraperitoneal portion of the omentum was left undisturbed. The peritoneum over the internal ring was now closed from within. I then removed the appendix which showed evidence of old inflammation, there being present adhesions passing off from it in various directions.

After closing the abdomen I made an incision over the tumor in the right inguinal region. This tumor was adherent to the skin. The skin was dissected back and the mass literally cut away from the fascia. There were numerous cysts, some filled with clear contents, others with a slightly turbid fluid, and quite a number with chocolate-colored fluid, strongly suggesting adenomyoma. Adenomyoma was considered probable, some stress being laid upon the declaration of the patient that the lump appeared to increase in size at each menstrual period. After dissecting away the lower portion of the tumor, which was also adherent to the fascia, I now lifted up the omentum from the hernial opening. The hole left near the internal ring was slit-like in form, about 1 cm. long and 4 mm. broad. It was closed with kangaroo tendon. To dissect back the fascia, and do an orthodox operation was out of the question, because of the large defect that would have been left. At most points good firm scar-tissue existed. I closed the wound with through-and-through silkworm-gut sutures; accurate skin approximation was made with fine black silk. The lower angle of the wound was drained with protective. The patient made a good recovery.

On December 8, 1915, Dr. Trout wrote me, saying that he had just spoken to the patient. She had had no return of the trouble, was free from pain, and had gained twenty-pounds.

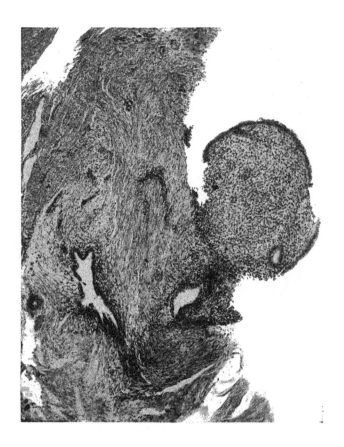

FIG. 3.—Adenomyoma of the round ligament. Gyn.-Path. No.
19,018. The solid portion of the specimen consists of non-striped
muscle and fibrous tissue. A little below the centre of the field is a
gland lined with one layer of cylindrical epithelium. In some places it
is separated from the tumor proper by a definite stroma. Projecting
from the surface on the right of the specimen is a dome-shaped mass
of tissue very rich in cells with oval nuclei. This tissue is identical in
every way with the characteristic stroma of the uterine mucosa. In
the lower part it contains a small gland lined with one layer of cylindrical epithelium. The surface of this dome-shaped mass of stroma
is covered over with one layer of cylindrical epithelium. The entire
picture is that of a typical adenomyoma. The dome-shaped mass of
mucosa evidently projected into one of the cyst cavities noted macroscopically.

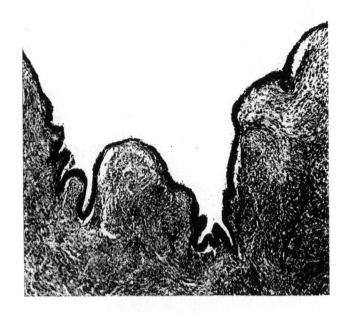

FIG. 4.—The lining of a cyst in an adenomyoma of the round ligament. Gyn.-Path. No. 19,018. The tumor consists of fibrous tissue
and non-striped muscle. The inner surface of this cyst was undulating
and had numerous depressions running off from it. These depressions
may with equal propriety be described as glands. The cyst is lined with
one layer of cylindrical epithelium, which at the more prominent or
exposed points has become cuboidal.

Gyn.-Path. No. 19,018. The outlying portion of the tumor consisted of fat with here and there yellowish or brownish pigmentation, suggesting the pigment of old hemorrhage. The central portion of the tumor closely resembled fibrous tissue. It had cystic spaces scattered throughout it. The contents of these varied, as noted above, some being clear, others turbid, and some being filled with chocolate-like material.

Histological examination. The outlying portion of the specimen consisted of adipose tissue. As one passed toward the tumor, the fat was gradually and irregularly replaced by fibrous tissue, which in many places had undergone almost complete hyaline transformation. Scattered here and there throughout the fibrous tissue were large or small areas of non-striped muscle. Several very small discrete myomata were also noted (Fig. 2). At numerous points in the tumor were glands, tubular or round, and lined with one layer of cylindrical epithelium (Fig. 3). Some of the glands lay in direct contact with the fibrous tissue or muscle; others were separated from the tumor by the characteristic stroma of the mucosa. The cyst spaces noted macroscopically were lined with one layer of cylindrical epithelium (Fig. 4).

From the description it is perfectly clear that this was an adenomyoma of the round ligament associated with a large amount of fibrous tissue. From a clinical standpoint the coexistence of a small inguinal hernia with incarcerated omentum and an adenomyoma of the round ligament is very interesting. The increase in size of the inguinal nodule at the period naturally made me suspicious of adenomyoma, and the indications supplied by the presence of old pigment in the fat at operation, coupled with the fact that some cysts contained chocolate-like material, justified a tentative diagnosis that the tumor was an adenomyoma even before the microscopic examination. I have not as yet gone over the recent literature, but do not know of any other case in which an inguinal hernia and an adenomyoma were found in the same hernial protrusion.

DISCUSSION

Dr. William R. Jackson, Mobile, Alabama.—Personally, I wish to thank Dr. Cullen for relating these two interesting cases, one of adenomyoma of the round ligament, and the other tuberculosis of the cervix. Adenomyoma of the round ligament is one of the most unusual forms of. tumor we have in this locality. We can understand how we can have a myoma of the round ligament because the round ligament primarily and histologically consists of myomatous tissue, or muscular tissue. Is not that so, Dr. Cullen?

Dr. Cullen.—Yes.

Dr. Jackson.—Therefore, we can understand the matrix of the cells of the myomatous but not of the adenomatous part. We have to take it for granted that the matrix was displaced from some portion of the epithelial cells of the intestine in early embryonic life according to the theory of Cohnheim. The matrix was primarily an adenomatous cell from the intestinal tract or the genito-urinary tract with muscular cells that are non-striated. This also tends to prove—many authors to the contrary notwithstanding—that Cohnheim's theory does explain the origin of many of these tumors.

The first case is more interesting than the one of secondary tuberculosis of the cervix, which may come from other parts of the body by embolic infection.

CYSTS OF THE APPENDIX

By John T. Moore, A.M., M.D., F.A.C.S.

Houston, Texas

During the present year (1914) I have operated upon a patient with a cyst of the appendix, of the pseudomyxomatous type, that I thought might possibly be of sufficient interest to place upon record.

I had previously operated upon two others which I shall also record. Through the courtesy of Dr. Gavin Hamilton I am enabled to report a fourth case operated upon by him. This is one of the largest cysts reported. This year (1915) I have had a fifth case of the type mentioned by Matas (*Trans. Southern Surgical and Gynecological Association,* 1915).

One would be inclined to think that cysts of the appendix ought to be of very frequent occurrence, but if we are to judge from our own experience, and that of the reported cases, the condition is not very common. Castle (*Annals of Surgery,* 61, p. 582) says that in the analysis of 13,158 postmortems, 29 cases of cystic appendix were found—0.2 per cent.

The literature on appendicitis is voluminous, yet up to 1909 J. A. Kelly was able to collect and report only 68 cases of cyst of the appendix.

Quite a number of other cases[1] have been reported since

---

[1] Through the courtesy of Dr. George E. Dodge, who has made a complete study of the cases in the literature, I am permitted to present 142 cases collected by him, and our own cases and that of Dr. A. B. Small, making in all 148 cases to date.

then and I desire, if possible, to present the complete number up to 1916.

The earlier descriptions of cysts of the appendix seemed to have considered them a hydrops of empyema.

Virchow is said to have been the first who described and directed attention to the cystic conditions of the appendix; he having reported a case of colloid degeneration of the organ.

Ferre, a French writer, was the first to apply the term *retention cyst* to these chronically occluded, sacculated appendices.

While the later writers use various terms in speaking of the condition they all have the same condition in mind, *i. e.*, a cystic one.

I think they may be considered according to Adami's view, as true retention cysts, *i. e.*, they are glandular cysts of postnatal origin.

These cysts all arise through the obstruction of the ducts of tubular glands.

The same character of cyst is found where the intestinal follicles become blocked from any reason, and the cells continue to secrete a mucoid material which may more and more enlarge the size of the tumor. The cyst wall thickens by hypertrophy of the muscle, or by the addition of the inflammatory material.

Matas suggests that the cyst reported by him as a retroperitoneal cyst attached to the appendix was an outgrowth of an embryologic relic connected with the mesentery. Possibly the development of an original lymphangioma cavernosum of the mesentery.

The structure and behavior of the appendix are strongly suggestive that this organ has a function to perform in our economy even at this stage of our development.

Most physiologists and anatomists are agreed that the appendix did at one time in our development occupy a very important position in the digestive tract. Though the human being seems to get along quite well without it, yet it might be that we do better with it.

Its glandular structure suggests the addition of a secretion to the contents of the cecum, while its richness in lymphoid tissue argues for some protective function.

Radiologists have demonstrated that it receives and expels such emulsions as are used in x-ray examinations of the intestines. It evidently fills and empties itself of the intestinal contents provided the lumen is normal in size, or there are no kinks of any kind to cause an obstruction. It is evident that it has the same or similar peristaltic waves as the intestines, hence the appendiceal cramps when it is trying to expel a concretion or a foreign body.

Its present size, shape and relation to the ileum and colon make it especially weak in its own defense.

The small canal, its abundant secretion, its rich lymphoid tissue, its strong musculature, and its shortened mesentery, render its own existence full of hazard.

Hence, if it escapes destruction by the usually acute processes that cause gangrene or suppuration it may receive such wounds that it becomes a hard, fibrous cord, or it may have its lumen blocked and give us a cyst.

Were it not that the retained material in a blocked-up appendix so frequently becomes infected, resulting in suppurative processes, cysts of the organ would be much more frequently found.

Hydrops and empyema of the appendix are more frequent than are the true cysts.

From the above discussion it is seen that two conditions seem to be necessary to cyst formation. (1) A partial or complete blocking of the lumen; (2) the content must be sterile or almost so.

The lumen may be only partly blocked to allow a sufficient pressure to destroy the lining epithelium. But with a communication with the intestines the material is apt to become infected, and thus lead to the formation of a pus appendix with necrosis of its walls. Such cases, as a rule, are too acute to allow cyst formation. The process must be a slower one. The epithelium must be only slowly impaired so that the cells are allowed to functionate somewhat.

These epithelial cells secrete a watery fluid, serum, and mucus which gradually dilate the appendix, causing hypertrophy of its muscular coats, and a degeneration of its mucous coat.

Finally most of the epithelium is destroyed, or possibly only the mucous cells are left and these keep up the secretion of mucus, thus enlarging the cyst until all of the epithelium is ultimately destroyed.

These appendiceal cysts reach quite a large size in a few cases. Most of them, however, rarely reach a size greater than a pecan nut.

SYMPTOMS. A large number of the reported cases of cyst of the appendix were found either at autopsy or while operating for other conditions.

The symptoms are more those of a chronic appendix mischief, or of a slowly growing tumor which can be felt in the region of the cecum.

In Case 1 of our series the marked anemia was the most striking in the patient's condition. There was indigestion, pain and belching of gas, and weakness, but these symptoms are common in chronic appendix mischief.

The symptoms in Case 2 were distinctly those of an acute or subacute appendicular attack.

Case 3 was decidedly the most interesting of these. The history was distinctly that of a slowly growing carcinoma of the colon or cecum. The most prominent symptoms were of obstruction.

Although the gelatinous material had escaped into the abdomen through rupture of the cyst wall, there had been no symptoms of a peritonitis, nor was there any evidence of such a condition. Treves regarded this as a dangerous complication. I am inclined to think that the material is entirely harmless where it is sterile, and most of the cases evidently are so.

In Case 4 (Dr. Hamilton's case) we had a diagnosis made of appendicitis, and the cystic condition of the appendix was not suspected until the tumor was removed. This is a particularly interesting case on account of the cyst being one of the largest of its kind.

Then, again, the case is unusual on account of the death of the patient following an operation so carefully done in a short time, and with but little ether.

Case 5 we feel sure could hardly have been diagnosed anything other than an appendiceal abscess. I did not even suspect a retroperitoneal cyst while operating, as the abscess was clearly caused by a ruptured appendix, and there was no connection between the cyst and the appendix.

Dr. Matas reported the largest cyst of this character, of which I have been able to find a record. It weighed 1580 grams, was multilocular, retroperitoneal and retrocecal, and was not in any way connected with the appendix, only attached to it.

Dr. Willy Meyer (*Annals of Surgery*, lvii, p. 271) reports a giant mucocele which infiltrated the cecum. He resected the lower end of the ileum and one-half of ascending colon.

Dr. Small, of Dallas, showed a specimen smaller than mine, but very similar, in which he resected the colon and part of the ileum (personal communication).

The study of my own case and that of Dr. Small showed such an extensive operation unnecessary, but J. A. Kelly (*Annals of Surgery*, xlix, p. 574) calls attention to the fact that four of the 68 cases collected by him showed carcinomatous areas present in the walls of the cysts.

CASE 1.—Miss B., aged eighteen years. Menstrual function normal. For three or four months has been in poor health. Indigestion, some pain in the lower right abdomen; not severe. Has never had fever nor attack of cramps.

Has belching of gas. Has grown weak and pale. Poor appetite.

Examination. Rather plump, but very pale young woman. Waxy complexion.

Nothing found abnormal except slight thickening in appendix region, suggesting a small mass. No rigidity of muscles. Hemoglobin 60 per cent. From the history and examination a diagnosis of some trouble with the appendix was made.

The removal of the appendix was advised. This was done and an appendix, rather oval in form, quite regular in outline and about 7 cm. long by 3 cm. in diameter was found.

Upon section the appendix showed a clear mucoid material in the interior—a pseudomyxomatous cyst.

This patient's improvement was most remarkable. Her condition changed from that of a very pale, anemic young woman to that of a clear-complexioned and rosy-cheeked girl.

CASE 2.—M. N., aged thirty-four years. Nothing important in history, except that he has had several attacks of cramps in the abdomen. He had an attack like appendicitis August 30, 1910.

Examination unimportant except that a thickening in region of appendix and cecum was felt. The operation was done September 22, 1910.

The appendix was 10 cm. in length, and the outer surface roughened. The distal two-thirds of the appendix is occupied by a mass 4 x 2 cm., which is a cyst, filled with a slightly turbid, thick, mucus-like material. The inner wall of the cyst seems to be free from papillomata.

Microscopic. Sections from the cyst wall show chronic fibrous changes in the muscular and serous coats. The mucous membrane is represented by small clumps of epithelial cells, remnants which seem to be undergoing degenerative changes. There is no evidence of any tendency toward proliferation of these isolated clumps of epithelial tissue.

CASE 3.—Miss A., aged fifty-five years. Family history negative. Menstrual history negative. Menopause established four years ago; no trouble. Previous health always good.

Present Sickness. She says that for the past twelve years she has suffered from constipation. During all that time she has had some pain in the appendix region. Has some nausea before breakfast. Thinks she is losing strength, though she is gaining weight. Has no diarrhea, though the stools are apt to be thin. Says she thinks she has some obstruction in the bowels or the rectum. Has had some burning in the vagina for the last six weeks. Feels hot all over. Feet burn. Has abdominal cramps.

Examination. Large, rather dark-skinned woman. Skin jaundiced a little. General examination negative, except there is found to be a general abdominal distension. Gas in the colon and the small intestines. There is felt a small nodular tumor in the region of the appendix or cecum. Slightly tender to pressure. The tumor is very slightly movable. Nothing abnormal felt in the rectum, nor could anything abnormal be seen by examination with a long proctoscope.

The x-ray examination gives evidence that there is an annular stricture in or near the ileocecal junction. A diagnosis of probable carcinoma and its removal advised.

Laboratory Findings. Urine normal. Blood: hemoglobin, 80 per cent.; white blood cells, 4500; polymorphonuclears, 58 per cent.; small lymphocytes, 4 per cent.; large lymphocytes, 1 per cent.

Operation. A right rectus incision was made, and upon examination of the mass we decided to resect the ascending colon and make an end-to-side anastomosis of the ileum and colon.

I could not feel but that we might be dealing with a combined carcinoma and cyst of the appendix.

While freeing the colon there was found lying to its outer side quite a lot of jelly-like material which had escaped from the ruptured extremity of the appendix. The material was carefully cleared away, but there seemed to be no evidence of a peritonitis.

All of the ascending colon up to and a little beyond the hepatic flexure and about nine inches of the ileum were resected, an end-to-side anastomosis, without clamps, was done, and the whole suture line covered by omentum. A careful closure was made of the peritoneum over the line of the cut mesentery, so that no adhesions might follow.

The patient showed little disturbance from the operation and her convalescence was without incident. She is now hearty and well.

Description of Specimen. A mass 9 cm. long by 4.5 cm. at the largest diameter, and 2 cm. at its smallest diameter which was at the extremity. The mass was seen to be lying to the right and a little posterior to the ascending colon. This mass was quite firm; at the outer surface smooth, and of whitish color. The distal end for a distance of 2 cm. was roughened and inflamed, and reminded one somewhat of the appearance of the fimbriated end of the Fallopian tube. There was lying just above this roughened end about a tablespoonful of a whitish gelatinous material. The whole mass was closely attached to the wall of the ascending colon. At the base the tumor jutted into the caput cecum in such a manner as to almost completely close the valves of the ileum.

Section through the mass revealed an appendiceal cyst, tensely filled with a gelatinous substance of a grayish-white color. The wall of the cyst was smooth for the most part. and covered with a soft white material resembling white brain matter. A few small areas in the wall had small masses of gelatinous material adherent to them.

The distal end of the cyst was dilated into several pockets with thin walls. One of these pockets had a small hole entirely through its wall, through which the gelatinous material had escaped.

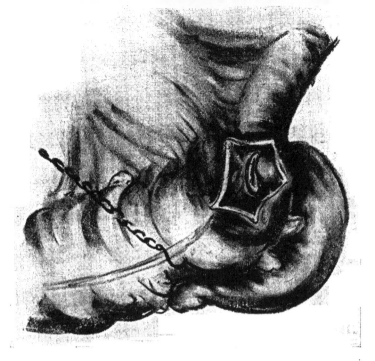

FIG. 1.—Cyst of the Appendix. Case III. Size, 9 cm. long x 4.5 cm. at largest diameter and 2 cm. smallest diameter. (Drawing by Prof. Wm. Keiller.) (Medical Department, University of Texas.)

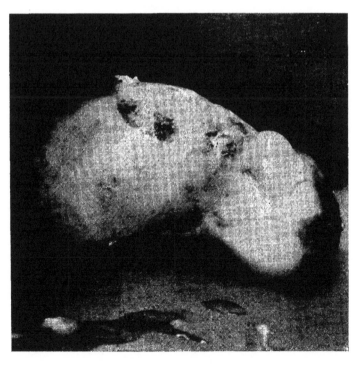

FIG. 2.—Cyst of the Appendix. Size, 14.3 cm. long x 7 cm. greatest diameter and 5.6 cm. smallest diameter. (Dr. Hamilton's case.) Photograph about one-half natural size.

Microscopic. Sections through the wall of the cyst at various levels showed fibroid changes in the muscular and serous coats, with an almost complete loss of the epithelial elements of the inner surface.

There was no evidence of a carcinomatous change of the tissues at any point.

CASE 4 (Dr. Gavin Hamilton's case. Personal communication.)—J. J., male, aged forty years; traveling salesman; very fat; weight, 240 pounds. Was seen by Dr. Hamilton June 6, 1914.

In last ten years has had two attacks of pain in back and in the right sacro-iliac region, which were diagnosed as lumbago. He never had any abdominal pain, gastro-intestinal symptoms, except gas on the stomach. Was suddenly taken with pain in the right iliac region, without nausea.

Urine negative. Temperature, 100° F.; pulse, 80. He had right iliac tenderness and rigidity.

A diagnosis of appendicitis was made, and immediate operation advised. The appendix was removed without difficulty through a gridiron incision. Patient given ether anesthesia for about thirty minutes. The patient's condition was very satisfactory for about fifty-four hours. He complained neither of nausea or pain. At the end of this time he became restless and nauseated. He had great abdominal swelling. By stomach-tube about a gallon and a half of dark green fluid was removed. This was repeated several times at two-hour intervals. In spite of the emptying of the stomach, and posturing the patient, he died about seventy-four hours after operation from acute dilatation of the stomach. The absence of pain or discomfort, following the operation was marked. The late onset of the gastric symptoms was unusual.

The following is the pathological report of the appendix made by Dr. E. L. Goar. Specimen from Dr. Gavin Hamilton.

Pseudomyxomatous cyst of the appendix. Tumor consists of an irregular potato-shaped mass, 14.3 cm. long by 7 cm. in its greatest diameter, and 5.6 cm. in its shortest diameter. The long circumference was 34.7 cm. and its greatest transverse circumference 20 cm., while the least transverse, 2.5 cm. from its cecal attachment, was 15.3 cm.

The weight was 11¾ ounces.

The outer anterior surface of the tumor is, for the greater part, smooth, whitish, and gives the appearance of dense fibroid tissue.

The posterior surface shows a mass of fat attached, and a roughening from adhesions; the bloodvessels are prominent in this area, and some parts are dark from the presence of blood in the tissues.

Two small openings in the wall, show the wall to be about the thickness of adhesive plaster, and the contents to be a clear gelatinous substance which filled the cyst very completely.

CASE 5.—Clara M., child, aged thirteen years, weight about 75 pounds, good health up to October, 1914, when she was taken with a sudden sharp pain in the abdomen. She had fever, was nauseated and had to remain in bed for several days. She got up and did well until about December 1 she had a similar attack of pain in the side while at school. She was nauseated and had fever. Was put to bed on account of the fever and after some days the family called a physician, Dr. L. W. Bain, who made a diagnosis of appendicitis and referred her to me for operation.

I saw her on December 24, 1914, and found a thin, somewhat pale, dark-complexioned child, who complained of pain and soreness in her right side. On examination showed nothing abnormal about her, except the mass in the appendix region about the size of a medium-sized orange. This mass was firm, but slightly fluctuating and was diagnosed as an appendiceal abscess and operation advised. Blood count at this time was: white blood cells, 20,000; polymorphonuclears, 92 per cent.; small lymphocytes, 7 per cent.; large lymphocytes, 1 per cent. No malarial parasites. The operation was performed under ether through a gridiron incision and a perforated appendix surrounded by an abscess containing about 2 ounces of thick, creamy pus. Just behind the cecum was noted quite a thickening which I took to be an exudate beneath the peritoneum and I did not attempt to do anything with it. I put in a gauze drain with three cigarette drains surrounding the gauze. The drainage was free and the patient did well for several days. About the fifth day I removed the drains except the gauze, and upon making a little pressure around the womb about 6 or 8 ounces of white gelatinous substance, which proved to be pseudomucine, came out. This material continued to discharge for several days along with the pus, and was observed upon the third or fourth day to be quite offensive in odor. Her temperature rose and she continued with fever up to the time of her death. She gradually declined in strength and the abdomen filled with a fluid which was withdrawn January 20, 1915, and was found to be alkaline, turbid, pale greenish-yellow, with some whitish flakes. The specific gravity was 1010 and showed much albumin almost solid with nitric acid. No tubercle bacilli were present, but there were a number of bacilli and diplococci.

There appeared about the abdomen, chest and thighs a number of pyemic abscesses which were opened and drained. She, in spite of all we did, continued to decline, and on February 6, 1915, we did a direct transfusion from the mother, amount of blood not being determined, except the hemoglobin rose from 50 to 70 per cent. She improved temporarily, but the abdomen again filled with fluid. Her appetite grew worse and she died on February 6, 1915, of what we thought to be a chronic peritonitis and pyemia, due to the infection of this ruptured retroperitoneal pseudomyxomatous cyst. No postmortem was permitted, hence I lost the opportunity of seeing exactly the conditions present.

No.	Author	Source	Sex	Age	Reference	Condition
1	Baillet	Op.	F.	.	Bull. de Soc. Aat. de Paris, 1891, v, 66, p. 67	Mus gt.
2	Baldwin	Op.	F.	40	Brooklyn Md Jour., B, 1904	fus gt.
3	Barber	Op.	.	.	Referred to by Baldwin	fus gt.
4	Berry	Aut.	.	.	ollr. of Pth., April, 95	Mus gt.
5	Bierhof	Aut.	M.	77	Pat. Aah. f. kin. Md., 1880, xxvii, 3, s. 248	fill mus yst.
6	Bierhof	Aut.	.	.	Pat. Aah. f. klin. Md., 1880, xxvii, 3, s. 248	Small cyst, us
7	Bf	Aut.	.	.	Pat. Aah. f. klin. Md., 1880, xxvii, 3, s. 248	M us t.
8	Bierring	Op.	.	.	Pan of all's ae	M Mus gt.
9	Biggs	Aut.	.	.	Med. Rc., vl. iii, p. 36	Mus gt.
10	Biggs	Aut.	.	.	Md. Rec., vd. xliii, p. 36	Sud lix.
11	Boody	Aut.	F.	70	Am. Med., Agt 16, 02, p. a	Lid us
12	Gto	Op.	M.	33	ous Archiv, B. 98, H. 2, s. 193	Gs gt.
13	Ge	Op.	M.	30	As of Surgery, My, 915, p. 582	Gs gt.
14	Chevrier	Aut.	.	.	La Revue Md. du Canada, 1903–1904, p. 15	Md us yst.
15	Combemale	Aut.	.	.	Bull. Md. du ord, a, p. 23	Lid us.
16	fe	Aut.	.	.	Bull. Md. du Nd, a, p. 23	Lid us.
17	Gs	Aut.	.	.	Glasgow Md. ollr., 1875, p. 26	Gs gk.
18	Gs (from Stengel)	Aut.	.	.	Gd by Kelynack, Ml d Path, 2d ed., 173	Gs gt.
19	ig	Op.	M.	16	Aby M Aas, Br, 95, cvi	Gs cst.
20	ig	Op.	F.	50	By Med. Annals, Br, 95, cvi	Gs cst.
21	ig	Op.	M.	36	By M Annals, Br, 905, cvi	Gs gt.
22	ig	Op.	F.	60	By Med. Aas, B, 95, cvi	Gs gt.
23	ir	.	F.	.	Ts. Gyn. Sc., Go, 1911, p. 23	i.
24	Crawford	Op.	M.	63	Iowa Med. Jour., September, 1909, p. 129	r of	ns not	d.
25	Crouse	.	M.	.	Surg., Gyn. and Obs., November, 1910, p. 457	Gs nd	y.
26	Crowell	Aut.	F.	40	Philippine Jour. of Science, February, 1912	Gs gt.
27	Deaver	Aut.	M.	29	Treatise on Appendicitis, Philadelphia, 1900	Mus gt; se of	ge.
	Dodge	Op.	M.	29	Described in this paper	Hydropic cgt.
	Draper	Aut.	M.	65	Bost. Med. and Surg. Jour., 1884, 110, vi, p. 131	Gd na.

Pseudomyxoma   Described as colloid.

No.	Name		Sex	Age	Reference	Remarks
28	Eden	Op.	.	.	Lancet, 1912, p. 1498	Gelatinous cyst. Pseudomyxoma peritonei.
29	Elting	At.	M.	81	Annals of Surgery, 1903, xxxvii, p. 549	Colloid carcinoma.
30	Fenwick	.	.	.	Cited by Kelynack	Milky contents; a hydrops.
31	Feré	Aut.	M.	55	Le Prog. Méd., Paris, 1877, v, p. 73	"Mucocele."
	Finklestein	.	.	.	Described under Guttman.	
32	Förster	.	.	.	Cited by Wölfler as having had a case. Reference not given.	
33	Fraenkel	Aut.	M.	79	Münch. med. Woch., 1901, xxiv, s. 965	Pseudomucinous cyst. Pseudo-
34	Garrow and Keenan	Op.	F.	21	Annals of Surgery, Mar, 1908	Cubical-celled cancer.
35	Gildersleeve	Op.	M.	43	Brooklyn Med. Jour., August, 1904, p. 318	... frothy contents.
36	Glassmacher	At.	.	.	Cid by Van Hook	Empyema.
37	Guttman	Op.	F.	70	Deut. med. Woch., 1891, s. 260	Described as a hydrops.
38	Hartman and Kindley	.	F.	.	Jour. Am. Med. Assn., 1904, p. 1795	Pseudomucinous cyst.
39	Hawkins	.	.	.	Diseases of ... Appendix, London, 1895	Empyema.
40	Hawkins (from Stengel)	Op.	F.	.	Diseases of ... Appendix, London, 1895	Empyema.
41	Hammesfahr	Op.	F.	.	Deut. ... Wch., July 31, 1913	Pseudomucinous ystc
42	Hammesfahr	Op.	.	.	Deut. ... Wch., July 31, 1913	Pseudomucinous cyst.
43	Hammesfahr	.	.	.	Deut. ... Wch., July 31, 1913	Pseudomucinous y ts ... peritonei. Pseudo-
44	Heckteon	Aut.	.	.	Described under Jaggard.	Large diverticulum.
45	Herb	Op.	.	.	Tr. Chicago Path. Soc., 1907	Mucous cyst. Possible pseudomyxoma peritonei.
	Hirst	.	.	.	Referred to by Stengel	
46	Hueter	.	.	.	Ziegler's Beitrage, 1907, Bd. 41, s. 517	Gelatinous cyst. Pseudomyxoma peritonei.
47	Jaggard	Op.	F.	.	Am. Jour. Obs., 1893, xxviii, p. 226	Empyema.
48	Jong	Op.	F.	47	Mitt. ... Grenz d. Med. u. Chir., 1907, xviii, No. 3.	Spheroidal-celled cancer.
49	Kelly, J. A.	Aut.	M.	43	... Say, April, 909, p. 524	Large gelatinous cyst.
50 65	Kelly and Hurdon (16 cases)	At.	.	.	Verm. Appendix and its Diseases. Philadelphia and London, 1905, p. 250	All small mucinous or gelatinous cysts.
66	Kelynack	At.	F.	.	Path. of the Verm. Appendix, London, 1893	Gelatinous cyst.
67	Kennedy	.	.	.	N. Y. Med. olr., March 22, 1913	Mucinous cyst.

No.	Author	Source	Sex	Age	Reference	Condition
68	Klm	Op.	F.	16	Münch. med. Woch., 1905, N o.4	Small empyema.
69	Klm	Op.	M.	37	Münch. med. Wch., 1905, N o.4	Small empyema.
70	Klemm	Op.	M.	26	M"mh. med. Wch., 1905, N o.4	Small empyema.
71	Lafforgue	Aut.	F.	50	Gaz. des Hôp., Paris, 1904, lxxvii, p. 33	Small granular mucous masses.
72	Ihm	Op.	F.	33	Nothnagel's Encl. of Med., New Am. ed.	Cyst filled with shot-like bodies.
73	Landau	Op.	M.	32	Berl. klin. Wch., 1906, December 10	Spheroidal-celled cancer.
74	?ager				N. Y. Med. Rec., 1904, lcvi, p. 856	Hydrops.
75	Leube	Op.	M.	23	Ziemssen's Encyclopedia, vol. vii.	"Colloid" cyst.
76	?sch	Op.	M.	69	N. Y. Med. Jour., 1903, lxvii, p. 233	Pseudomyxoma peritonei.
					Ergebn. d. Agn. Path. u. Path. Anat., 1903, xviii, s. 847	
77	M Arthur	Op.	M.	50	Ith. Jour. Obs., Gust., 1893, xxviii, p. 275	Small cyst in il sac.
78	McConnell	Aut.	F.	25	Int. Clis., 1907, iv, Series 17	Ga in nga fei.
79	MacCarty and McGrath	Op.			Als of Surgery, lix, 1914	ic appendix.
80	MacCarty and McGrath	Op.	F.	36	As of rep. i, 1914	Gd a.
81	MacLean	Op.	M.	20	Mh. med. Wh. st. 1908, s. 1746	Eja.
82	Maylard (from Stengel)	Aut.			Tr. Glasgow Clin. and Par. Med. Sc., June 6, 69 p., 822	Gs nd st. y.
83	Mas Merkel	Op. Aut	M.	69	Ergebn. d. Allgem. An. Med. An., 93, 3 i, iii ah. 1 Path. At., At. 2, vol. 1 s. 329	Gs nga hi.
84	Montgomery	Op.	F.	27	Jour. A. Med. An., ix, p. 172	Gt vh nyl ai nt.
85	Montgomery	Op.	F.	60	Ur. A. Med. Assn., ix, p. 172	Ns. nga ui.
86	Moore	Op.	F.	44	Brit. Mr., 9, i, p. 89	Gs nga fi.
87	Nager				Ziegler's i g, 1904, Bd. 36, L I, s. 88	Described as a ngo-d-thel' aa.
88	Norris	Op.	F.	27	Univ. Pa. Med. Bull., November, 1903, No. 9	Very rge ia.
89	Neumann	Op.	M.	60	Berlin. klin. Woch., January, 1909, No. 1, s. 15	rge st; ds at gst.
90	Noble	Op.			Jour. Am. Med. Assn., March 9, 1912	ns of d-d.
91	Oberndorfer	Aut.	M.	69	Verh. der Deut. Path. Ges., 1906, s. 235	Small gelatinous gst.

No.	Name	Op./Aut.	Sex	Age	Reference	Notes
92	Oberndorfer	Aut.	M.	64	Verh. der Deut. Path. Ges., 1906, s. 235	
93	Oberndorfer	Aut.	M.		Verh. der Deut. Path. Ges., 1906, s. 235	
94	Oberndorfer	Aut.	M.	74	Verh. der Deut. Path. Ges., 1906, s. 235	
95	Ogilvie	Op.	M.	22	Jour. Am. Med. Assn., February 20, 1915, p. 657	calcareous
96	Pauchet	Op.	F.	15	Gaz. … de …	
97	Perkins, I. B.	Op.	F.		… 1900, xviii, p. 146	
98	Phemister	Op.	F.		Med. … My 29, 1 95	
99	Rathe	Op.	F.	31	Mf. … Gyn., 1913, xxxvii	Large
100	Ribbert	Aut.	F.	30	… xii, s. 66	
101	Ribbert	Aut.	M.	19	… xii, s. 66	
102	Ribbert	Aut.	M.	55	… xiv, s. 66	
103	Ribbert	Aut.	M.	26	… xii, s. 66	
104	Ribbert	Aut.	M.		… xii, s. 66	
105	Ribbert	Aut.	F.		… xii, s. 66	
106	Roberg	Op.	F.	70	Tr. … Soc., 90, p. 80	
107	… (from	Aut.			… xiii, s. 179	
10	…				… iii, s. 184	
11	…	Op.	M.	60	… July, 1911	
112	…	Aut.	M.	28	… 1892, vi, p. 387	Possible
13	…	Op.		19	… 1 9, 3, s. 82	
14	…	Op.			… 1 9, 3, s. 82	
15	…	Op.	F.	50	Discussion of …	
16	…	Aut.	F.	30	Jour. An. … Assn., … xli	
117	…	Aut.			Referred to by …	
18	…	Aut.			Referred to by …	
19	…	Aut.			Referred to by …	
20	…	Aut.	F.	55	Als of Surgery, … p. 186	
21	Stone, I. S.	Op.			… u … 1907, s. 89	gities.
22	…	Aut.			Gt. f. allg. … 1 05	
23	…	Op.				Escape of … to meso-

No.	Author.	Source.	Sex.	Age.	Reference.	Condition.
124	ffes	Op.	.	.	From Van H dk	Mus cyst.
125	Treves	.	.	.	From Van H dk	Gelatinous cyst.
126	Treve sard Swallow	.	.	.	Lancet, February 9, 1899	This cyst.
127	ffer	Op.	M.	36	British Med. Jour., Mh 9, 1910, p. 681	Pseudomyxoma ...mai.
128	Vaughn	Op.	.	.	Wash. Med. ...ls, Wash., D. C., May, 1911	Small cyst.
129	Vaughn	Op.	.	.	Observation	Large cyst.
130	Van H dk	Op.	F.	.	...me, Mh, 196	Cy t sin hernial sac.
131	Vim nt	Aut.	.	.	Bull. de la Soc. Anat., Paris, 1887, lxii, p. 608	"Mucocele."
132	Virchow	Aut.	F.	.	Die Krankhaften ...de, 1863, I, s. 250	Cy t ssize of a fist. "Hydrops."
133	Wald	Op.	F.	74	Monatsschr. f. Geburtsh. u. Gyn., April, 1909	Large pedunculated cyst. " ghtly turbid ...ents," ... ghly fluid.
134	Wehe Wizel-...ffer	Aut.	.	.	Archiv f. Coagak., 1884, 24, s. 100	Mus cyst.
135	Wier	Op.	M.	55	Virchows ...kv, Bd. 63, H. L., s. 98	Cyst drained by incision.
136	Wier	Op.	.	.	Md. Record, 1880, xvii, p. 44	Cyst drained by incision.
137	Wilks (from Stengel)	.	.	.	Refers to similar case . Quoted by Fagge, Tr. on Append., Lon., ii, p. 174	Large mucous y ts
138	Wilson	Op.	F.	68	Lancet, 1912, p. 1498	Small mucinous cyst.
139	Wilson	Op.	F.	52	Lancet, 912, p. 1498	Ruptured cyst.
140	Wood	Op.	M.	19	...th Jour. of Obstetrics, January, 1900, p. 15	Large hydr pic cyst.
141	Mer	Op.	.	.	Archiv f. ...kd Surg., 1879, xxi, s. 432	Cy t sin hernial sac.
142	Zdeker	.	.	.	Prag. med. Woch., 1888, xxvii, s. 340	An ...na.
143	Moore	Op.	F	18	Trans. Southern Surg. and ...G. Association	Large oral-shaped mcoid cyst (7 cm. x 3 cm.).
144	Moore	Op.	M.	34	Trans. Southern Surg. and Gyn. Association	Club-shaped appendix, uter end cystic (4 cm. x 2 cm.).
145	Moore	Op.	F.	55	Trans. Southern Surg. and Gyn. Association	Pseudomyxomatous cyst.
146	Moore	Op.	M.	40	Personal communication (Dr. Hamilton's case)	Pseudomyxomatous y ts
147	Moore	Op.	F.	13	Trans. Southern Surg. and Gyn. Association	Retroperitoneal pseudomyxomatous y ts
148	Moore	Op.	F.	55	Personal communication (Dr. Small's case)	Pseudomyxomatous y ts

EARLY TUBERCULOSIS OF THE CERVIX

By Thomas S. Cullen, M.B., F.A.C.S.

Baltimore, Maryland

A FEW weeks ago, when taking up diseases of the cervix with my class in Gynecological Pathology at the Johns Hopkins Hospital, we encountered the following striking example of very early tuberculosis of the cervix: Gyn. Nos. 19,534 and 20,660. The patient, a healthy looking colored woman, aged twenty-five years, was admitted to the Johns Hopkins Hospital on October 16, 1914, complaining that she had been discharging fecal matter through the vagina for two years. She had been married six years but had never been pregnant. Her menses had begun at nineteen, but for the last five years she had had no periods.

At operation, Dr. J. Craig Neel, the resident gynecologist, found the uterus in retroposition and the bladder adherent to it above the internal os. The sigmoid was adherent to the vesico-uterine reflection just above the level of the internal os. The right tube and ovary had become twisted over the anterior surface of the uterus.

The bladder and tube were freed, and the fistula between the vagina and rectum was cut across. The small opening in the sigmoid was closed. The uterus which contained several myomata was now removed, a complete hysterectomy being done.

The laboratory diagnosis was: *bilateral follicular salpingitis, uterine myomata, tuberculosis of the endometrium, tuberculosis of the cervix.*

The photograph of an area from the section of the cervix shows at each outer portion of the picture normal squamous epithelium with a normal underlying stroma. In the centre, the superficial portion of the squamous epithelium is still intact; the underlying layers of epithelium are missing, and a crescentic space is seen filled with blood. Immediately beneath this is a tubercle, occupying partly the epithelial layer and partly the underlying stroma. It is sharply circumscribed, consists of epithelioid cells and contains several types of giant cells. The stroma on the left shows small round-cell infiltration.

Tuberculosis of the cervix is rare, and such an early stage as is here depicted I have never seen before.

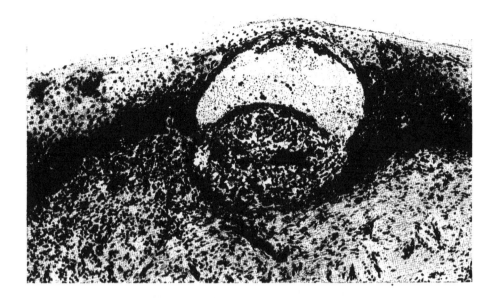

Gyn. Nos. 19,534 and 20,660; Gyn.-Path. No. 20,640.   The tuberculous process was much more advanced in the mucosa lining the cavity of the uterus than in the cervix.   The cervical mucosa is intact.   In the centre of the field is a well-defined tubercle consisting of epithelioid cells and containing giant cells of various types.   Between the tubercle and the overlying squamous epithelium is a crescentic space filled with blood.   The stroma to the left of the tubercle shows some small round-cell infiltration.

GENITAL ELEPHANTIASIS FOLLOWING EXTIR-
PATION OF INGUINAL GLANDS

By J. T. WINDELL, M.D., F.A.C.S.
Louisville, Kentucky

Two cases coming under my personal observation, in which genital elephantiasis developed subsequent to bilateral inguinal adenectomy, constitute the principal incentive for the preparation of this paper. In one the hypertrophy promptly subsided under conservative treatment, in the other it has persisted for several years. The fact that genital elephantiasis may occasionally follow inguinal adenectomy suggests the advisability of greater conservatism in the surgery of this region. When one considers the reckless manner in which the groin has hitherto been invaded by the surgeon and the large number of patients subjected to operation for inguinal lesions, it is remakarble that genital edema and elephantiasis have been so infrequent.

A brief survey of inguinal topology seems necessary to a proper understanding of the pathology of this region. Text-books and current literature contain meager information concerning the surgical anatomy of the groin, but the lymphatic distribution has been carefully studied during recent years. The latest classification limits the inguinal region to Scarpa's triangle, yet this small area contains several important structures, viz.: arteries, nerves, veins, lymphatic vessels and glands. The older anatomists described the groin as the lower portion of the abdomen, between the lumbar region above and Poupart's ligament

GENITAL ELEPHANTIASIS FOLLOWING EXTIR-
PATION OF INGUINAL GLANDS

By J. T. Windell, M.D., F.A.C.S.

Louisville, Kentucky

Two cases coming under my personal observation, in which genital elephantiasis developed subsequent to bilateral inguinal adenectomy, constitute the principal incentive for the preparation of this paper. In one the hypertrophy promptly subsided under conservative treatment, in the other it has persisted for several years. The fact that genital elephantiasis may occasionally follow inguinal adenectomy suggests the advisability of greater conservatism in the surgery of this region. When one considers the reckless manner in which the groin has hitherto been invaded by the surgeon and the large number of patients subjected to operation for inguinal lesions, it is remakarble that genital edema and elephantiasis have been so infrequent.

A brief survey of inguinal topology seems necessary to a proper understanding of the pathology of this region. Text-books and current literature contain meager information concerning the surgical anatomy of the groin, but the lymphatic distribution has been carefully studied during recent years. The latest classification limits the inguinal region to Scarpa's triangle, yet this small area contains several important structures, viz.: arteries, nerves, veins, lymphatic vessels and glands. The older anatomists described the groin as the lower portion of the abdomen, between the lumbar region above and Poupart's ligament below, and between the hypogastrium and the inferior iliac spine. Thus, in addition to the structures already mentioned, the right groin contained the cecum, the appendix, the ureter and the spermatic vessels; the left including the sigmoid flexure of the colon, the ureter and the spermatic vessels.

The inguinal region is abundantly endowed with lymphatic structures, the superficial and deep glands, constituting one of the most important glandular centers of the body. The deeper glands are few in number and of minor consequence so far as this paper is concerned. The superficial glands are infinitely more important; they are variable (seven to twenty) in number and size, and occupy the area defined as Scarpa's triangle, i. e., limited above by Poupart's ligament, externally by the anterior inferior iliac spine, internally by the pubic spine, extending downward in triangular shape approximately two and a half inches.

The superficial inguinal glands are situated in the deeper layers of the superficial fascia, in close proximity to the superficial circumflex iliac and superficial external pudic arteries, the corresponding veins, the terminal portions of the internal saphenous vein, and the crural branch of the genitocrural nerve. A horizontal line drawn through the saphenous opening divides the superficial glands into two groups: (a) the superior, and (b) the inferior; a vertical line similarly placed separates these groups into (a) external, and (b) internal. A more elaborate classification would be: (a) the superexternal, (b) the supero-internal, (c) the inferointernal, (d) the infero-external, and (e) the central group of glands. However, such divisions, being purely arbitrary, are of interest only for the purpose of anatomical study.

The superficial inguinal glands receive the cutaneous lymphatics of the lower limb, the perineum, the scrotum, the penis, the anus, and the subumbilical portion of the abdominal wall. As the afferent penile and urethral branches discharge their contents through trunk vessels into the superficial glands, the frequency of infective lymphadenitis in this situation is not difficult to understand. The pathology of genital elephantiasis is peculiar in that irrespective of its cause the resulting changes are invariably the same. Lymphangiectasis is a constant feature; enlarged lymphatic vessels are apparent everywhere in the involved area, from immediately below the epithelium to deep within the corium and subcutaneous tissues; they contain no erythrocytes but are found adjacent to the bloodvessels. Local obliterative endarteritis is commonly observed, and collections of round and so-called plasma cells are noted near the bloodvessels; cell proliferation and hypertrophy invariably involve both the superficial and deeper structures. Increase in fibrous tissue is the most prominent feature and constitutes the bulk of the enlargement; the process involves the skin, the bloodvessels, the lymphatics, also the nervous and muscular structures; the various layers of the skin become indistinguishable because of the enormous increase in fibrous tissue fascicles; the corium is thickened and indurated; the fascia and intermuscular septa are augmented and present evidence of fatty degeneration; section shows the hypertrophic tissue to be fibrous, lusterless, sclerotic, homogeneous, and a lymph-like fluid exudes.

The fact that genital elephantiasis infrequently follows radical inguinal surgery renders its occurrence none the less unfortunate. In many instances the local pathology for the relief of which the operation is undertaken owes its origin to infection (Neisserian, tuberculous, syphilitic, streptococcic, etc.) with resulting lymphadenitis and obstruction. As a rule the obstruction is temporary, and if infiltration be not extensive, recovery ensues under conservative treatment. Even when the glandular enlargement and infiltration are considerable, surgical extirpation is seldom justifiable; obstruction from pressure of the enlarged glands usually disappears with restoration of the circulation, and elephantiasis rarely follows when conservative measures are employed. It must be remembered that genital elephantiasis may be produced by any pathology which markedly interferes with the inguinal lymphatic circulation, even without previous infection, e. g., pressure from adjacent neoplasms, partial obliteration of the lymphatic vessels from external trauma, mechanical obstruction from any cause. However, not all external traumatisms, surgical operations, and pathological lesions of the groin which interfere with lymphatic circulation are followed by genital elephantiasis; in fact, experience has demonstrated that it is an exceedingly infrequent sequel. This is further emphasized by the fact that in experiments upon animals, no one has yet been able to produce genital elephantiasis by resection of the inguinal glands.

The clinical history sometimes suggests an infection entirely independent of operative or mechanical factors which might interfere with the circulation of lymph; in such instances repeated chills, fever, swelling, itching, redness, etc., noted as concomitant manifestations, indicate that an erysipelatous infection ("recurrent erysipelatous lymphangitis") may be the determining causative factor. "It is not unlikely that the obstruction is secondary to the infection in many cases, and that the recurring cellulitis is to a large degree responsible for the hyperplasia of tissue constituting the main element in these singular cases; in other instances, the infection occurs following operations which interrupt the continuity of the lymph channels." (Le Count.)

It is the contention of Shattuck and others that the essential characteristics of acquired elephantiasis in any situation are: (a) lymphangiectasis, (b) hyperplasia of connective tissue, and (c) chronic edema. The inter-relation of these phenomena, however, in the production of genital elephantiasis is not clear. The tissue changes may be attributed to the interaction of lymph stasis and inflammation; stasis always occurs early and persists; inflammation may precede or follow stasis, or it may not be manifest at any stage of the pathology; when present it may be acute or chronic, and is generally traceable to bacterial invasion. While either chronic stasis or inflammation from any cause may predispose to elephantiasis, even when occurring together, hypertrophy does not always result. Congenital weakness or anomalies of the lymphatics may play an essential part in the production of elephantiasis.

The researches of Bayer on the pathology of genital elephantiasis following inguinal adenectomy direct renewed attention to the importance of greater conservatism in the surgery of this region, *i. e.*, of preserving the periglandular and areolar tissues, as these structures contain an extensive system of lymph spaces from which regeneration of the glands and vessels quite frequently occurs. If the periglandular fatty tissue is removed or otherwise destroyed, regeneration is impossible and a condition favorable to the development of genital elephantiasis exists. "These conclusions are all the more important because when once genital elephantiasis is established, nothing can be done for its relief, except wide excision which is unsatisfactory. As a very unpleasant pitfall in the way of surgeons operating in this region, this complication deserves very careful consideration."

Unfortunately there has yet been devised no satisfactory method of treating genital elephantiasis which is applicable to all cases. When the hypertrophy is moderate, however as occurred in one of my cases, conservative local treatment by the application of a suitable suspensory apparatus will sometimes be of benefit. "The injection of fibrolysin (Castellani) has proved disappointing, as have also the methods devised by Carnochan (ligation) and Handley (lymphangioplasty). Radical operative intervention, contemplating extirpation of the elephantiasic tissue with preservation of functionating genital organs, will usually be futile although a few successful cases have been recorded in the literature. In the majority of instances the hypertrophy gradually progresses as in the endemic type, and amputation of the genital organs may become necessary to relieve the patient of the tremendous weight.

"The scope of this paper precludes consideration of endemic elephantiasis due to lymphatic obstruction from systemic invasion by the Filaria sanguinis hominis, in which structures other than the genital organs are usually implicated in the pathology. So far as can be ascertained the filaria have not been demonstrated present in any case of genital elephantiasis following inguinal adenectomy.

"*Personal Observations:* I. Mr. N., aged thirty-seven years, single; date of first observation, June 25, 1911. The patient at that time presented an enormous elephantiasic enlargement of the entire scrotum and penis. The scrotum measured sixteen inches in circumference; the penis (at its largest part) was twelve inches in circumference and eleven inches in length. He gave the history of having contracted syphilis in 1903."

Two surgical operations had been performed for the removal of enlarged and infiltrated inguinal glands, one in 1905, the other in 1909, but for what character of pathology, the patient did not know. Dense fibrous tissue scars, adherent to the underlying structures, were present in both inguinal regions. The scar tissue was more abundant in the left groin, which probably explained the greater scrotal enlargement present on the corresponding side. The patient stated that he had been under antisyphilitic treatment continuously since 1903, and that thickening of the penile and scrotal tissues was first noted early in 1910.

"Several instances of moderate genital elephantiasis have been observed accompanying Hunterian chancre, probably due to the production of an exudate in the lymphatic glands by the action of the Spirocheta pallida, or from occlusion of the lumen of the lymphatic vessels by the organisms themselves. The hypertrophy soon subsided under active antisyphilitic treatment."

Local treatment consisted of an appropriate suspensory apparatus and antiseptic dressings. At no time while the patient was under my care was there any acute inflammation of the penile tissues; but the scrotum, owing to the continuous exudation of lymph from its surface, at times became infected and exhibited evidence of acute inflammation, which was relieved by suitable antiseptic applications.

On July 10, 1911, the Wassermann reaction was found to be three-plus. For several months the patient was treated by mercury in its various preparations and modes of administration, and later by salvarsan. The man suffered from periodic attacks of intense pain apparently involving the entire body, and lasting sometimes for two or three days. These attacks were relieved by the administration of iodide of potassium of which he was able to take very large doses, i. e., half an ounce of the saturated solution during twenty-four hours.

November 11, 1913, the Wassermann reaction was two-plus. Twelve days after the administration of salvarsan, December 7, 1913, there occurred considerable swelling, pain and redness of the left arm around the elbow-joint, which was sufficiently severe to cause the patient to remain in bed and require the constant attention of a trained nurse. Such manifestations following the injection of salvarsan must be exceptional, and are difficult of explanation excepting upon the hypothesis that there existed a local lymphatic or vascular abnormality preventing prompt elimination of the drug. The symptoms subsided within six weeks, and there was no similar recurrence following subsequent salvarsan injections.

Salvarsan was again administered on March 29, April 14, and May 10, 1914. On September 2, 1914, the Wassermann reaction was one-plus. There has been no reduction in the genital hypertrophy; the supportive bandage has been continued. The patient is in excellent physical health. At my suggestion he has consulted several eminent authorities, some of whom are Fellows of this Association, and all have agreed that surgery is not indicated.

II. Mr. B., aged thirty years, single. On September 10, 1912, three months after bilateral inguinal adenectomy for enlarged and suppurating glands probably of tuberculous origin, the patient presented an immense hypertrophy of the penis. It was unaccompanied by redness or pain, and the scrotal tissues were apparently uninvolved. Several deep scars were present in each groin from the previous operations.

Having in mind the unfortunate case just reported, it was thought this was another of similar character, and the diagnosis was made accordingly. An appropriate suspensory apparatus was applied, and the patient requested to report three days later for further observation and treatment. However, he failed to return, and from information subsequently received, it appears that the penile hypertrophy subsided within two or three months.

Collected Cases: Quite recently Hill reported a case of elephantiasic fever followed by genital elephantiasis in a patient, aged forty-three, developing six years after bilateral inguinal adenectomy. The penis measured nine inches, and the scrotum twenty inches, in circumference. The author states that the hypertrophied tissue was removed by extensive resection, the testes and penis being preserved, and the resulting anatomical defects overcome by plastic surgery. Perpendicular incisions extended from the abdominal rings downward, the testes and spermatic cords being dissected from the scrotum "where they were embedded in a mass of lax, blubbery, dropsical areolar tissue;" then the "sacred highway so essential to the perpetuity of the race" was liberated, and practically the entire scrotum removed. The testes were covered with adjacent skin, in the loosening of which the deep muscular lymph spaces were extensively

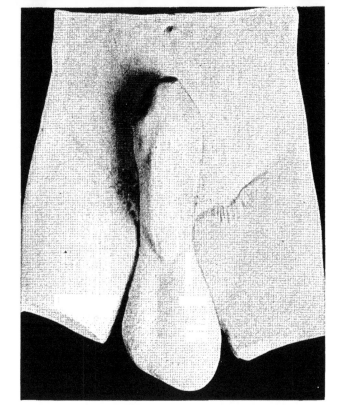

FIG. 1.—Photographs of a plaster cast of Case I.

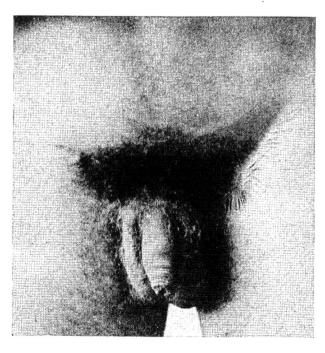

FIG. 2.—Inguinal cicatrices in Case II.

exposed. Upon the dorsal surface the incision extended the entire length of the penis which was freed of its covering "as you would a banana." After extensive dissection the pubic skin was sutured to the mucosa of the glands, practically covering the organ. The wounds readily healed, "and although the organ is whiskered and rather unsightly, it retains its reach when in action and the owner says it is more than satisfactory." The elephantiasic fever recurred after the patient left the hospital, which was relieved by the administration of polyvalent antistreptococcic serum according to the recommendation of Matas. The patient recovered and has since remained well.

Hamann encountered four cases of genital elephantiasis following extirpation of the inguinal glands, one of which is described in detail occurring in a female from whom the glands were removed during dissection of the sac of a femoral hernia. Six weeks after operation there occurred chills and fever accompanied by swelling and redness of the labium majus of the corresponding side, and during the succeeding four months seven or eight similar attacks were experienced, during each of which the labial induration increased. Diagnosis, lymphangitis accompanied by lymphatic edema due to interference with the lymph circulation, produced by removal of the fatty tissues and lymphatic glands and the succeeding cicatricial contraction. "There is small room for doubt that in cases of this kind infection added to the interruption of the lymph current bring about the hyperplasia of the subcutaneous tissues constituting elephantiasis."

Three cases of genital elephantiasis following inguinal adenectomy observed by Riedel, induced him to abandon the operation and substitute therefore incision and curettement. Bush (*Lancet*) records two similar cases, and another is reported by Baker. In his recent work on urology Guiteras cites four interesting personally observed cases of scrotal edema; in three the edema developed subsequent to radical removal of the inguinal glands, in the other it was apparently due to tuberculous epididymitis and subsided after orchidectomy.

Rubinstein observed a case of scrotal elephantiasis without immediate venereal precedent in a male, aged twenty-three years, who immediately after lifting a heavy weight noticed swelling of both sides of the scrotum. A week later the scrotum was four times its normal size, the penis and testes being uninvolved. Two years previously the right inguinal glands had been removed on account of acute inflammation. The author remarks that a few similar cases have been recorded, produced by sudden strain in persons suffering from chronic Neisserian infection, where bilateral inguinal adenectomy had been previously performed.

The following two cases are included in the series, although the elephantiasic enlargement did not follow inguinal adenectomy.

Campbell observed scrotal elephantiasis due to truss-pressure in a male, weighing two hundred and twenty-five pounds. For twenty-five and twelve years respectively, he had worn a single and then a double truss because of inguinal herniæ. The prolonged pressure where the scrotal lymphatics empty into the inguinal glands evidently produced obstruction. The author says when a truss is worn upon both sides compensatory lymphatic circulation is prevented.

In a case recorded by De L. Terrores genital elephantiasis owed its origin to the simple operation of posthetomy. A boy aged eight years had phimosis with preputial excrescences accompanied by anasarca. Complete relief followed circumcision and he remained well for three years, when lymphatic varices were noted in the inguinal regions and about the genitalia. A few months later he developed typical elephantiasis of the left lower extremity, the external genitals, and a semilunar zone of the lower abdomen, with slight involvement of the right foot.

REFERENCES

Baker.   Proc. Southern Surg. and Gynec. Assn., 1908.
Bayer.   Cited by Jour. Am. Med. Assn., loc. cit.
Campbell.   Brooklyn Med. Jour., April, 1905.
De L. Terrores.   Cited by Pediatrics, August, 1915.
Delamere-Poirier-Cuneo-Leas.   The Lymphatics, 1913.
Editorial.   Jour. Am. Med. Assn., July 8, 1899.
Gage.   Ref. Handbook of the Medical Sciences, vol. v.
Guiteras.   Urology, 1912, vol. ii.
Hamann.   Cited by Jour. Am, Med. Assn., loc. cit.
Hill.   Proc. Alabama State Med. Assn., 1915.
Le Count.   Ref. Handbook of the Medical Sciences, vol. v.
Rubinstein.   Cited by Med. News, April 15, 1899.
Sappey.   Cited by Gage, loc. cit.
Shattuck.   Boston Med. and Surg. Jour., November 10, 1910.
Riedel.   Cited by Jour. Am. Med. Assn., loc. cit.

A CLINICAL AND EXPERIMENTAL STUDY OF POSTOPERATIVE VENTRAL HERNIA

By Willard Bartlett, A.M., M.D.

St. Louis, Mo.

THE consensus of opinion gathered from the literature is that the causes of postoperative ventral hernia, as far as they come under our control, are: (1) incisions out of keeping with anatomic and physiologic principles; (2) improper wound closure; (3) needless drainage and tamponade. There is also (4) increased intra-abdominal (postoperative) tension which we can influence very largely; and (5) wound infection, for which we will rarely be to blame in this age of technical refinement.

In order to get light on the purely anatomical phase of the question, I made the following animal experiments, operating upon 23 dogs:

Ten had all but one layer of the wall destroyed, no hernia resulting where we preserved or restored (a) the anterior rectus sheath, (b) the posterior rectus sheath, or (c) where the recti muscles were sutured together in the midline.

On 2 dogs defects were produced in all the layers except the skin, and on 3 only the skin and peritoneum were restored; 4 of these developed hernia and 1 dog was lost.

In an attempt to restore the integrity of the wall in the above four resultant herniæ, 1 had the opposite sheath inverted with only partial success; 2 had both sheaths overlapped and fascia transplanted, with good results; and 1 had simply an overlapping of both anterior sheaths with cure. These dogs were under observation for 49 to 240 days.

Of 6 complete defects, 3 were repaired by immediate fascia transplants, with good results; in 2 immediate sheath transplantation was done, with a satisfactory result on 1 dog, the other being still under observation; and in 1 the opposite sheath was reflected with cure.

In these herniæ and defect repairs, one, two or, at most, three fibrous layers were depended upon to restore the wall, after finding that the original preservation of one layer prevented the occurrence of hernia.

The rarity of postoperative hernia in the dog after simple, faulty, and partial closure indicates that mere damage, no matter how extensive, to the abdominal wall of the dog does not produce hernia with any degree of regularity. In fact, no bulging at all has occurred in any instance in which one firm layer has been left intact, demonstrating conclusively that postoperative hernia depends on two general factors: (1) weak wall; (2) tendency to hernia, which was not produced experimentally. Clinical experience shows the same thing to be true in the human subject, since we find hernia occurring in those who have left the hospital well but who are subject to increased intra-abdominal tension due to obstruction in digestive, urinary, or respiratory passages, and in others who strain at lifting, etc. Any attempt at cure must consider two factors: (1) removal of hernial tendency, (2) and repair of the abdominal wall. The hernial tendency is corrected previous to operation both by reducing the patient's intra-abdominal fat and intestinal contents. One, a short plethoric man, who came under my care, exercised and dieted until he reduced his weight fifty pounds between the two operations. It was surprisingly easy, at the second sitting to overlap the tissues, a thing which would have been utterly impossible at the beginning of his preoperative treatment. It is an excellent idea to put such patients to bed a few days before operation, keep them on liquid diet, and practice liberal catharsis. This not only makes the plastic easier, but also decreases the likelihood of postoperative meteorism. It is absolutely essential in this connection that a chronic cough be attended to; that any tendency to chronic vomiting or undue straining at stool be rendered improbable, and especially that obstructive conditions in the urinary passages be relieved before one considers an operation for postoperative hernia.

During the operation it will at times be necessary to reduce the tendency to hernia by decreasing the abdominal contents. This is a comparatively simple matter as far as the omentum is concerned, but may take us into extreme technical difficulties, as was the case a few years ago when I resected practically the entire colon which "had lost its right of habitation." This operation was entirely successful, but will, of course, be very rarely necessary. As a matter of course, *undue tension* on a reconstructed abdominal wall is bound to result in failure of the operation, and it must be added that any interference with the movements of the lower ribs is likely to result in respiratory and circulatory derangement, which will end fatally.

The prophylactic use of local infiltration anesthesia in a few of these operations has, in my own hands I am sure, prevented coughing, vomiting, gas formation, and urinary retention.

Much experience has convinced me that an operation which does not open the sac has certain distinct advantages. It enables one to use to the best advantage all scar tissue and sac wall that may be present. The technical difficulties are greatly minimized if no omental or visceral adhesions are taken care of, to say nothing of peritoneal closure. But the chief gain in not opening the peritoneum is seen in the greatly decreased likelihood of recurrence due to distention, vomiting, coughing, and unrest, all of them expressions of the functional intestinal disturbance which I have seen follow extensive handling of these viscera. (Of course it will be necessary, in exceptional instances, to open the peritoneal cavity for a pathological condition which is entirely independent of the hernia.)

Having briefly disposed of the general considerations which should obtain in the treatment of this malady, it must be said before taking up the special forms of operation in detail that no one of them is generally applicable as best in all cases. A choice depends upon:

1. The site of the lesion.
2. The size of the opening and hernia.
3. The condition of the surrounding tissues.
4. The general condition of the patient.

Varieties of technic:

1. Overlapping is the simplest if there is enough tissue.
2. Reconstruction of the wall is anatomically ideal if there is no atrophy or destruction of the muscles.
3. Flap inversion is good if the hernia is in the mid-line above the semilunar fold of Douglas.
4. Filigree implantation is for emergency use only.
5. Free fascial transplantation is indicated if there is no other way to close the hernia. I thus obtained good results in two large hernias.

It is natural to suppose that every tissue possibility has been utilized in the effort to cover absolute defects of the abdominal wall, though distinctly the most successful is that of Kirschner, who is the father of free fascial transplantation. He prefers fascia lata because: (1) it is easy to get; (2) there is an inexhaustible supply; (3) it is strong and inelastic; (4) it shows marked tendency to heal in; (5) it is easy to adapt to any shape. With the appearance of this idea the surgery of the abdominal wall defects may be said to have taken on an entirely new aspect.

One fascia flap reinforcing suture a line, or one inside and one outside a complete defect practically insures success.

Two working teams are required to successfuly handle free fascial transplantation.

No.	Hernia.	Original operation.	Method of secondary repair.	Result.	Observation.
57	None	Left posterior sheath			
57	Yes	Suture of skin and peritoneum	Sutured ring; inverted left rectus sheath	Partial	49 days.
59	Yes	Suture of skin and peritoneum	Overlapped both rectus sheaths; transplanted fascia	O. K.	240 days.
58	None	Preserved left anterior rectus sheath	......	....	150 days.
8	None	Preserved recti	......	....	105 days.
27	None	Preserved recti	......	....	105 days.
19	None	Anterior sheath only overlapped	......	....	105 days.
56	None	Anterior sheath only overlapped	......	....	105 days.
47	?	Slide rectus muscle; suture of anterior sheath	......	....	Ether fatality.
49	None	Slide rectus muscle; suture of anterior sheath	......	....	70 days.
60	?	Skin and peritoneum	......	....	Lost.
37	None	Complete defect and immediate fascia transplant	......	O. K.	25 days.
21	None	Complete defect and immediate transplant of rectus sheath	......	O. K.	11 days.
42	None	Preserved posterior rectus sheath	......	....	90 days.
45	None	Preserved posterior rectus sheath	......	....	37 days.
40	None	Complete defect; reflect opposite sheath	......	O. K.	72 days.
41	None	Complete defect; reflect opposite sheath	......	O. K.	72 days.
63	None	Complete defect; immediate fascia transplant	......	O. K.	50 days.
10	Yes	Skin only preserved	Overlapped sheaths and transplanted fascia	O. K.	191 days.
39	None	Complete defect; immedate fascia transplant	......	O. K.	250 days.
12	Yes	Skin only preserved	Overlapped rectus sheaths	Under observation.	
29	?	Skin only preserved	......	Under observation.	
66	?	Complete defect; transplant of rectus sheath	......	Under observation.	

The after-treatment will concern itself chiefly with coughing vomiting, defecation, passage of gas, and urination, to say nothing of muscular violence; in fact, every form of insult to the wound and sutures. Of course, the convalescent patient is to be warned against occupation or recreation which unduly raises intra-abdominal tension. In many instances the after-treatment is of vital importance, but it must be dismissed with a word, since so many points have to be considered.

My own interesting experience in the treatment of post-operative hernia embraces a study of seventy-eight people on whom I have operated for this accident. In 26 cases the original operation was performed by me.

Out of the 78 we know definitely of success in 61 of them, the time elapsing between their operations and when last heard from ranging from one week to nine and one-half years, an average of about one year. In 7 of the cases we have been unable to learn the result; 6 were complete failures, in 2 of which a filigree was used, the overlapping method being employed in the remaining 4 instances.

The 4 following patients died: (1) a strangulated hernia, eight hours after operation; (2) cancer of the uterus, a few days after operation; (3) a cirrhosis of the liver after four days; (4) a second case of cirrhosis of the liver died very suddenly eleven days after operation, during my absence from the city.

There follows a diagrammatic classification of my animal experiments mentioned earlier in this article.

MOSCHOWITZ'S OPERATION—INGUINAL ROUTE FOR FEMORAL HERNIA

By J. D. S. Davis, M.D.

Birmingham, Alabama

———

In Moschowitz's recommendation of the inguinal route for femoral hernia he places this operation in the same relationship to femoral hernia that the Bassinni operation occupies to inguinal hernia.

The inguinal attack on femoral hernia has not come into general use because the authors who have recommended it have not given sufficient description to Cooper's ligament. In closing the femoral ring by the inguinal route one must of necessity suture Poupart's ligament to Cooper's ligament. Cooper's ligament is a very thick, very resistant, flat, fibrous cord extending from the pubic tuberosity to the ilio-pectineal eminence. It is formed by the fusion of various fascial layers: pectineal aponeurosis, Gimbernat's ligament, Colle's ligament, fascia transversalis, and the ligaments of Henle and Hesselbach, reinforced by the pectineal fascia. Cooper's ligament is principally developed from the pectineal fascia and consists in that part of the fascia that spreads over the pubic ramus and extends as a flat cord to the ilio-pectineal eminence.

If the same surgical factors were utilized in femoral hernia that are used in inguinal hernia, relapse would be rare. There are certain erroneous impressions regarding the crural route for femoral hernia that give rise to disaster. The opinion is prevelant that the repair of femoral hernia by the thigh route is a simple operation, that the technic does not require anatomical exposure of the field of operation and that recurrence is rare. The statement that femoral hernia does not tend to recur after high ligation of the sac is without foundation. Even with closure of the ring by the operation of Bassinni or Fabricius with high ligation of the sac, a funnel projection of the peritoneum is always left, which constantly tends to recurrence. If the same precautions are resorted to in femoral hernia that are utilized in inguinal hernia (high ligation of sac, secure closure of the internal ring from above, and asceptic wound healing) relapse would be as rare as in inguinal hernia.

The inguinal route or approach renders resection and anastomosis a very easy procedure compared to a resection in an operation by the crural route. The supplementary abdominal incisions so often necessary in resection when the crural operation is made, need not for a moment even be considered when the inguinal operation is made.

Moschowitz reports a case on which he had operated for femoral hernia by the thigh route and secured an apparently satisfactory result. About a year and a half later he did a laparotomy on the patient and examination within the abdomen revealed a sac two inches deep.

Pott analyzes 422 cases of femoral hernia operated on by the thigh route with 36.7 per cent. relapse in the cases that had simple ligation and 28.4 per cent. relapse in the cases with sac ligation followed by ring closure.

Bressét reported 395 cases of femoral hernia operated on by the thigh route. In 232 cases operated upon by simple ligation of sac, 29 per cent. recurred. In 163 cases operated on with ligation of the sac and closure of the ring 8.6 per cent. recurred.

The statistics quoted show that the crural route is not to be relied on as a satisfactory method of operation for femoral hernia.

When femoral hernia is attacked by a high incision

(inguinal route) anatomic exposure of the femoral ring can be made from above, bringing into view Cooper's ligament, which is utilized in the closure of the femoral ring. Cooper's ligament is a very important structure and I have utilized a drawing of Drs. Seelig and Tuholske for the purpose of illustrating the female pelvis with the description of the exact anatomic relationships at the femoral ring (Fig. 3).

In the operation for the cure of femoral hernia by the inguinal route, the skin incision is not unlike that made for the Bassinni operation, except when the sac is found adherent, when the incision may be extended down into the thigh so as to give room for extirpation of the sac.

The next step in the operation is that of dividing the aponeurosis of the external oblique in the direction of its fibers.

The upper flap of the external oblique aponeurosis, the internal oblique and transversalis are held up by a retractor while a second retractor is placed under the lower flap of the external oblique aponeurosis, which retracted downward brings Poupart's ligament into view. A tape or piece of gauze is passed beneath the round ligament or spermatic cord, and used to retract the round ligament inward, and in the case of a male, the spermatic cord is to be retracted outward, which gives a very good exposure of the field of operation, with its floor covered by the transversalis, a thin layer of fascia just over or next to the peritoneum. The transversalis fascia is bluntly divided along the line of the original incision, then picked up by the retractors and held with the other tissues, upward and inward, and downward and outward. This retraction brings the peritonium with the constricted neck of the sac into view (Fig. 4).

If the deep epigastric artery should run an anomalous course, it will at this stage come into view, which may be retracted or cut between ligatures.

The sac is retracted with its contents, or if this is impossible, Gimbernat's ligament, which forms the sharp margin of the constricting ring, may be cut with a blunt pointed

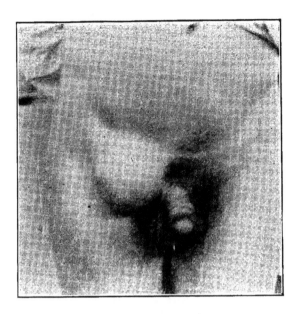

Fig. 1.—Femoral hernia in male on right side.

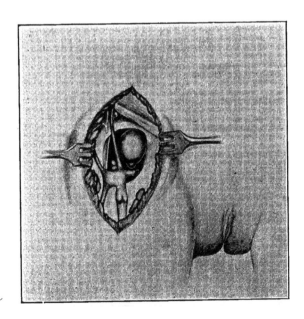

Fig. 2.—Represents a dissection, showing a protruding femoral hernia beneath Poupart's ligament.

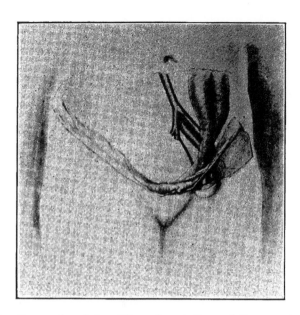

FIG. 3.—Femoral pelvis with a description of the exact anatomic relations at the femoral ring with peritoneum removed, by Drs. Seelig and Tuholske.

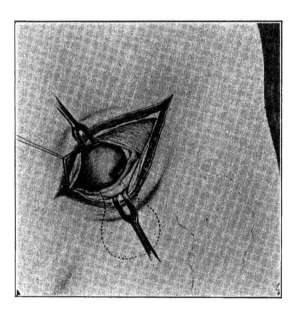

FIG. 4.—A sketch illustrating a femoral hernia with its peritoneal covering, by Drs. Seelig and Tuholske.

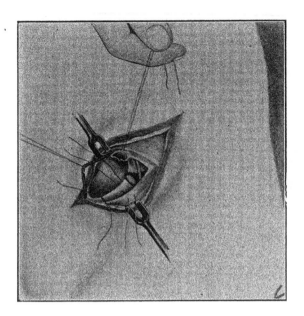

FIG. 5.—Showing relation of Cooper's ligament to Poupart's ligament
with sutures in place for closure, by Drs. Seelig and Tuholske.

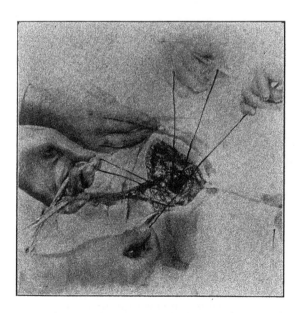

FIG. 6.—Sutures in place for closing the femoral ring.

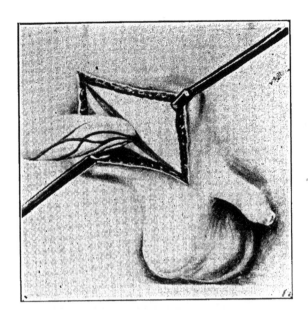

FIG. 7.—Illustration of sac after pulling out of femoral bed.

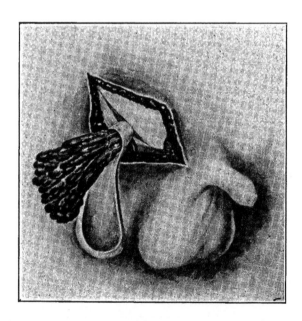

FIG. 8.—Showing sutures placed in omentum preparatory to removal.

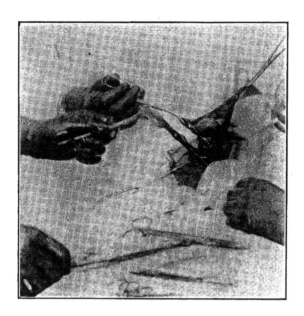

FIG. 9.—Showing sac opened with the gut exposed for resection.

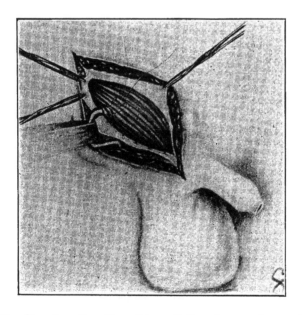

FIG. 10.—Showing the disposition of the stump of sac after it is ligated and amputated, fastened well up under the internal oblique and transversalis muscles.

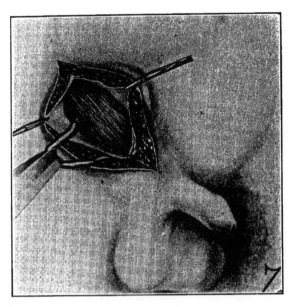

FIG. 11.—Showing the closure of the internal oblique, transversalis
and conjoined tendon below the cord to Poupart's ligament.

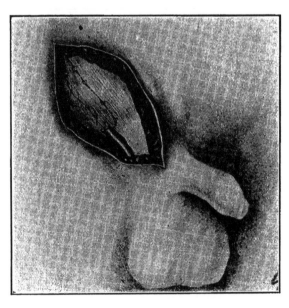

FIG. 12.—-Showing the embrication of external oblique.

herniotomy knife. The ligament is in full view which makes it practically impossible to encounter an anomalous obturator artery. If so, it is in view and the hemorrhage can be promptly controlled. But in an operation by the crural route or by the thigh, Gimbernat's ligament may be cut blindly, endangering the obturator artery, from which a hemorrhage may occur that is very hard to control, or the sac may be opened just where it converges to the neck, through which opening the hernial contents may be retracted and placed in the peritoneal cavity.

If the hernial contents are adherent to the sac loose in its bed, the sac and contents can be pulled out of the hernial bed, converting a femoral hernia into an inguinal hernia, which makes it convenient and an easy task to deal with sac and contents (Figs. 7, 8, and 9).

If the sac is adherent to its bed a pair of artery clamps should be introduced down to the lowest point in the sac, then closed and withdrawn. If the sac does not evert on account of adhesions to the bed in which it lies, the lower skin flap may be retracted down over the thigh, or the inguinal incision may be extended downward on the thigh over the hernial protrusion, thus enabling the operator to dissect the sac free of adhesions.

Fig. 7 shows the hernial sac and contents elevated before opening the sac and reducing the contents.

Fig. 8 illustrates the transfixion of omentum preparatory to its removal.

Fig. 9 illustrates the gut exposed for a resection.

The inner and upper flap is retracted inward and upward, and the outer and lower flap outward and downward, which exposes to full view the femoral ring, bounded externally by the external iliac vein, femoral and internal epigastric arteries; anteriorly by Poupart's ligament; internally by Gimbernat's ligament covered by a reflection of the transversalis fascia; and posteriorly by Cooper's ligament.

With a small curved blunt pointed needle, threaded with

catgut suture No. 2, Cooper's ligament which can be seen—
a dense, tough, white glistening, fascial membrane—covering
the horizontal ramus of the pubis is pierced just internal
to the iliac vein, and then the needle is carried through the
lower flap of the transversalis fascia, and the edge of Poupart's
ligament. Two or three sutures are now similarly placed
internal to the first. The last one and most internal suture
picks up Gimbernat's ligament. Tying all these sutures
approximates Cooper's ligament which effectually closes the
hernial orifice (Figs. 5 and 6).

The operation is to be completed as in inguinal hernia by
the Bassinni method.

Fig 10 represents the stump of the sac transfixed beneath
the transversalis and internal oblique muscles. It is drawn
up under the transversalis and internal oblique muscles so
as to provide against leaving a protrusion, or dimple, or
projection of the peritoneum, and safeguards against relapse.

The internal oblique and transversalis muscles and the
flap of the divided transversalis fascia are sutured in mass
to Poupart's ligament, making a bed for the spermatic
cord in the male (Fig. 11). The round ligament in the female
is never transplanted. The external oblique is next closed
over the cord—lapped or embricated—(Fig. 12), and the
skin is closed with buried cat-gut No. 1 suture or with a
silk or horsehair button hole suture.

DISCUSSION ON THE PAPERS OF DRS. BARTLETT AND DAVIS

Dr. John Young Brown, St. Louis, Missouri.—In 1906,
in a paper read before the Mississippi Valley Medical Association, I reported a series of cases where it was necessary to
resect gangrenous bowel found in the sac of femoral hernias.
In that report, I advocated a supplementary abdominal incision
for two reasons: In the first place, it is absolutely mandatory
where a gangrenous resection is made, that the proximal bowel
be drained of its highly septic contents. In the femoral types

of hernia operated on by the usual technic, it is impossible to properly accomplish this. In the second place, wide resection is essential, well back into healthy bowel and as the femoral ring is small, there is danger, in returning the bowel to the peritoneal cavity, of undoing the anastomosis whether made by suture or button, thereby causing fatal leakage.

I have had occasion to do the operation described by Dr. Davis only once, and I agree with him fully that it does away with the necessity of the supplementary abdominal incision. By this method we are able to get a wide opening, we can resect the bowel well back into healthy tissue and can drain the proximal bowel and make any type of anastomosis that may be indicated. In addition to these advantages, we are able to secure a much more accurate closure of the hernial ring than has been possible under methods adopted heretofore.

I had occasion a week ago to operate on a case of strangulated · hernia by this method with a most satisfactory result. I consider the method outlined by Dr. Davis, a marked step in advance.

DR. THOMAS S. CULLEN, Baltimore, Md.—I would like to ask Dr. Bartlett in what percentage of cases the hernia was due to a diverticulum. These are occasionally found in the region of the umbilicus and also above and below the umbilicus.

I have reported in the *Journal of the American Medical Association* a case where an ovary passed out through a diverticulum in the abdominal wall. Later this ovary developed into an ovarian cyst. This cyst lay just beneath the skin and totally external to the abdomen.

Recently, I operated on a femoral hernia that was of interest. The patient had had indigestion for years and also suffered from the hernia. In recent years the hernia had become very painful.

As the patient had definite pelvic symptoms as well, I first made a median incision and attended to the pelvic condition. I then examined the right femoral ring through the abdominal incision and was surprised to find the cecum drawn over and firmly fixed to the ring. This led me to suppose that the appendix was in the hernial sac. I now made an incision over the femoral hernia and deliberately cut across Poupart's ligament. This allowed me to gently push the hernial sac up into the abdomen.

I then again went through the median abdominal incision and transversely severed the peritoneum of the right abdominal wall downward until the ring of the right femoral hernia was reached. The peritoneum around the ring was severed. I could then lift the cecum and the unopened hernial sac out of the abdomen as one piece and carefully walled the tissues off. Thus what would have been a tedious operation was converted into a very simple one.

The appendix was now removed in the usual manner. During the operation nothing but the base of the appendix was seen. The hernial sac and its contents were not opened until the specimen had been thoroughly hardened. Poupart's ligament was united, the hernial space obliterated and both the hernial and median incisions closed. The patient made an uneventful recovery.

In the handling of umbilical hernia, and where employing the method of Dr. Will Mayo, Dr. Charles P. Noble and others, I have recently adopted a procedure which has proved very satisfactory. In the Mayo method the lower flap is slid up in under the upper flap, mattress sutures being used. The edge of the upper flap is then fastened down by a second row of mattress sutures. In placing this second row of sutures in the lower flap one fears to take a good bite on account of the danger of going too deep and piercing the underlying intestines. The method I employ obviates the danger. This second row of sutures is placed in the lower flap before the first have been tied. Thus with the finger as a guide one can go through almost the entire thickness of the flap if necessary. These sutures are now clamped and turned down toward the symphysis. As soon as the first row has been tied the ends of each mattress suture are re-threaded and carried through to the edge of the upper and free flap. In this way the maximum bite of the suture may be obtained without there being the slightest danger of injuring the bowel.

DR. J. GARLAND SHERRILL, Louisville, Kentucky.—There is one point in connection with Dr. Bartlett's paper I would like to emphasize, and this may explain the causation of postoperative hernia, and that is, interference with the nerve supply to the abdominal wall. It should be recognized that damage to the nerve trunks tends especially to the production of hernia, in primary operations this should be avoided, as far as possible, because muscle or fascia that is not supplied with nerve force will always be weak.

Some ten years ago I began the treatment of strangulated

femoral hernia according to the plan described by Dr. Davis and found it to be of great value. In other words, in releasing a hernia from the sac, it can be done from above without damaging or injuring the intestine. If the gut is strangulated, is blackened or weakened, an attempt to push it forcibly through the constricted part is liable to cause material to escape from the lumen into the abdominal cavity. Again, if you make a blind cut, as mentioned by the doctor, you may cut the abnormally placed epigastric artery or its communicating branch with the obdurator, and get a serious hemorrhage, so that in strangulated femoral hernia I find the operation described by Dr. Davis of great value.

Perfect result can be obtained in femoral hernia by making the incision in the thigh. The operation will be greatly facilitated by making a semilunar cut, reflecting back the flap toward the median line, and making the convexity of your incision toward the outer side of the thigh. In this way good access to the hernia is obtained; we can release it, suture the peritoneum and also suture the fascial layers according to the method of Bassini, with very good results. I limit the use of the upper incision to cases of strangulated hernia, and in these it will prove very valuable.

The point made by Dr. Cullen relative to incorporation of the appendix which is inflamed in such a sac, also demonstrates its value.

DR. CHARLES H. MAYO, Rochester, Minnesota.—Dr. Bartlett called attention to the repair of ventral hernias that occur in fat people. In experimenting on dogs, an animal rarely subject to hernia, you are working on a type of animal that is not subject to the conditions which bring about hernia in the human being. Horses and cows are subject to hernias without rupture of the skin. The next animal subject to fat and hernia is the hog. In doing such experimental work the hog should be selected.

The point brought up by Dr. Davis with reference to the inguinal route in the cure of femoral hernia is important in certain cases of strangulation; still the old methods of treating femoral hernia are very successful. Going back to the cause of femoral hernia. It is probably a traction hernia caused by a bolus of preperitoneal fat coursing along the femoral vein, making traction upon the attachment of the fat and peritoneum at that point. It may not contain abdominal contents even up to a late age.   Because of anatomical reasons these hernias occur more frequently in the female than in the male.   In doing low abdominal operation on a patient with femoral hernia the hernia may be cured by taking a closed, blunt forceps, pushing them into the hernia from inside the abdomen, then spreading them, pushing against the sac, closing the forceps, bringing the sac inverted into the abdomen.   Put a mattress suture through the neck, spread over the sac about the opening and catch the parietal peritoneum with four or five sutures.   We have used this method for years.

Dr. Herman J. Boldt, New York City.—Dr. Mayo has brought out the essential features with regard to the reduction of obesity before operating on such patients.

So far as the technic of the operation is concerned, there is nothing which will equal overlapping of the fascia from above downward, as advised by Mayo, but which subsequently was claimed as a new procedure by a foreign surgeon.   However, I believe the Mayos are entitled to the credit.   It seems to me, that our primary incision through the skin should always be made in those patients, particularly when we have a large postoperative ventral hernia, in a transverse direction.   Instead of making the incision in a longitudinal direction, we should make a transverse incision, work down to the muscles, and after we bring the muscles and posterior fascial sheath of the rectus together, then we can close the fascia.   In that way, by making a quite large transverse incision, we can get good muscular and fascial union in the majority of patients, without the necessity of transplantation.

Dr. V. P. Blair, St. Louis, Missouri.—Had Dr. Bartlett more time he might have said in transplanting fascial lata, it is of advantage to put the fibers transverse to the line of suture of the abdominal wall.   Fascia is strong one way and very weak in another.   By watching the results of removing fascia lata some eight by twelve inches, I find it can be done without apparent damage to the thigh.   In one case, in which a woman had a fecal fistula with a very large hernia, it was treated in this fashion.   The fat broke down superficially, the wound opened to the extent of eight inches, and for six weeks we were able to watch the healing of the fascia.   It turned a little yellow; granulations came through it, and just how much fascia was retained, I do not know, but no part was thrown off *en masse*. Six months later the woman was seen with a strong abdominal wall.

Dr. WILLARD BARTLETT, St. Louis, Missouri (closing).—I have nothing further to say except to answer the question of Dr. Cullen. I do not know whether diverticula existed in any of the postoperative hernias in my cases or not.

I would say in reference to the remark made by Dr. Mayo that there are other animals better suited for studies of this kind, we considered that question fully in the discussion of another subject at the time. We were doing experimental work on gastric and duodenal ulcer, and we considered trying it on animals better suited, the digestive tract of which is more like our own than dogs and cats, but the insurmountable object was the keeping of these animals. We could devise no means of keeping them.

THE ADVANTAGE OF SEPARATE SUTURE OF THE MUCOUS MEMBRANE IN GASTRIC SURGERY

By Richard A. Barr, M.D., F.R.C.S.

Nashville, Tennessee

It has unfortunately been proved to the satisfaction of most observers that simple gastrojejunostomy, with its low mortality of 1.5 to 2 per cent., will be definitely curative in less than half the cases of chronic gastric ulcer and in hardly more than two-thirds of the cases of chronic duodenal ulcer that come to operation.

That many ulcers do not yield to medical treatment, and yet are permanently and completely cured by surgery (simple or complicated) is a fact as firmly established as that gastro-jejunostomy is not a cure-all. More than this, that properly applied surgery can cure every existing ulcer of this region is a reasonable expectation, though the cure may be effected at a great risk.

Leaving out all consideration of cancer, actual or potential, the cure of ulcer by surgery can only be *positively* assured by resection or permanent exclusion of the involved area. Drainage and the admission of alkaline secretions into the stomach may give temporary relief of symptoms. This much may be and often is accomplished by gastrojejunostomy. An opening at the usual site of the posterior gastro-jejunostomy does, under some conditions (pylorospasm for instance or in case of very large stoma), hasten the emptying of the stomach and does admit the bile and pancreatic juice into the stomach. Animal experiments, x-ray observations, and average clinical results all go to prove, however, that to act advantageously a moderate-sized artificial opening must be assisted by spasmodic or organic closure of the pylorus. Nature ignores to a greater or less extent the artificial opening unless obstruction exists at the natural one. This is an established fact, and many ills besides recrudescence of ulceration result from the presence and disuse of the new opening.

My own idea of the proper way to view a gastrojejunostomy is merely as a new channel for food. This new channel is necessitated by reason of the fact that cicatrization (or operation) has caused closure of the pylorus. In other words it bears somewhat the same relation to the surgery of ulcer of the stomach and duodenum that colostomy does to the surgery of cancer of the rectum.

To exert a *certainly* curative influence on an ulcer of the stomach or duodenum, surgery must either remove the ulcer or exclude the area occupied by it not only from the passage of food but even from contact with the acid gastric secretion.

These objects can be accomplished in duodenal ulcer by closure of the pylorus, in pyloric ulcer by pylorectomy or closure on the proximal side, in all others by resection of more or less of the stomach, including the pylorus in suitable cases. When the resection does not include the pylorus it might be wise at least to occlude it for prophylactic purposes. The reasonableness of this would be more assured if we knew the etiology of ulcer more definitely. However, prompt emptying of the stomach and the admission of alkaline secretion are doubtless beneficial (experimental ulcer cannot be produced in the absence of acidity), and these can be assured by gastrojejunostomy when done as an adjunct to pyloric closure.

This statement of the case sounds extreme, and yet if we are to do anything definite for non-perforating and nonstenosing ulcers this is almost the irreducible minimum. Fortunately most ulcers are so situated that closure at or near the pylorus will meet the indications. When pylorectomy or resection elsewhere is required, the surgical risk will not be out of proportion to that of the pathology.

In doing the limited work I have had in stomach surgery I have been torn between the conviction that only radical measures would get results, and the fear of the mortality associated with these radical measures.

The technical difficulties of resection of the stomach are not a negligible matter to the surgeon who does not do stomach operations every day. The satisfactory application of clamps, the thickness of the stomach wall, and the exposure of the inner surface of the mucous membrane have been among my greatest difficulties in doing the technic as I think it should be done. By splitting the stomach wall, so to speak, and using the mucous and submucous coats as one layer, and the serous and muscular coats as another, I have avoided these difficulties to an appreciable degree. This technic has been used to a greater or less extent by others, but I do not believe its advantages have been duly appreciated.

This use of the mucous membrane is most satisfactory in occluding the pylorus. For this purpose an incision is made on the anterior surface of the stomach, or of the duodenum, according to conditions. This incision is carried down to the submucosa, which in all succeeding description will be included in the term mucous membrane. The incision should be preferably transverse to the long axis of the organ, and should extend from border to border.

When the mucous membrane is reached the overlying tissues are removed from its anterior surface for at least an inch, and for as much more as may be desirable. Then the posterior surface is freed by blunt dissection with a narrow knife-handle or some similar instrument (Fig. 1). A cylinder of mucous membrane is thus gotten up which is clamped at its centre. The mucous membrane is closed just on either side of the clamp by a chain ligature of linen, tied in two or more sections as required by the width of the cylinder of mucous membrane (Fig. 2). The clamp is then removed and the mucous membrane divided along the groove left by the clamp.

When the length of the cylinder of mucous membrane permits double clamping with incision between the clamps, this should be done, as it simplifies suture or ligation of the stump. When double clamping is done, I always prefer suture to ligation and use linen, which is put in with two needles just under the clamp after the fashion of a harness stitch (Fig. 3).

As the next step of the operation a purse-string of catgut or linen is thrown around the base of each stump (Fig. 4). This purse-string is put in the angle of tissue where the exposed mucous membrane terminates, and it may be placed in the mucous membrane itself, but preferably should be in the muscular tissue. The stumps are inverted and the purse-string tightened. When the width of the stomach makes a purse-string undesirable, as may readily happen on the proximal side, a continued suture, approximating the anterior and posterior walls, in the inner surface of the overlying muscular coat will serve the same purpose. The seromuscular tissues are then closed, the edges of the wound being inverted so as to bring the peritoneum in contact with the muscle of the posterior wall, or the edges of the seromuscular wound may be brought together by sutures which also catch the posterior wall.

Instead of inverting long stumps of mucous membrane the stumps may be ligated (or preferably sutured) close to their bases and then cut short. This makes the inversion less satisfactory, but is necessary when, on account of the location of the ulcer, the dissection has to be carried across the face of the ulcer, leaving possibly an opening in the membrane corresponding to it. Inversion of the stump gives an additional sense of security, and yet is probably not of any special value provided the mucous membrane is trimmed short.

When the ulcer is of suitable size and located on the anterior wall it may be surrounded by crescentic incisions, running from curvature to curvature, down to but not through the mucous membrane, and the dissection and ligation of this structure completed as just described (Fig. 5).

It would appear at first glance that an incision in the long axis midway between the borders would be most satisfactory, but there are several objections to this. First the ulcer would be more difficult to avoid or to include by encircling. Then the closest attachment of the overlying structures to the mucous membrane is found at the borders, and here we get the most hemorrhage in separating them. At the extremities of the transverse incision we have immediate access to these borders and also to the posterior surface of the mucous membrane.

In doing this little operation it will not usually be necessary to ligate the omenta at the upper and lower borders of the viscus, but this can be done if hemorrhage is at all troublesome.

The advantage this method of occlusion has over the Biondi method and various other methods with or without dissection of the mucous membrane is that it is more apt to be permanent, and is equally as simple as any, except the ligature methods which are least reliable.

The advantage of the procedure over von Eiselberg's exclusion is that the omenta do not have to be divided and the pylorus does not have to be mobilized. Further than this, the cavity of the viscus is not opened up and the inner surface of the mucous membrane is not exposed to the same extent. Closing a seromuscular wound on the anterior surface of the stomach or duodenum is a very much less difficult job than closing the two openings left by division of all tissues.

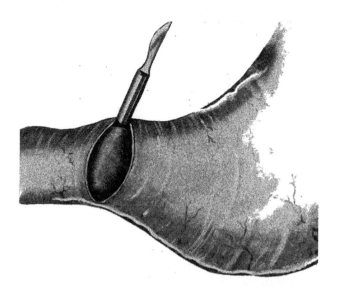

FIG. 1.—The posterior surface is freed by blunt dissection with a
narrow knife-handle or similar instrument.

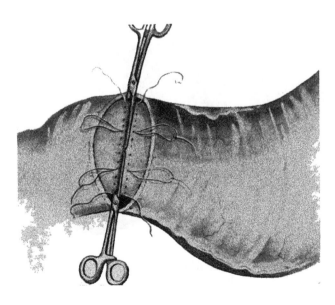

FIG. 2.—Showing the ligatures of the mucous membrane about clamp.

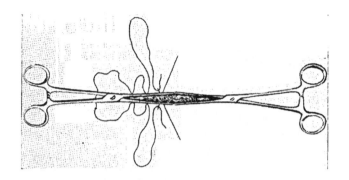

FIG. 3.—Showing method of suturing when it is possible to double
clamp the cylinder of mucous membrane.

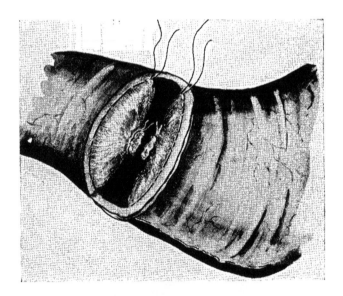

FIG. 4 —A purse-string suture of catgut or linen is thrown around the
base of each stump.

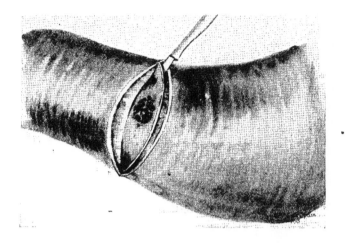

Fig. 5 —Method of resecting an ulcer of suitable size on the anterior wall.

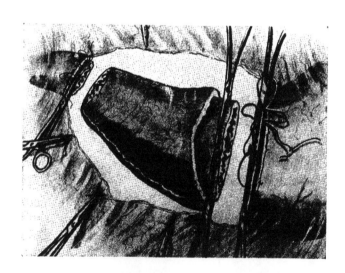

Fig 6.—Showing technic used in pylorectomy.

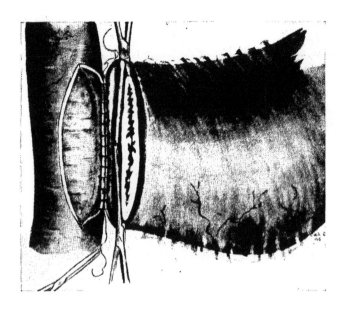

FIG. 7.—Cavity of stomach held closed by clamps on mucous membrane until posterior seromuscular suture line is completed in gastrojejunostomy.

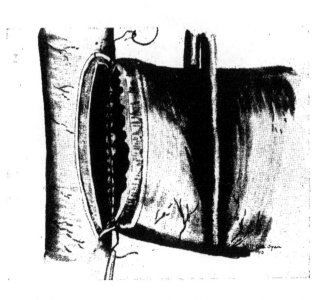

FIG. 8.—Posterior seromuscular suture line completed and rubber-covered clamps in place.

There is small choice in technical difficulty between unilateral exclusion and Rodman's pylorectomy, and between these two procedures I would choose pylorectomy. The only advantage the procedure just described has over pylorectomy is that it is more easily performed, and it serves almost the same purpose so far as getting rid of the ulcer and cancer-bearing area is concerned, for the pyloric mucous membrane is removed. It can be made a submuscular resection of the ulcer and cancer-bearing, and even of what, according to recent teaching, is the acid-producing area of mucous membrane.

Should the location and extent of the ulcer at or near the pylorus or the presence of adhesions prevent the use of this technic, and yet cicatrization should not have produced an efficient and permanent stenosis, pylorectomy at some later date primary or secondary to the gastrojejunostomy is of course indicated.

In doing pylorectomy the mucous membrane can be handled in much the same way as just described. After the omenta have been tied and you are ready to divide the viscus, with or without clamping the duodenal end of the area to be resected, cut down upon the mucous membrane anteriorly and posteriorly and dissect up a short area of it as already described, for pyloric occlusion. Double clamp this mucous membrane, cut between the clamps, suture or ligate the distal end (Fig. 6), and then suture the seromuscular structures over this stump inverting the serous coat carefully.

The incision through the stomach at the opposite end of the resected area is handled in the same way (Fig. 6). The mucous membrane is closed by the harness stitch of linen already mentioned, which is drawn snug as it is placed (Fig. 3). The mucous membrane may be sutured close up to its line of reflection from the muscle and cut short, but the overlying structures are more easily and smoothly closed if the mucous membrane is long enough for its suture line not to hold the anterior and posterior stomach walls too rigidly in contact.

I have found this method of closure technically much easier than the ordinary one, and that the line of closure is much smoother and less bulky. Hemorrhage can be accurately and permanently disposed of as you proceed. Rubber-covered clamps may be used for the temporary control of hemorrhage, and being used for this purpose alone may be loosened at any time for the detection and control of vessels that would bleed.

In performing gastrojejunostomy I use no clamps except a small Murphy clamp at either end of the proposed incision in the jejunum. It is at times difficult to get room on the stomach for a gastro-enterostomy clamp, and once applied the clamps necessitate a blind method of controlling hemorrhage.

In the absence of clamps the viscera are held in contact and supported outside the abdominal wound by sutures which catch a good bite on each organ just beyond the limits of the proposed lines of incision. The incisions are made down to the mucous membrane, and this structure cleared for a space half an inch wide at the centre of each incision and tapering to the angles. The posterior cut edges of the seromuscular layers are united by a continued suture, the mucous membranes are then incised down the centre of the exposed areas, the cut edges are united all the way round with a whip-over suture, and the seromuscular suture completed anteriorly. Catgut is used throughout. The inner layer of sutures placed in this way is a more simple procedure to accomplish than the usual through-and-through suture, and the suture line when complete is more flexible and more readily pushed out of the way for the seromuscular suture to follow. A third line of sutures may be used if desired.

If in doing a primary pylorectomy it is considered desirable to anastomose the cut edge of the stomach into the jejunum after the method of Polya, the resection of the stomach is carried out as already described. The union betweed the stomach and jejunum is made as in ordinary gastrojejunostomy (Figs. 7 and 8), except that the cavity of the stomach is kept closed by the clamps on the mucous membrane until the posterior seromuscular suture line is completed (Fig. 7), and when these are removed by rubber-covered clamps as ordinarily used.

In the *Journal of the American Medical Association* of September 25, 1915, Dr. W. J. Mayo described a method of excision of ulcers of the body of the stomach, accessible from the serous surface and not extensive enough to demand more radical measures. A seromuscular flap is raised, the ulcer cauterized, the opening closed by sutures placed in the mucosubmucous coat, and the flap replaced with over-lapping. Dr. Mayo advises gastrojejunostomy, but says that blocking the pylorus has not seemed to have added anything to the operation. He gets results without blocking, but many of us cannot.

I have been experimenting on dogs with a wire snare for dividing the mucous membrane in gastrojejunostomy after the inner line of sutures has been completed both posteriorly and anteriorly except for the small space required by the snare. The snare has worked very well so far as results in dogs are concerned, but such a strain is thrown upon the sutures when the tissues are drawn upon during the crushing action of the snare that I have not tried it upon a human subject.

I will say in conclusion that unless you have given the matter special attention you probably have no idea what a tough substantial structure the mucous and submucous coats of the stomach make. The peritoneum and muscle are much more readily divided, it is easy to cut down to the submucosa and leave it intact, and the overlying structures are readily detached from it.

DISCUSSION

DR. WILLIAM R. JACKSON, Mobile, Alabama.—I wish to thank the doctor for his paper. He has given us a new idea, but the criticism I would make is as to the friability of the mucosa. It is easy to separate the seromuscular coat from the mucous membrane and make a tubular mucous canal. I think in many cases, when we commence to apply crushing forceps we will have laceration of the mucosa. I have tried it in one or two cases, and as he says, particularly, it is impossible with the jejunum of dogs, and the same is true of some delicate female anemic patients. However, the operation seems to be a very good one.

I notice that the doctor uses catgut throughout for his gastrojejunostomy, and silk for his end closures in blocking the pylorus.

DR. RICHARD A. BARR, Nashville, Tennessee (closing).— In handling the pylorus it is not necessary to put on a clamp. You use finger control. I do not put any instrument on the mucous membrane; I find you can hold the pylorus with two fingers and control hemorrhage and roll out the mucous membrane sufficiently for dissection without putting an instrument on it at all.

SARCOMATA IN UNUSUAL SITUATIONS

By Hubert A. Royster, A.B., M.D., F.A.C.S.

Raleigh, N. C.

SARCOMATA occurring in unusual situations may well engage our attention, not only on account of their pathological interest, but also because of their diagnostic importance. If sarcomata always invaded organs and regions in which we expected to find them, their recognition would be comparatively easy and their disposal more certain. But when they are situated where benign growths are more apt to be found, not to suspect their presence would be productive of serious harm.

It is not necessary to discuss the general nature of sarcomatous tumors. It is enough to recall that they are atypical cellular tumors of the connective-tissue group, neoplasms which in their structure closely resemble embryonic or immature connective tissue. In common they present the following characteristics: their cells have no wall and are in constant relation with the stroma; vessels ramify among the cells and are very thin walled; dissemination by bloodvessels and not by lymphatics is the rule; local recurrence is common; their rate of growth is not slow, but varied and spasmodic; they usually attack young active organs and tissues; they contain no juice; they often result from injury.

The truth of the last statement has been recently assailed by Schepelmann,[1] who believes that no one has succeeded in proving experimentally that trauma produces new growths, and quotes Lubarsch to the effect that not a single authentic case has been reported in which a lone trauma gave rise to a malignant neoplasm. He admits that continued mechanical irritation is a factor in their production, but thinks that not more than 2 per cent. of tumors show a history of preceding injury, and that in many of the cases it is probable that the trauma only revealed the presence of a tumor that already existed. He lays down the dictum that "there is no possibility of a neoplasm having been caused by injury if the inter-. val between the accident and the development of the tumor is more than three or four weeks." Schepelmann further says it is not known whether trauma is capable of changing a benign into a malignant tumor, but if Cohnheim's theory is true that all tumors are benign at first and only become malignant from the removal of inhibiting influences, this would seem very probable.

Schepelmann's paper has been reviewed somewhat at length because it bears directly upon some of the points for discussion in the cases about to be presented. The views expressed seem to be at variance with those of many other authors. At best the question is difficult to prove one way or the other.

The seats of predilection for the different types of sarcoma may be stated as follows:

(a) The round-celled variety in periosteum, bone, lymph glands, testicle, eye, ovary, uterus, lungs, kidneys, and skin (rare). Subvarieties, such as glioma, lymphosarcoma, and psammoma occur always in a particular tissue.

(b) The spindle-celled variety in skin and subcutaneous tissue, fasciæ and intermuscular septa, periosteum and interior of bones, eye, breast, and testicle. Mixed cells are seen chiefly in bone.

(c) The giant-celled variety in the lower jaw, lower end of the femur, and the head of the tibia.

Among my records I have found six cases in which sarcomata were discovered in unusual locations, either growing from tissue rarely the seat of such growths or exhibiting other characteristics out of the ordinary. In addition I have abstracted from the literature certain reports of cases corresponding to them and, as far as they go, I have grouped these under separate headings.

1. FIBROSARCOMA OF THE SHEATHS OF THE MUSCULO-SPIRAL AND MEDIAN NERVES.

Miss B., aged seventeen years; July 7, 1899. Tumors of right upper arm and left wrist, both the size of golf balls; hard, movable, and not tender, but accompanied at times by shooting pains. Duration about six months. Operation showed that the growths developed from the sheaths of the right musculospiral (three inches above the elbow) and the left median nerves (two inches above the wrist) respectively. The nerves themselves were not involved in the growths. The tumors were removed without resection of the nerves, but on the right pressure had been sufficient to cause atrophy of the nerve at one point and a partial wrist-drop had developed. This persisted for some time, and is not yet entirely relieved. The girl declined any further procedure to remedy this condition. She is living and is in good health, with no recurrence of the growths. The pathological report was fibrosarcoma.

Tumors of nerve tissue itself (glioma or gliosarcoma) are not uncommon; sarcomata of the connective tissue covering the nerve bundles are very rare. The only case found in the literature showing a similar origin is a sarcoma of the carotid sheath reported by Spicer and Collier[2]. They removed the growth with portions of the carotid artery, internal jugular vein, and pneumogastric nerve. Much shock attended the operation, but the patient soon rallied and recovered.

2. RHABDOMYOSARCOMA OF THE TRAPEZIUS MUSCLE.

Mrs. M., aged twenty-eight years; March 22, 1900. A flat ulcerating growth on the upper posterior aspect of the left shoulder. It covered an area 2 by 2 1-2 inches. She had noticed the lesion for three years. She complained of severe pain. A wide excision was made, deep enough to remove a strip of fibres from the left trapezius muscle. The resulting raw surface was allowed to granulate. Healing took place rapidly and the patient has not seen the slightest evidence of return. The pathologist pronounced the growth rhabdomyosarcoma.

According to Adami "the existence of this type renders it possible that a group of large spindle-celled tumors of muscle showing also great irregularity and some polymorphism may be sarcomata derived from muscle elements." They exhibit large and very long imperfectly formed muscle fibres. This tumor is less frequently seen than similar growths in the unstriped muscles (leiomyosarcomata). The muscles of the extremities show the largest number of sarcomata of the rhabdo variety. A peculiar feature of these tumors is their predilection for the kidneys, especially in early life, showing that embryologic causes play by far the greater part in their determination. A look through different libraries reveals no sarcomata occurring in the trapezius muscle save the one herein reported.

3. FIBROSARCOMA OF THE BREAST.

Mrs. S., aged twenty-nine years; September 5, 1911. A large solid tumor of the right breast (Fig. 1), comprising the whole gland and hanging away from the chest wall, as if it were pedunculated. The tumor had existed for twelve months or more, and had grown slowly until the last three months. It was not very painful; there were no enlarged glands in the axilla and no discharge from the nipple. Under local anesthesia the breast was raised and severed from the chest. Enough skin was left to make a good closure. The patient easily recovered and is now perfectly well. No recurrence has been noted. Fibrosarcoma was the pathologist's report.

Undoubtedly this growth was originally benign and later underwent a so-called sarcomatous degeneration—a customary process. Attention is called to the case for the purpose

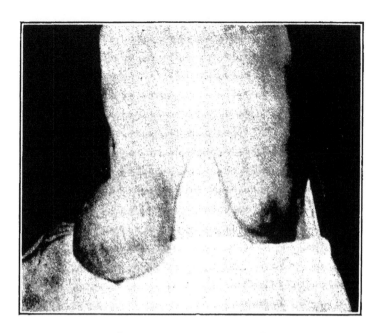

FIG. 1.—Sarcoma of right breast (Case III).

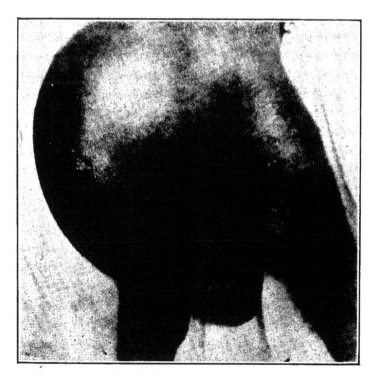

FIG. 2.—Huge sarcoma of left buttock (Case VI).

of emphasizing the fact that, though rare, sarcoma does occur in the breast and we must be ready and able to distinguish it. We have had two other cases but their records are incomplete and they are, therefore, not included. In Rodman's compiled list of 5000 mammary tumors 16.5 per cent. were benign and 2.7 per cent. sarcomatous. A recent investigation by Geist and Wilensky[3] disclosed 22 sarcomata (3.9 per cent.) among 558 cases of breast tumors. Following is a summary of their findings: The growths were chiefly fibromyxosarcomata and spindle celled; as a rule rapidly growing with fixation of the skin and dilatation of the veins in one-third of the cases. Lymph-node metastasis was rare. Heredity seemed to play small part in the etiology. A history of trauma existed in 10 per cent. Nipple retraction and cachexia were uncommon. Cystic tumors presented a more favorable aspect, being suitable for simple excision, while the round- and spindle-celled varieties gave the worst prognosis. Altogether the outlook is better than in carcinoma of the breast, 63 per cent. of all cases being cured. Radical operation is advised, but even then one-third of the patients show local recurrences.

Accumulated experience seems to demand that the same thorough operation should be done for sarcoma as for carcinoma of the breast. We are beginning to believe that glandular involvement in sarcoma is almost as frequent as in carcinoma and it would be unwise, therefore, not to clean out the axilla in operating, whether the glands are palpable or not.

Numbers of instances might be cited to illustrate the rapidity of sarcomatous change in previously benign breast tumors and the certainty of recurrence in many cases in spite of radical procedures. Duchamp[4] saw a woman of twenty-four with fibrosarcoma of the breast which grew to a great size. It had been noticed for three years, but had just recently taken on very rapid growth. The axillary glands presented no enlargement and the growth did not adhere to the pectoral muscles. It was easily removed, but two years afterward returned in the scar. The patient refused a second operation and soon died. Malherbe[5] speaks of a breast sarcoma, a third recurrence upon fibroma. The patient rapidly succumbed. He also lays stress upon the earliest possible removal of a fibroma of the breast and mentions the case of a woman 60 years old who had a breast tumor for fifteen years, enlarging progressively, hard and lobulated, not adherent to the skin or chest wall. Ulceration took place later. It was removed with difficulty owing to the extensive area involved. Two months after operation the pectoral muscles became infiltrated along with the axillary glands. A second operation proved fatal. Mosher[6] did a radical operation on a sarcoma of the breast and recurrence came after three years in the upper arm, involving the humerus; the patient dying the fourth year from brain complications. The x-ray relieved the pain but appeared to hasten death.

The woman whose case I have reported here, owes her life so far to the fact that the sarcomatous change had probably just begun and not to the character of the operation performed. It is another example of the advantage of a simple operation in the early stage over any extensive operation in the later stage.

4. SPINDLE–CELLED SARCOMA OF THE ABDOMINAL WALL.

Mrs. H., aged forty years; August 27, 1912. Sixteen years previously a small growth appeared under the skin of the abdomen just above the pubes. Four years ago it was removed under local anesthesia but promptly recurred. It grew larger and two years ago was again removed, this time under a general anesthetic. Rapid recurrence took place and again it increased in size. The mass, about the size of a large cocoanut, was situated in the lower midabdominal region, raised above the surface and glazed, but not ulcerated. It was attached only to the abdominal wall, somewhat movable and showing little tenderness. The tumor was excised widely and deeply down to the sheath of the rectus, the bleeding points ligated and the wound closed with some tension. This patient recently reported that there is no sign of the tumor's return. The laboratory diagnosis was spindle-celled sarcoma.

Sarcomata of the abdominal walls usually results from malignant transformation of originally benign tumors. The commonest of these are the fibromata, formerly referred to as desmoid tumors, on account of the arrangement of their constituent elements. They differ in no respect from fibroid tumors elsewhere in the body. Also lipomata, papillomata and cysts occur here, as well as tuberculosis and syphilitic myositis and actinomycosis. Cancer is seen generally in association with the involvement of some intra-abdominal organ. The prognosis of sarcoma in this region is not encouraging. Bouffleur[7] reports the successful removal of a fibrosarcoma of the abdominal wall involving the iliac vessels and requiring the removal of a portion of the external coat of the iliac artery.

5. LYMPHANGIOSARCOMA OF THE COCCYGEAL REGION.

Mrs. C., aged seventy years; February 4, 1915. A tumor in the region of the coccyx, rather toward the left buttock, slightly movable. It was barely elevated above the general surface, but encroached perceptibly upon the rectum. Three years before she fell down some steps, striking forcibly, as she said, on the end of her spine. She thought no more of it until six months ago when she noticed the enlargement and felt the pressure on the rectum. It was impossible to be sure of the nature of the tumor. The x-ray, however, showed it was not a bony growth. It was with difficulty excised and found to spring from the periosteum and fascia covering the tip of the coccyx, which was also removed. The rectal wall was freely exposed in the dissection. The tumor of the, size of a large orange, was bi-lobed and soft and covered by a fibrous sheath. Laboratory finding lymphangiosarcoma. The patient bore the operation well.

She reports that she is still in good condition, but it is too early yet to draw any conclusions.

The age of the patient, the type and location of the tumor and the history furnish the interesting features in this case. The growth could easily have been mistaken for a lipoma (as it was) and it was also very naturally at first thought to be of bony origin. In spite of the views of Schepelmann and Lubarsch, previously quoted, a suggestion of trauma even at the age of seventy will be ignored by few.

Malherbe[5] records a sarcoma of the ischio-rectal fossa in a woman of fifty years. There were five or six separate small tumors between the rectum, vagina and left tuberosity of the ischium, the deeper ones being free, but the superficial ones adherent to the skin. The patient had been twice operated upon. The same author also speaks of a sarcoma in the coccygeal region, a recurrence upon one removed ten years before. No history is given. Again, he describes a tumor of the sacro-coccygeal region, which was removed from a woman sixty years of age. The appearance of the growth dated from a fall twenty-five years before. It was a sarcoma with mucoid degeneration, cystic, resembling a dermoid. Its contents were a gelatinous material, traversed by fibrous bands and containing cavities with hemorrhagic foci. The whole neoplasm was enclosed in a distinct fibrous capsule. This case tallies closely with the one herewith reported.

6. MYXOSARCOMA OF THE BUTTOCK.

James T., colored, aged twenty-one years; April 7, 1915. An enormous growth of the buttock. He first noticed a swelling on the left hip in 1905, but it did not grow much until a year ago, when it began to enlarge rapidly. There are small masses also on the right shoulder and thigh and on the right leg. The growths are all semifluctuating. There was no history of tuberculosis or of syphilis. The man complained of no pain, but he was greatly emaciated and anemic. On account of the size of the tumor (Fig. 2) he was unable to walk and when he stood without support he fell toward the left from the tumor's weight. It was an inoperable case, but the patient constantly implored us to remove at least a portion of the mass, being perfectly sensible of the risk. Accordingly an excision of the tumor was attempted. After making a very long incision I found that a part of the growth was too deeply imbedded to remove. From this part about a pint of yellowish fluid was evacuated. The basal attachment was the intermuscular septum of the gluteal region. The patient's condition became critical on the table and the operation was not completed. He died an hour afterward. The tumor was a typical myxosarcoma.

Not a few sarcomata of the buttocks have been observed and some of them attained to large size. A huge one is pictured in the *American Text-book of Surgery.*[8] The enormous tumors are usually seen in patients of the lowest class, who through ignorance and neglect allow them to grow to these proportions. Almost invariably such tumors in the beginning were small, of slow growth and nonmalignant, but assumed sarcomatous change after a long period of quiescence. Injury or irritation may play an important rôle either before the original growth develops or after it becomes large enough to be vulnerable.

In a concluding paragraph it may not be out of place to mention some other rare cases of sarcomata collected from the bibliography. Primary sarcoma of the tongue of which there are very few cases on record, is referred to in *Guy's Hospital Gazette*[9] in which one case is reported and elsewhere by Downie[10] who presents two cases. The same number of the *Gazette* contains notes on a sarcoma of the esophagus, growing from the anterior wall and dilating the lumen instead of contracting it, and also a large sarcoma of the neck, involving the larynx—both with interesting autopsy findings. MacDonald[11] and LeConte[12] each report a sarcoma of an undescended testicle, the former case appearing in the groin and weighing over six pounds; the latter situated retroperitoneally and mistaken for a peritonitis of appendicular origin. Healy[13] relates a case of primary sarcoma of the pancreas with extension to the liver, while Jores[14] contributes an angiosarcoma of the spleen and liver. Malherbe's[5] remarkable list contains a sarcoma of the plantar aponeurosis, and one of the dura mater. Boldt[15] extirpated a primary melanotic sarcoma from the posterior vaginal wall, which proved to be very malignant, evidences of recurrence being present in two weeks.

BIBLIOGRAPHY

1. Schepelmann. Med. Klin., Berlin, 1915, xi, 741.
2. Spicer and Collier. Lancet, August 5, 1899.
3. Geist and Wilensky. Annals Surg., 1915, lxii, 11.
4. Duchamp. Loire Méd., November 15, 1898.
5. Malherbe. Recherches zur La Sarcome, Paris, 1904.
6. Mosher. Brooklyn Med. Jour., 1904, xviii, 226.
7. Bouffleur. Annals Surg., November, 1899.
8. American Text-book of Surgery, Edition 1892, Opp. p. 198.
9. Guy's Hospital Gazette, London, 1889, iii, 186.
10. Downie. Brit. Med. Jour., October 21, 1899.
11. MacDonald. Albany Med. Jour., 1893, xiv, 65.
12. Le Conte. Int. Clinics, 1907, 17 series, iv, 125.
13. Healy. Jour. Roy. Army Med. Corps, Lond., 1905, iv, 362.
14. Jores. Centralbl. f. Allg. Path. u. Path. Anat., 1908, xix, 662.
15. Boldt. Trans. New York Obstet. Soc., 1906–7, 153.

DISCUSSION

DR. ALEXIUS MCGLANNAN, Baltimore, Maryland.—Dr. Royster, in his paper, spoke of the relation of sarcoma to trauma, and of cases in which the trauma was subcutaneous. Sarcoma does show some similarity to the cellular reaction on part of the tissues to subcutaneous trauma. The subcutaneous trauma which does not heal rapidly, or which ends in tumefaction should be regarded as a foundation for or a beginning sarcoma. This includes all cases except ossifying myositis, probably because bone is an end-product in the development of connective tissue cells, and having reached the stage of bone there is no tendency for the cells to migrate and develop pathological conditions elsewhere. The benign tumor of the heart, which develops into sarcoma when it becomes malignant is the intracanalicular myxoma. Multiple tumors never become malignant, but a single intracanalicular myxoma becomes sarcoma, especially after it has grown to a size where it replaces the breast tissue. A fibroma in which sarcomatous change is prominent is the fibromyxoma of the nerve sheath, so that the presence of myxomatous change in the connective tissue apparently makes the tumor more likely to undergo malignant degeneration than the other forms of connective tissue tumors. Laboratory experience proves conclusively it is the character of the tumor and not the extent of operation, that is the important factor in the cure of the patient. Complete excision of the local tumor is all that need be done for sarcoma because if the tumor is not cured by complete excision alone, it cannot be cured by a local wider operation on account of widespread and disseminated metastasis. In our breast cases we have not taken out the glands because we have never noted metastasis in the glands of the axilla in our breast sarcoma. It does not add particularly to the difficulty of the operation which takes away the pectoralis major with the tumor, but we have not noticed metastasis and therefore have not removed the glands.

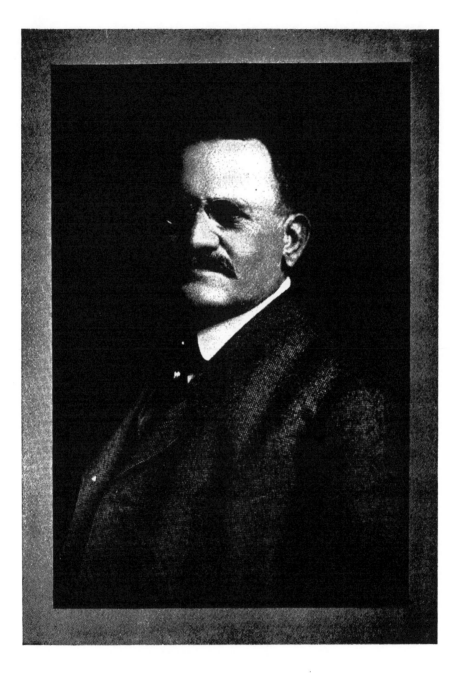

WALTER BLACKBURN DORSETT, M.D., F.A.S.

IN MEMORIAM

WALTER BLACKBURN DORSETT, M.D., F.A.C.S.

1852–1915

In the death of Dr. Walter B. Dorsett, of St. Louis, on July 27, 1915, the profession of the country lost one of its ablest and most substantial members, and our Association one of its most cherished Fellows.

While Dr. Dorsett was scholarly in his attainments, studious and diligent in his habits, sincere in a laudable ambition to succeed in his life's work, an air of cheerfulness and of real humor lightened his personality.

He was devotedly loved by friends, patients, and students, and was welcome in every circle in which he moved.

He was staunch and true to his friends, outspoken in his beliefs, well-balanced in his creeds.

While he made no pretense of affection for those not held in his esteem, he was ever frank and fair with them, and malice had no place in his makeup.

His decease at the age of sixty-three years followed a prolonged illness from nephritis with cardiac complications, accompanied by much suffering. Although he knew before the end what the outcome must be, he never lost courage nor abandoned hope. The brightest moments of his illness were those lightened by the calls of his professional friends.

To Dr. Dorsett had been given the realization of a most successful surgical career. Capably assisted by his son, he had been able to dispose of a large amount of operative work. The bitterest disappointment connected with his illness, no doubt, was the necessity of abandoning the work that had proved his life's achievement.

He will be remembered pleasantly by many who attended the meeting of the American Medical Association in St. Louis in 1907 as its genial host and as the efficient chairman of the Committee of Arrangements.

Dr. Dorsett was born in St. Louis County, Missouri, June 13, 1852. He was the son of Henry L. Dorsett, born in Louden County, Virginia, and Georgia Ann Dorsett, *nee* Blackburn, born in Versailles, Kentucky. His first college course was in civil engineering at the Washington University. Later he took up the study of medicine at the old St. Louis Medical College, now the Medical Department of Washington University. March 4, 1878, he graduated with the degree of M.D. For a year he served as an interne in the St. Louis City Hospital. In the summer of 1879, during the epidemic of yellow fever, he was made superintendent of the St. Louis Quarantine Hospital.

Dr. Dorsett married Miss Eleanor C. French, at Olney, Ill., in 1880. One son was born, Dr. E. Lee Dorsett, who is now a practising physician in St. Louis. From 1880 till 1887 he was chief dispensary physician and from 1887 to 1892 was superintendent of the St. Louis Female Hospital. He was a Fellow of the American Medical Association and chairman of the Section in Obstetrics and Diseases of Women in 1908; he was a member of the House of Delegates at seven annual sessions. He has been president of the St. Louis Medical Society, Missouri State Medical Association, St. Louis Obstetrical and Gynecological Society, and the American Association of Obstetricians and Gynecologists. Dr. Dorsett was a member of the Medical Society of St. Louis City Hospital Alumni; of the St. Louis Surgical Society; of the St. Louis Medical History Club; of the Surgeons' Club of St. Louis; of the St. Louis Academy of

Science; of the American Association of Railway Surgeons; of the Western Surgical Society; of the Southern Surgical and Gynecological Society, and of the Medical Association of the Southwest. He was also delegate from the State of Missouri to the International Congress of Tuberculosis.

Dr. Dorsett's hospital service included the positions of attending gynecologist to the Missouri Baptist Sanitarium and the Evangelical Deaconess Home and Hospital. He was consulting gynecologist to St. Mary's Infirmary, the Rebekah Hospital, and the Alta Vista Hospital, at De Soto, Missouri. He had been for many years Professor of Gynecology and Pelvic Surgery in the St. Louis University School of Medicine.

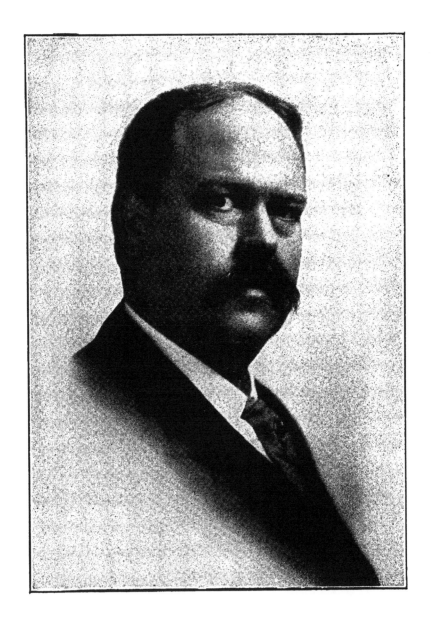

AP MORGAN VANCE, M.D.

AP MORGAN VANCE, M.D.

1854–1915

THE profession of Louisville and Kentucky lost one of its most illustrious and honored members in the death of Dr. Ap Morgan Vance, December 9, 1915. The Southern Surgical and Gynecological Association of which he was Vice-President in 1913, will miss his genial presence and his frank personality.

He had been in declining health for the past two years, suffering from chronic nephritis with a greatly enlarged heart, but he kept up until six or eight weeks before his death.

Dr. Vance was born in Nashville, Tenn., May 24, 1854. He was a son of Morgan Vance, a planter, and Mrs. Susan Preston Thompson Vance. With his parents he moved to New Albany, Ind., when a child, and his boyhood days were spent there, he being a resident of that city from 1868 until 1880. He attended the public schools and also received educational training at Moss's Academy.

In 1878 Dr. Vance was graduated from the old medical department of the University of Louisville. He then entered the office of the late David W. Yandell, one of the most noted surgeons of his day. Several years later he became house surgeon at the Hospital for Ruptured and Crippled, on Forty-second Street, New York City. He remained there two years.

During his early practice, which has always been limited exclusively to surgery, Dr. Vance did much orthopedic work, and with his wonderful mechanical skill did much for many

sufferers.   Because of the need for a special hospital for the
care of these children, Dr. Vance was instrumental in found-
ing and was the chief benefactor of the Children's Free
Hospital, and later in building the new wing of this hospital.
Later, Dr. Vance entered the field of general surgery.

Perhaps his broad training was shown best in his work as
a member of the Hospital Commission, which erected the new
Louisville City Hospital with the proceeds of the $1,000,000
bond issue voted by the people.   The Jefferson County
Medical Society voted by a large majority to recommend the
appointment of Dr. Vance to the Mayor as a member of this
commission.

Dr. Vance was the retiring President of the Jefferson
County Medical Society, was elected President of the
Kentucky State Medical Association at the 1915 meeting in
Louisville.   He was for years a member of the American
Orthopedic Association.

For many years Dr. Vance was a member of the visiting
staff of the Sts. Mary and Elizabeth Hospital and of the
John H. Norton Memorial Infirmary.

Dr. Vance was married in 1885 to Miss Mary Huntoon,
daughter of Prof. B. B. Huntoon, for many years superintendent of the Kentucky Institute for the Blind.   Eight
children survive him.

Dr. Vance was a man of tender heart.   The sight of
human suffering always affected him, and he was ever willing
to offer his able service to alleviate pain and affliction.   He
carried with him something more than the certainties of
science; his mind and character inspired hope and faith and
made the weak strong again.   Gentleness may be part of
power, "but only strenth makes gentleness divine."

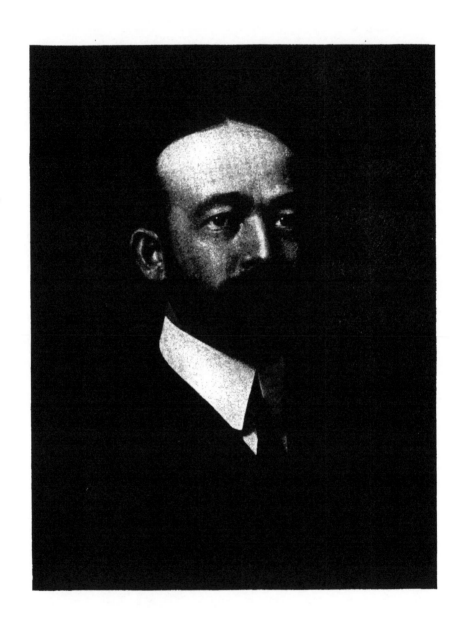

JAMES SCALES IRVIN, M.D.

JAMES SCALES IRVIN, M.D.

1868–1915

DR. JAMES S. IRVIN, of Danville, Va., was born at Reids-
ville, N. C., June 9, 1868, and died at his home at Danville,
April 13, 1915.

Dr. Irvin was well known in Virginia and much beloved by
his professional colleagues, to whom he was always sociable
and much attached. Prior to the study of medicine he
graduated in pharmacy and practised it long enough to enable
him to educate himself in medicine. He studied at the
University of Virginia and was graduated in 1893. He then
became house surgeon to the New York City Hospital in
1894, and subsequently served a year's internship at the
New York Maternity Hospital in 1895. In Danville he was
engaged in the general practice of medicine until 1910, when
he began to do special work in surgery. He was a skilful and
painstaking surgeon, and his success was due not alone to
his acumen but to his close personal attention to his patients
after operation.

He was always more than fair and generous to his
colleagues, and stood ever ready to give them the benefit
of his experience and mature judgment. Dr. Irvin was a
member of the local, State and county society, and also of
the Tri-state Medical Society of Virginia and the Carolinas.
He was surgeon to the Southern Railway.

Dr. Irvin joined the Southern Surgical and Gynecological
Association in 1908. He was always a regular attendant,
and in the charm of his delightful personality drew many
members to him.

INDEX

S Surg · 32

Lightning Source UK Ltd.
Milton Keynes UK
UKHW012127290119
336431UK00008B/435/P